Leadership in Nursing Practice

Changing the Landscape of Health Care

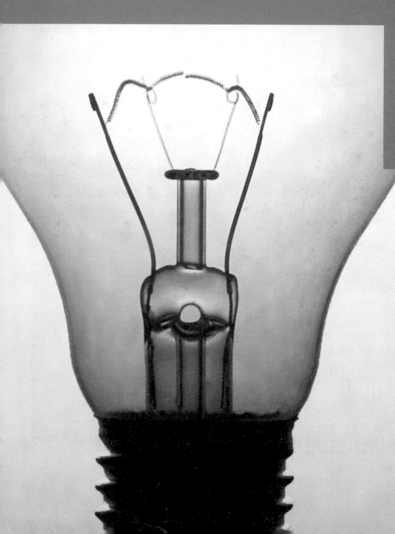

The Pedagogy

Leadership in Nursing Practice: Changing the Landscape of Health Care drives comprehension through various strategies that meet the learning needs of students, while also generating enthusiasm about the topic. This interactive approach addresses different learning styles, making this the ideal text to ensure mastery of key concepts. The pedagogical aids that appear in most chapters include the following:

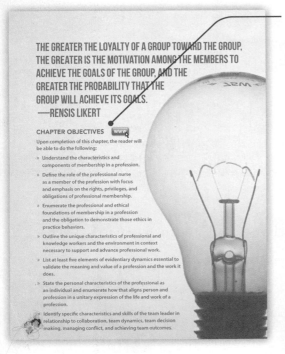

Chapter Objectives

These objectives provide instructors and students with a snapshot of the key information they will encounter in each chapter. They serve as a checklist to help guide and focus study. Objectives can also be found on the companion website at **http://go.jblearning.com/leadership**.

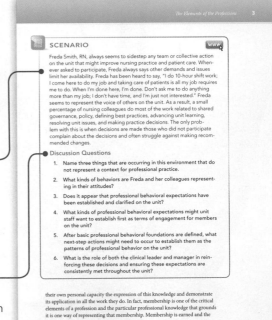

Scenarios

Scenarios encourage active learning and promote critical thinking skills in learners. Students can read about real-life scenarios, and then analyze the situation they are presented with. Scenarios can also be found on the companion website at **http://go.jblearning.com/leadership**.

Discussion Questions

Discussion questions focus on how the information in the text applies to everyday practice. Students can answer questions in a group or as individuals.

Critical Thought Boxes

Each chapter includes critical thought boxes to introduce new concepts to students and encourage them to reflect on concepts.

expectation of membership is fully exemplifying its knowledge and demonstrating participation in the life of the profession. It is expected that the professional, by virtue of his or her membership and work, is committed to advancing the role and contribution of the profession.

Because knowledge is a centerpiece of the character of a profession, there is emphasis on the continuing relevance of the professional and that person's commitment to expanding the personal knowledge base and in participating in continuing the development of knowledge over the life of membership in the profession (Steiger & Steiger, 2008). This idea that knowledge development continues and grows for the professional supports the profession's commitment to those it serves, ensuring that they will experience the most relevant service that represents the latest state-of-the-art information or skills in a way that advances their interests and meets their needs.

The Profession Becomes Identified with the Person

A key element of the life of a profession is the understanding that for the professional, the role becomes closely identified with the person, such that the profession becomes a part of the person and the person identifies who he or she is through the lens of the profession. In this way the profession and the person become one and cannot be differentiated from each other. For the professional, his or her work is not simply a job. It is, instead, an expression of his or her identity, a representation of his or her ownership of the work and life of the profession that operates at all times and in all places. For the professional, work is not codified in hourly increments and prescribed only within the context of a job category

CRITICAL THOUGHT

Professions are a social mandate and thus receive their power from the society they serve. For nursing, as with any licensed profession, it is against the law for institutions to unilaterally control the profession. Such controls are defined by state legislatures and regulated by the state's professional board. Professions and professionals are members of an international discipline, which responds to a social mandate that is broad and universal. Nurses must keep in mind that this mandate responds to a greater call than is expressed in simple institutional employment. Nurses must therefore express their accountabilities to the public, which empowers them, not just the institutions within which they practice.

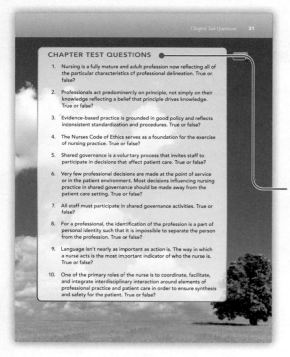

CHAPTER TEST QUESTIONS

1. Nursing is a fully mature and adult profession now reflecting all of the particular characteristics of professional delineation. True or false?

2. Professionals act predominantly on principle, not simply on their knowledge reflecting a belief that principle drives knowledge. True or false?

3. Evidence-based practice is grounded in good policy and reflects inconsistent standardization and procedures. True or false?

4. The Nurses Code of Ethics serves as a foundation for the exercise of nursing practice. True or false?

5. Shared governance is a voluntary process that invites staff to participate in decisions that affect patient care. True or false?

6. Very few professional decisions are made at the point of service or in the patient environment. Most decisions influencing nursing practice in shared governance should be made away from the patient care setting. True or false?

7. All staff must participate in shared governance activities. True or false?

8. For a professional, the identification of the profession is a part of personal identity such that it is impossible to separate the person from the profession. True or false?

9. Language isn't nearly as important as action is. The way in which a nurse acts is the most important indicator of who the nurse is. True or false?

10. One of the primary roles of the nurse is to coordinate, facilitate, and integrate interdisciplinary interaction around elements of professional practice and patient care in order to ensure synthesis and safety for the patient. True or false?

Chapter Test Questions

Review key concepts from each chapter with these questions at the end of each chapter. More questions can be found at **http://go.jblearning.com/leadership**, where students can submit their answers and instantly review their results.

contribute to the local level in a role that can have a broad impact on the quality of health and community.

- Testifying for boards, committees, and commissions regarding specific elements of care and service provides a notable and effective way of having an impact by educating and deepening understanding of specific issues, policies, or changes necessary to advance the health and quality-of-life issues of the community.

REFLECTIVE QUESTION

Does membership in the profession not also imply obligation to the community? Does that not mean that members of the profession have an obligation to demonstrate their commitment by also serving their community in a wide range of public and personal efforts?

- Equally, serving on specific health-related boards, committees, and commissions can expand the option of the nurse to be able to influence policy and strengthen advocacy for particular health causes through the action of collective wisdom in a way that can strongly influence changes in policy, practice, and education.

- Serving in elective office provides a more definitive and specific process in advocating and legislating advancing public policy and law. Full engagement in the political process ensures stronger ownership, direct political accountability, ability to establish law, and the capacity to drive meaningful and sustainable change.

In every level of professional life, from local agency advocacy to representation of broad-based political roles and legislation, nurses have an opportunity to significantly influence the quality of life of the community, the political and social role of the profession, and the passage of law and regulation that can establish firm standards upon which quality, safety, and health can be advanced and assured. Each nurse should be fully aware of the personal obligation the professional has for addressing issues of advocacy and public policy. Making a difference in the life of the community, individual patients, and the profession itself is a fundamental obligation of membership in the professional community (Cowen & Moorhead, 2011). This obligation should not be taken lightly. Each nurse must reflect individually on his or her level of commitment and specific role in addressing personal professional advocacy in a way that advances the interests of those each nurse serves. Such advocacy need not be widely publicized;

Reflective Questions

Students can work on reflective questions individually or in a group after reading through the material. The "www" icon directs students to the companion website **http://go.jblearning.com/leadership** to delve deeper into concepts by completing these exercises online.

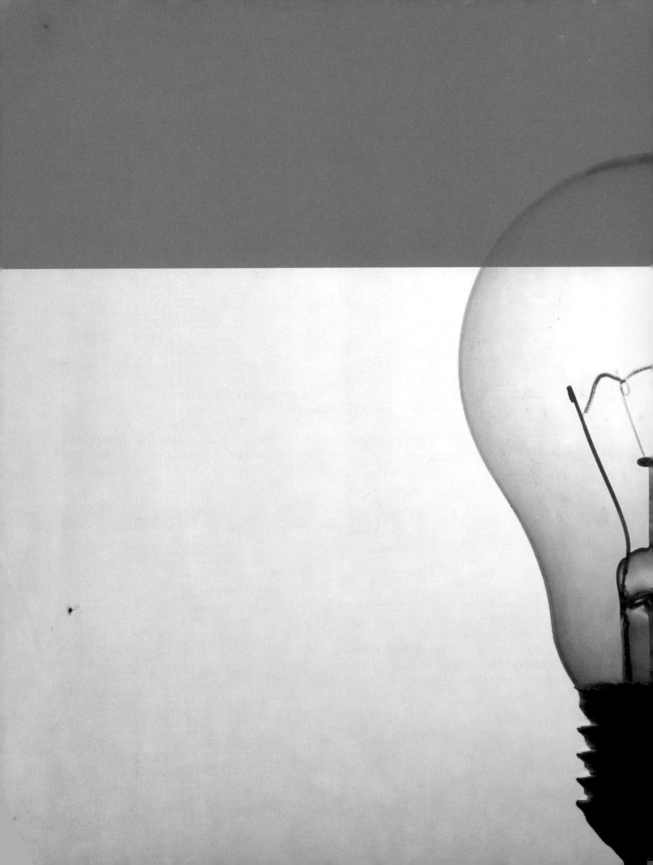

Leadership in Nursing Practice

Changing the Landscape of Health Care

Tim Porter-O'Grady, DM, EdD, ScD, APRN, FAAN

Senior Partner, Tim Porter-O'Grady Associates, Inc.
Atlanta, Georgia

Associate Professor, Leadership Scholar
College of Nursing and Health Innovation
Arizona State University
Phoenix, Arizona

Kathy Malloch, PhD, MBA, RN, FAAN

President, Kathy Malloch Leadership Systems, LLC
Glendale, Arizona

Associate Professor
College of Nursing and Health Innovation
Arizona State University
Phoenix, Arizona

Clinical Consultant, API Healthcare, Inc.
Hartford, Wisconsin

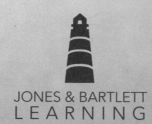

JONES & BARTLETT
LEARNING

World Headquarters
Jones & Bartlett Learning
5 Wall Street
Burlington, MA 01803
978-443-5000
info@jblearning.com
www.jblearning.com

Jones & Bartlett Learning books and products are available through most bookstores and online booksellers. To contact Jones & Bartlett Learning directly, call 800-832-0034, fax 978-443-8000, or visit our website, www.jblearning.com.

Substantial discounts on bulk quantities of Jones & Bartlett Learning publications are available to corporations, professional associations, and other qualified organizations. For details and specific discount information, contact the special sales department at Jones & Bartlett Learning via the above contact information or send an email to specialsales@jblearning.com.

Production Credits

Publisher: Kevin Sullivan
Acquisitions Editor: Amanda Harvey
Editorial Assistant: Sara Bempkins
Production Editor: Amanda Clerkin
Marketing Manager: Elena McAnespie

V.P., Manufacturing and Inventory Control: Therese Connell
Composition: Publishers' Design and Production Services, Inc.
Interior Design: Michael O'Donnell
Cover Design: Scott Moden

Cover and Chapter Opener Image: © Paulus Rusyanto/ShutterStock, Inc.
Printing and Binding: Courier Kendallville
Cover Printing: Courier Kendallville

To order this product, use ISBN: 978-1-4496-7358-1

Library of Congress Cataloging-in-Publication Data

Porter-O'Grady, Timothy.
    Leadership in nursing practice: changing the landscape of health care / Tim Porter-O'Grady and Kathy Malloch.
        p. ; cm.
    Includes bibliographical references and index.
    ISBN 978-1-4496-6746-7
    I. Malloch, Kathy. II. Title.
    [DNLM: 1. Leadership. 2. Nurse Administrators. 3. Nursing--organization & administration. 4. Professional Competence. WY 105]
    610.73068--dc23
        2011052546

6048

Printed in the United States of America
16   15   14   13   10   9   8   7   6   5   4

Contents

3   The Person of the Leader:
        The Capacity to Lead   81

4   Conflict Skills for Clinical Leaders   121

11   Policy, Legislation, Licensing, and Professional Nurse Roles   405

12   Delegation and Supervision: Essential Foundations for Practice   429

15   Integrating Learning: Applying the Practices of Leadership   537

Reviewers

Sharon E. Beck, PhD, RN
Educational Consultant

A. Maria Fisk, DNP, APRN, BC
Professor of Nursing
Piedmont College
Demorest, Georgia

Therese A. Fitzpatrick, PhD, RN
Assistant Clinical Professor
Department of Health Systems Science
University of Illinois, Chicago
Chicago, Illinois

Roy A. Herron, RN, MSN
Adjunct Faculty
University of Texas, Brownsville
San Antonio, Texas

Vonnie Pattison, MSN, RN-BC
Assistant Professor
Montana State University, Northern
Havre, Montana

Georgianna M. Thomas, EdD, MSN, RN
University Lecturer
Governors State University
University Park, Illinois

Foreword

I have taught courses in professional issues and leadership to prelicensure students in schools of nursing in both the United States and Canada for over a decade. The content in these courses tends to be broad. Normally, around a dozen topics are tackled touching on a few major themes related to the idea of nurses being citizens of their work groups, organizations, professions, and societies—it's a bit of a flyover because whole courses could be devoted to nearly every topic. Many students start off the semester a little apathetic or even suspicious of the material; by the end, nearly everyone is clear that the course content is essential to their career success. And with good reason. On the surface, many of the topics are "high level" abstractions, but scratch beneath that surface and it's obvious that the themes in such courses permeate day to day life in healthcare settings and that an understanding of them is critical to making the most of jobs and careers in nursing, whether a titled manager or not.

Healthcare systems around the world are facing financial constraints, demographic upheavals, along the with rising public expectations and fears, and overwhelming evidence in terms of population health measures and assessments of quality and safety of services that the status quo in health care is both unsustainable and unacceptable. Today's nurses, nursing students, and nurse educators are working in an environment that is changing much faster and in so many ways that few could have imagined even a mere decade ago—and those changes keep coming. Never has there been a greater need for nurses who have clear professional identities and the necessary habits of mind to work with colleagues and leaders in steering and reinventing health care in their communities.

What tends to help senior students make the leap to becoming well-informed, accountable professionals is a text written with a clear vision and voice that serves as a guide through new terminology and approaches to thinking about nursing work and its organizational contexts. For the diverse student body coming into nursing these days, the approach must be straightforward but challenging, clear but not oversimplified. Fantastic articles are written every year in many disciplines that touch on the core ideas in these courses, new ways of thinking about them, and current developments in the practice—some are in the nursing literature, others are written in related fields. But few are targeted at upper-level nursing students, and selecting and assembling them into a coherent package, let alone an up-to-date one is a task beyond most instructors' time and resources. And while there are many textbooks that introduce leadership and management concepts for a variety of other purposes, or attempt to ease the transition of students from apprentice to professional on a very concrete plane, no texts have been written at a consistently high level, without condescension, and have been geared towards helping students adopt a mature professional outlook. Kathy Malloch and Tim Porter-O'Grady have prepared exactly such a resource.

This text will challenge and provoke. It asserts nursing's rightful legacies of social justice and service, but does not airbrush some of the past failures of nurses to assume accountability as individuals, as leaders, or as a profession. Nevertheless, the approach is forward-looking and the tone is heartening and hopeful. It will help nurses, especially early career ones, realize that leadership is their business no matter where they work or will work, and that taking social and historical context into account is critical to understanding the present and building the future of nursing. Equally vitally, it clearly shows new nurses how they are partners in the settings where they practice who need to take charge of their professional lives and engage in the improvement of their organizations as a matter of duty, rather than expecting personalized invitations to do so.

An introduction to some of the freshest and best ideas in nursing and health care management and leadership, prepared by two of the leading minds in our field, is in your hands. Whether you're reading it as a newcomer to the profession, picking it up later in your career for whatever reason, or are reviewing it to prepare for guiding others into their roles as nurses, you're in for a treat. Anchored in a sense of nursing as a professional practice discipline, the authors are about to walk you through clear discussions of teamwork, leadership, staffing, and a host of other core topics. You are sure to walk away with many new ways of talking and thinking about nursing and for contributing to the future of health care.

Sean P. Clarke, RN, PhD, FAAN
RBC Chair in Cardiovascular Nursing Research and Deputy Director
Nursing Health Services Research Unit (Toronto site)
Bloomberg Faculty of Nursing
University of Toronto and University Health Network

Preface

It is always a challenge to write a book on leadership. Because of the dynamic nature of leadership, it is difficult to maintain currency and to assure that the most contemporary and relevant notions of leadership are provided to the learner. Both the theory and application of leadership are dynamic, and therefore, in the constant throes of transformation and change. It is important, therefore, to ensure that the teaching and learning of leadership concepts and applications are just as dynamic and reflective of the state-of-the-art.

No text, no matter how detailed, can provide all of the insights and information to adequately address the foundations of leadership. The learner must recognize that each attempt to explicate leadership simply provides another one of a wide variety of resources that must be included in the library of learning for every person who approaches the subject. We consider this text as one small but seminal resource that we hope will generate further interest in leadership learning and development and comprise a part of the larger resource base of the ever-emergent and learning leader.

This text is designed to address the foundations of leadership. It is not a management text. So many of the textbooks and resources used for leadership courses in nursing are overwhelmed by the management content and many of the core concepts of leadership get lost in the minutia of management. Less than 1% of graduating nurses will ever play a management role. In consideration of this reality, we have focused on those foundations of leadership that are essential for the clinical practitioner making up the 99% of professional nurses. We hope to provide insights and tools that are relevant to the clinical leadership role in a way that challenges thinking and yet provides the foundation for translation and application in the practice setting. While necessarily incomplete, we hope that the essential and foundational leadership skills necessary to thrive in a complex clinical environment are addressed in a way that provides both meaning and understanding. Learning leadership content has no value if it cannot be successfully incorporated into patterns of behavior that have a meaningful impact on everyday practice. At the same time leadership learning must challenge current thinking and confront leadership notions, practices, and behaviors that do not reflect the science and lead to expressions which may not be appropriate or effective.

The chapters in this text purposely focus on foundational concepts, elements, and practices of contemporary leadership. Contemporary understanding of the complexity of organizational cultures is used as a contextual framework for the discussion of leadership in each chapter. The emerging "complexity leader" must recognize that the leadership of organizations, systems, and how people work in networks and communities of practice is different from our previous understanding. With these newer concepts influencing complex organizational clinical and work networks, the leader applies a new frame to the expression of the leadership role. This understanding forms the backdrop of the content of each of the chapters in this text.

At the same time, it is important to integrate the obligations of the profession with the actions of the professional. Professions are a social mandate and address a significant social need. There is no greater social trust than that of nurses for the communities they serve and the health they advance. It is within this context of a social mandate that the professional nurse serves the health needs of the community. This understanding of nursing's social mandate provides the framework for meaning for each chapter. From discussion of the professional role to the incorporation of change and innovation and its application, focus has been on the unique character of the professional nurse in the clinical setting. Chapters that focus on foundational issues representing resource obligations provide an essential understanding of the operational mechanics of the systems within which the professional nurse will practice. Social issues related to the professional's obligation for ethical behavior and participating in policy and legislation affecting social health, have also been emphasized. Functional skills related to conflict, team-based leadership, negotiation, collective action, and personal relationships all emphasize the individual's responsibility for effective professional behavior and relationships. Since professional practice is a lifelong pursuit, issues related to role accountability, career management, and the personal leadership learning journey have been particularly emphasized in this book. The final chapter attempts to collate and synthesize the leadership information covered in each of the chapters in a way that provides linkage and integration of leadership learning.

The content of the chapters and the learning associated with this text includes contemporary notions of development and learning practices. Relevant questions, scenarios, and online resources have all been developed in support of the learning activities associated with the leadership concepts of this book. The student of leadership is encouraged to use the full multimodal learning applications associated with this text as an opportunity to facilitate development and to translate concepts into leadership practices. Each of the tools attempt to provide reinforcement of learning and opportunities for leadership practice and personal expression of leadership skills.

As always, the authors acknowledge that this text is a work in progress. Learning material and support associated with this book will be continually refined and developed as will the content of each of the chapters during future additions, refinements and revisions. In addition, we encourage the reader to use a wide variety of leadership learning resources to supplement the foundations laid in this text. As we are all a part of the leadership learning journey, the authors expect to grow and develop influenced by students of leadership and other readers who will challenge our own thinking and writing and participate in the improvement and advancement of leadership learning. In the final analysis, it is our hope that through this work, we will contribute in a small way to the development of future leaders in a way that provides a growing assurance of the maturation of nursing as a profession and the impact it will continue to have in making a difference in the health and lives of those we serve.

Tim Porter-O'Grady

Kathy Malloch

Acknowledgments

As always, I am thankful for the scholarship, colleagueship and friendship of my co-author Kathy Malloch. She continues to challenge my own leadership learning and role and serves as a role model for the caring component of the good leader for me and the profession.

My thanks to my life partner and best friend of 35 years, Mark Ponder, RN, for his lifelong support of my own learning journey and his tolerance for my times away in the work of the profession across the globe and his personal modeling to me of living the experience of caring for self and others.

Finally, I want to express my appreciation to the many colleagues, mentors, learners, and partners who have advanced my own learning and growing as a person, professional nurse, and leader. They have made my lifelong journey an endless joy, challenge, and exploration that has enriched me in ways both understood and reflective of the mystery that drives learning. I am in deep debt for the many gifts they have given me.

Tim Porter-O'Grady

Working with Tim Porter-O'Grady is an incredible gift that life has given to me. Tim's dedication to nursing, excellence, and advancement of the profession continues to provide me with a beacon that never dims. Most of all, I am thankful for Tim's friendship as a kindred soul in this very complex world.

I am especially grateful to my husband Bryan for his unqualified support of me and the work I have chosen to do. As we celebrate our 25 years of marriage this year, I can only hope the next 25 years are equally special and rewarding.

Finally, leadership never occurs in isolation and this work would not have been possible with all of the very special friends and colleagues who have contributed to my journey of lifelong learning. I continue to be inspired by your accomplishments, dedication to excellence in patient care, and your never-ending challenges.

Kathy Malloch

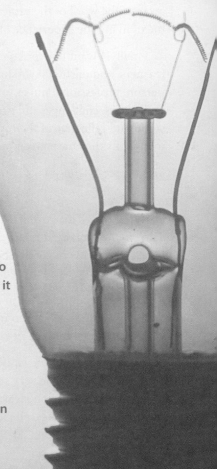

THE GREATER THE LOYALTY OF A GROUP TOWARD THE GROUP, THE GREATER IS THE MOTIVATION AMONG THE MEMBERS TO ACHIEVE THE GOALS OF THE GROUP, AND THE GREATER THE PROBABILITY THAT THE GROUP WILL ACHIEVE ITS GOALS.
—RENSIS LIKERT

CHAPTER OBJECTIVES

Upon completion of this chapter, the reader will be able to do the following:

» Understand the characteristics and components of membership in a profession.

» Define the role of the professional nurse as a member of the profession with focus and emphasis on the rights, privileges, and obligations of professional membership.

» Enumerate the professional and ethical foundations of membership in a profession and the obligation to demonstrate those ethics in practice behaviors.

» Outline the unique characteristics of professional and knowledge workers and the environment in context necessary to support and advance professional work.

» List at least five elements of evidentiary dynamics essential to validate the meaning and value of a profession and the work it does.

» State the personal characteristics of the professional as an individual and enumerate how that aligns person and profession in a unitary expression of the life and work of a profession.

» Identify specific characteristics and skills of the team leader in relationship to collaboration, team dynamics, team decision making, managing conflict, and achieving team outcomes.

Transitioning to the Professional Role

As a professional nurse, you are about to embark on one of the most significant careers anyone could experience. As a member of the nursing profession, there are few places in the healing community that you do not have a role to play. One of the most important realities applied to any career is the flexibility and opportunity it provides to fulfill meaningful goals and personal meaning. Nursing is one of the very few professional choices that meets both the conditions of value and of meaning (Daly, 2005).

At the same time, nursing brings with it many challenges for its members. While nursing is certainly one of the oldest healing practices in human history, it is one of our youngest professions (McDonald, 2010). The scientific foundations and the codification of the art associated with its practice have only recently been affirmed and expanded upon since the time of Florence Nightingale. When compared with the other professions such as medicine and the law, nursing is still in its formative stages and is just beginning to mature in a way that can be compared with other disciplines (Marriner-Tomey & Alligood, 2002).

 REFLECTIVE QUESTION

What are six ways in which a professional (knowledge) worker is different from any other employee work group?

The journey to a **profession** and as a professional has required a great deal of effort by a number of nurse leaders who have devoted their work and lives to advancing the foundations, science, and practice of the profession. However, this effort can be considered a work in progress both at the personal and collective levels. This chapter will emphasize the conditions and characteristics of a profession and the personal behavior that reflects the action of a profession, and it demonstrates membership in the professional body. Furthermore, the social mandate and characteristics of professionals will be outlined along with the tools and insights necessary to embed professionalism into the role of each professional person.

The Elements of the Professions

There are several components that define the unique character of a profession. Throughout history attributions and accolades have been generated to those who characterize wisdom or great knowledge. The notion of collective knowledge associated with an identified group has been a consistent theme throughout human history. The idea of a knowledge group morphed into the format of a profession generating from associating a particular arena of knowledge to a specific kind of practice (Bennet & Bennet, 2004). Professions were identified with not just having great knowledge but with doing something important with that knowledge that made a difference in the world. The practice or the use of particular knowledge is what can be associated with the emergence of professions.

CRITICAL THOUGHT

Being a member of a profession is not just a different way of doing work; it is a different way of being, an expression of the role and its relationship to the world, representing a social contract and reflecting high expectations for its exercise from those who will depend on it.

Professional Work Is Knowledge Work

The centrality of knowledge is critical to the existence of professions. In fact, knowledge is one of the characteristics that is an identifier or distinguishing feature of professions from other groups. A central assumption of a profession is that some unique body of knowledge must be obtained prior to becoming a member of the profession. The body of knowledge is specific and unique to the profession and is sanctioned by the profession as the foundation of the expression of its work in the world. All members of the profession are obligated to demonstrate in

SCENARIO

Freda Smith, RN, always seems to sidestep any team or collective action on the unit that might improve nursing practice and patient care. Whenever asked to participate, Freda always says other demands and issues limit her availability. Freda has been heard to say, "I do 10-hour shift work; I come here to do my job and taking care of patients is all my job requires me to do. When I'm done here, I'm done. Don't ask me to do anything more than my job; I don't have time, and I'm just not interested." Freda seems to represent the voice of others on the unit. As a result, a small percentage of nursing colleagues do most of the work related to shared governance, policy, defining best practices, advancing unit learning, resolving unit issues, and making practice decisions. The only problem with this is when decisions are made those who did not participate complain about the decisions and often struggle against making recommended changes.

Discussion Questions

1. Name three things that are occurring in this environment that do not represent a context for professional practice.

2. What kinds of behaviors are Freda and her colleagues representing in their attitudes?

3. Does it appear that professional behavioral expectations have been established and clarified on the unit?

4. What kinds of professional behavioral expectations might unit staff want to establish first as terms of engagement for members on the unit?

5. After basic professional behavioral foundations are defined, what next-step actions might need to occur to establish them as the patterns of professional behavior on the unit?

6. What is the role of both the clinical leader and manager in reinforcing these decisions and ensuring these expectations are consistently met throughout the unit?

their own personal capacity the expression of this knowledge and demonstrate its application in all the work they do. In fact, membership is one of the critical elements of a profession and the particular professional knowledge that grounds it is one way of representing that membership. Membership is earned and the expectation of membership is fully exemplifying its knowledge and demonstrating participation in the life of the profession. It is expected that the professional, by virtue of his or her membership and work, is committed to advancing the role and contribution of the profession.

Because knowledge is a centerpiece of the character of a profession, there is emphasis on the continuing relevance of the professional and that person's commitment to expanding the personal knowledge base and in participating in continuing the development of knowledge over the life of membership in the profession (Steiger & Steiger, 2008). This idea that knowledge development continues and grows for the professional supports the profession's commitment to those it serves, ensuring that they will experience the most relevant service that represents the latest state-of-the-art information or skills in a way that advances their interests and meets their needs.

The Profession Becomes Identified with the Person

A key element of the life of a profession is the understanding that for the professional, the role becomes closely identified with the person, such that the profession becomes a part of the person and the person identifies who he or she is through the lens of the profession. In this way the profession and the person become one and cannot be differentiated from each other. For the professional, his or her work is not simply a job. It is, instead, an expression of his or her identity, a representation of his or her ownership of the work and life of the profession that operates at all times and in all places. For the professional, work is not codified in hourly increments and prescribed only within the context of a job category

CRITICAL THOUGHT

Professions are a social mandate and thus receive their power from the society they serve. For nursing, as with any licensed profession, it is against the law for institutions to unilaterally control the profession. Such controls are defined by state legislatures and regulated by the state's professional board. Professions and professionals are members of an international discipline, which responds to a social mandate that is broad and universal. Nurses must keep in mind that this mandate responds to a greater call than is expressed in simple institutional employment. Nurses must therefore express their accountabilities to the public, which empowers them, not just the institutions within which they practice.

or an institutional position. Instead, the profession is something the professional occupies and lives 24/7/365. The professional understands that society expects him or her to represent their best interests at all times and will respond to their call for services any time the need arises.

Professional Work as a Social Mandate

One of the unique characteristics of professionals is the recognition that they provide a socially sanctioned or mandated service. Professions, in fact, are often a response to a social mandate or trust that provides a social good or fulfills a social obligation for their role. In this classification of the professional role, licensing regulations usually enumerate the conditions of membership and the statutory requisites for membership and practice (United States Congress, House Committee on Veterans' Affairs, Subcommittee on Economic Opportunity, 2011). The language usually enumerates the nature of the social mandate and the obligations that represents. For nurses and physicians the mandate usually includes language about the service that is provided, the necessary competence necessary to hold membership in the profession, and the social requisites for legitimate expression of that membership in a way that meets the demands of the license.

The social mandate usually also expresses penalties for nonperformance or professional wrongs. Because the expectation for contribution is so clearly enumerated and the failure to do so causes severe social deficits, the penalties are usually severe. A profession is a social trust; the breach of this trust results in considerable cost to the profession and the person. Society needs to be assured that its professions do not take their obligations lightly or fail to demonstrate responsiveness to the call for service in a way that minimizes risk and advances outcomes and fulfills the interests of the user (Roux & Halstead, 2009).

CRITICAL THOUGHT

If you are a professional, you may be an employee of an institution, but you are always a member of your profession.

Knowledge Work Always Changes

Besides establishing a knowledge foundation for the profession, an additional obligation for the profession is its ability to advance and change those expectations as new knowledge informs the actions of the professionals (Megill, 2004). This continual generation of knowledge is so critical to the professions that they invariably have mechanisms that take the professional beyond the foundation to demonstrate new levels of understanding and contemporary **research** that alters expectations and changes behaviors. This knowledge generation continually assures society that the professional continually fulfills the obligation to advance the interests of the profession in a way that ensures the best interests of the client will always operate as the centerpiece of the work of the profession.

Evidence, Improvement Science, and Translation of Knowledge and Best Practices

The digitalization of data in the 21st century has advanced the quality and effectiveness of the management of data and its utility in informing practice behavior (Becerra-Fernandez & Leidner, 2008). The fluidity, flexibility, portability, and mobility of data and data systems now make it possible to use just-in-time tools to quickly inform clinical decisions and actions. This evidence-based process has now become the fundamental expectation of clinical practice and is growing as the foundational frame of reference for the future of the clinical professions and the work they do.

Although it is not in the scope of this text, **evidence-based practices** in the **evidentiary dynamics** (referring to evidence as a system) upon which they are based are critical characteristics of the behavior of professionals. Ostensibly, professionals make judgments in a way that reflects facts and truth. Because of the highly variable nature of persons, conditions, and circumstances related to clinical practice, building an evidentiary foundation for deliberation and **decision making** is important to best inform clinical judgment, choices, and actions (Rapp et al., 2010).

 ## REFLECTIVE QUESTION

What is the difference between a knowledge worker and an employee work group? Are there performance expectations different for knowledge workers and for regular employee work groups?

Every contemporary knowledge-based profession such as nursing needs to be able to demonstrate its commitment to fact and value-based choice making and clinical action. Whatever variety of approaches to evidence-based practice are used by the professional, the result must reflect the best evidence of what is both viable and effective in advancing the health and safety of the population that is served (Melnyk & Fineout-Overholt, 2010). Evidence-based practice is both a science and a discipline. In every approach to demonstrating the use of evidentiary dynamics there are five components:

1. Formulating a critical clinical question using a **PICO approach** (P: patient or problem; I: intervention; C: comparison; O: outcomes).

2. Searching for and gathering data regarding integrated and relevant evidence using a variety of information resources (general, filtered, and unfiltered). Officially sanctioned and integrated clinical systems databases must be used in order to ensure that officially sanctioned information is used that is relevant, comparable, and rigorous, such as those shown in the following table.

Background information	Filtered resources	Unfiltered resources
UptoDate	ACP Pier	OVID MEDLINE
Harrison's Online	Cochrane	PubMed
E-books	Natural Standard	CINAHL
	InfoPOEMS	PsycINFO
	MDConsult (First Consult)	BIOSIS
	Natural Medicines Comprehensive Database	
	OTseeker	
	Physiotherapy Evidence Database (PEDro)	
	National Guideline Clearinghouse	

3. Determining the validity of the data. This requires critical deliberation of the relevance of the data to the clinical situation and ensuring that the specific data to which practice is being compared is used as a reference source.

4. Using the evidence for a particular clinical scenario. Determining the

efficacy and closeness of the relationship to the diagnosis, treatment or intervention, therapeutic impact, potential, and possible outcomes within a particular or specific patient situation or clinical scenario.

5. Evaluating the impact of evidence-based choice(s). Evaluation questions relate to successful impact of the choice on diagnosis, intervention, clinical change, practice processes, or patient condition. This critical fifth stage is what informs the most relevant up-to-date practices. When consolidated with other information related to the same clinical circumstance or scenario, this information serves to aggregate the database and inform future practice.

The reader is encouraged to pursue evidence-based practice principles in greater detail using the many other available resources. One of the lingering characteristics of good professional reflection, interaction, and communication is the ability to base the conversation on evidence that has been well researched, clarified, and formed into a legitimate presentation or communication. The professional nurse should look at this process as a foundational framework for practice by the nurse so that communication within the discipline and with other disciplines is informed by the understanding of evidence-grounded principles. Translating these principles into specific patient applications and effectively and rationally communicating their purpose, reason, and the clear logic of nursing action informed evidence represent the ground of professional practice.

CRITICAL THOUGHT

Evidence-based practice suggests that practice competence is constantly in motion, reflecting the latest just-in-time information that guides patient care. Therefore practice knowledge is always changing, and professionals change with it. The professional makes sure that every element of practice reflects the latest understanding of the best standards of patient care in everything he or she does.

With regard to professional work, the professional nurse has no accidental conversations. Every opportunity for dialogue and interaction includes the requisite of careful thought and planned communication. Evidentiary dynamics (the system of evidence) provides a systemic and scientific format that frames the logic, which drives effective clinical decision making. Within the context of the PICO process and its faithful execution, the professional nurse provides a continual format within which the deliberations of practice and clinical application unfold in a confident, informed, and rational manner. The ability to express this model of communication and the disciplines embedded in it projects a professional character of the nurse in relationship to those he or she communicates with and generates a sense of clarity, personal confidence, accuracy, and trust in the validity of the clinical, patient care content expressed in the conversation.

Such a discipline of these evidentiary dynamics (systematic/scientific approach to clinical judgments and actions) cannot be understated. The professional decision-making mechanism and clinical relationship reflect a scientific manner of conversation and interaction. Furthermore, good clinical decision making is diminished to the extent that any of the elements of care have been poorly constructed or badly thought out or not expressed in a conscious, intentional, and scientific manner (Bennet & Bennet, 2010). It is unfortunate that this discipline of communication is not formalized in the classroom as a particular capacity of competence so the framework of the communication dynamic itself becomes the tool set with which the professional nurse demonstrates great skill and accuracy in presenting a perception of clarity, confidence, and understanding about practice and patient care that is palpable to those with whom he or she is communicating. Effective, clear, confident, precise, and accurate generation of information in a focused presentation yields effective response, trust, and value of both the informant and the information.

The Ethical Foundations of a Profession

Professions generally represent their trust with society in a strong **code of ethics**. This code generally assures others that their best interests will not be jeopardized by members of the profession, that members will act within the parameters of the code and the law, that they will enforce their code with all members, and that they will update that code in ways that reflect the latest understanding of appropriate behaviors and practices.

The Nursing Code of Ethics

The nursing profession, like all professions, has a code of ethics that enumerates the expectations of members of the profession and the personal and performance standards that represent what is best in the work of the profession. The code specifically spells out the role and relationship of the nurse with individual patients and with issues that advance the health needs of society as a whole. The code further defines the behavioral expectations of members of the nursing profession in terms that relate to who and how they serve the public and advance the social good.

The American Nurses Association (ANA) has historically enumerated the professional code of ethics and conduct for professional nurses in the United States (Hain, 2009). This code of ethics reflects a strong foundation in ethical theory and principles and in the establishment of a culture of virtue and value. The code of ethics focuses on the specific and individual role of the nurse as a professional and key provider and enumerates ethical foundations of the individual and collective action of the professional in relationship to patients' health and the health of the community. The code of ethics is promulgated on the understanding that the profession and the individual nurse will use the code as the foundation for ethical analysis, decision making, and professional behavior. There are nine specific provisions of the code of ethics, each with detailed explication of their interpretation in the application of related principles. The nine provisions of the ANA Code of Ethics for Nurses are as follows:

1. The nurse, in all professional relationships, practices with compassion and respect for the inherent dignity, worth, and uniqueness of every individual, unrestricted by considerations of social or economic status, personal attributes, or the nature of health problems.

2. The nurse's primary commitment is to the patient, whether an individual, family, group, or community.

3. The nurse promotes, advocates for, and strives to protect the health, safety, and rights of the patient.

4. The nurse is responsible and accountable for individual nursing practice and determines the appropriate delegation of tasks consistent with the nurse's obligation to provide optimum patient care.

5. The nurse owes the same duties to self as to others, including the responsibility to preserve integrity and safety, to maintain competence, and to continue personal professional growth.

6. The nurse participates in establishing, maintaining, and improving health care environments and conditions of employment conducive to the provision of quality health care and consistent with the values of the profession through individual and collective action.

7. The nurse participates in the advancement of the profession through contributions to practice, education, administration, and knowledge development.

8. The nurse collaborates with other health professionals and the public in promoting community, national, and international efforts to meet health needs.

9.   The profession of nursing, as represented by associations and their members, is responsible for articulating nursing values, for maintaining the integrity of the profession and its practice, and for shaping social policy. (American Nurses Association, 2001)

SCENARIO

A young man was admitted to your nursing unit with severe infectious complications caused by acquired immune deficiency syndrome (AIDS). He was very sick with a broad number of opportunistic infections and required continuous complex medical and nursing care.

Sarah, one of the staff licensed practical nurses on the unit, had made it clear about her religious and personal feelings related to AIDS and homosexuality, often stating that it was "a sentence from God." She was often heard to say that those who get such diseases were receiving the "wrath and punishment of God." Although many of the nursing staff did not hold the same beliefs as Sarah did, they avoided scheduling Sarah as a caretaker for this patient and simply did not discuss the issue further.

Discussion Questions

1.   Does the ANA Nurses Code of Ethics address this clinical scenario as an ethical issue?

2.   Should there be nursing code of ethics policies related to these kinds of patient care issues?

3.   How should the ANA Nurses Code of Ethics be implemented at the point of service by the professional nurse(s)?

A code is generally adopted by a profession to assist professionals in making appropriate decisions in a way that helps the individual differentiate between right and wrong and helps the individual apply this understanding to critical decision making. What differentiates a profession is that a code of ethics is considered as a part of the regulation of the profession. It outlines a defined frame for professional responsibility, guides **critical thinking** especially related to difficult decisions, and provides as clear a framework as possible regarding what behavior meets the criteria for ethical behavior guiding the individual or discipline to make a correct or right decision within a particular set of circumstances. From the perspective of the profession, failure to comply with the code of ethics for practice can result in questions regarding the appropriateness of the individual's behavior and its impact on continuing membership in the profession.

Strong moral and ethical foundations are an essential element of the behavior of all professionals. Because the professions act in trust for the society they serve, the social expectation that professionals maintain a high level of ethical behaviors is itself considerable. Adherence to a strong code of ethics exemplifies confidence by society with regard to personal trust toward the professional and the belief on the part of society that this individual will always act in the best interests of those they serve. It is incumbent upon each professional nurse to be familiar with the profession's code of ethics and the ethical principles articulated by the organizations within which the nursing professional practices. It is always expected when questions related to ethical nursing behaviors arise in the practice environment that the professional nurse will explore these issues and work to resolve ethical challenges in a way that best addresses the standards of the profession and the needs of those it serves.

Shared Governance and Creation of a Professional Infrastructure

It has been more than 30 years since the early vestiges of professional governance were outlined and applied to the institutional structures framing the professional practice of nursing (Allen, Calkin, & Peterson, 1988). Over that time within the principles of **shared governance**, many approaches have attempted to demonstrate the appropriate applications of professional governance in a wide variety of international settings (Porter-O'Grady, 2009). Whether many of these models of professional governance (within the concept of shared governance) legitimately represent the principles grounding professional governance or not is the subject of much question, their claims notwithstanding.

The structures of professional governance are not much of a mystery. Law, medicine, engineering, architecture, academics, etc. have exhibited common characteristics of self-governance for generations, in spite of modifications reflecting professional and cultural differentiation. Notions of self-governance applied to nursing and nurses, on the other hand, have emerged more recently and have been approached more tenuously and with a level of reticence not generally experienced by other professional disciplines. Although much of this uncertainty can be attributed to the relatively recent emergence of the idea of self-governance as applied to an almost completely employed profession such as nursing, the following issues demonstrate at least as much influence:

- Self-governance is historically a masculine exercise with no prevailing mechanisms for modification to a predominantly feminine application.

- Nursing has almost always been an employed profession; the nurse is generally an employee and therefore subordinated to traditional employment conditions and legal requisites.

- Historic power relationships in nursing are predominantly vertically derived and directed, while the historic power relationships in the major professions are much more classically horizontally delineated.

- Much of the social and legal framework for the traditional professions is designed to protect the public and the independence of the discipline to control its right to practice with little external or regulatory constraint. Much of the social and legal language applied to nursing is also designed to protect the public and to more carefully circumscribe nurses' practice boundaries and to limit its scope in a way that keeps it fully within defined parameters.

- The definitive character of the requirements of professional membership in the traditional professions is succinct, crisp, and definitive related to education, certification, and experience. In nursing, it is diffuse, often undifferentiated, and frequently broadly described and relative.

A Profession Is as a Profession Does

The journey of nursing to professional maturity has been slow and challenging. Unbundling its historic gender challenges has been a significant undertaking. Because of the social discomfort and the public challenges of institutionalized sexism and oppressed group syndrome, nursing's capacity to break out of traditional models of institutional control and to function as a viable profession has met with highly variable degrees of success. As well, nurses have themselves been a great source of the problem in limiting the achievement of full professional delineation.

Constructing a Structure for Professional Practice

The initial purpose of implementing shared governance models within nursing was to provide a structural format for the profession to implement the more horizontal loci of control and practice power enablers so essential to professional self-governance (Figure 1-1). Taking into consideration the historic social and employment structures impacting the practice of nursing, shared governance provides a model where shared **accountability** serves as the frame for partnering practicing nurses with their institutions in ways that would provide for mutual obligation and advantage in the interest of advancing shared interests in patient care excellence. The four cornerstones of a profession's ownership and account-ability—practice, quality, competence, and knowledge management—serve as the structural frame for the exercise of staff accountability over these professional requisites and the institutional partnership necessary to incorporate resource and institutional stewardship.

- Ninety percent of decisions are local.
- Decisions are made where they are implemented.
- The work is knowledge work.
- Quality is achieved by the owners of the work.
- Decisional competence is required.
- Clinical decisions require ownership and investment by clinicians.

Figure 1-1 Shared governance basic principles

Building the structural forms and constructing bylaws that enumerate them has provided much evidence of the success of such models to distribute own-ership and enumerate accountability in the profession. Although there is little evidence that the power balancing necessary to true professional behavior has come anywhere near fruition, the infrastructure for it has certainly been well established. This, of course, raises the question, why has so little professional empowerment and interdependence emerged even in organizations where signifi-cant progress toward real professional status has been evidenced?

The Four Requisites in Professional Governance

Much contemporary leadership research now demonstrates the importance of differentiating the patterns of behaviors in knowledge workers from those of employee work groups. Although this is considerably more difficult for nurs-ing and for the more historic and masculine traditional professions, work has progressed to make this possible. Since the early 1980s, considerable effort has been undertaken to challenge traditional organizational constructs and their legitimacy in light of constructing an organizational framework for professional behaviors. Much of the research has suggested that professional (knowledge work) behaviors can neither be obtained nor sustained in an employee work group structure where the expectations for performance are defined and con-trolled by the workplace and predominantly functional in orientation; where few peer-driven performance and evaluation processes operate; where work value is on volume, time, and motion determinants; and where work is highly subordinated to others and essentially management controlled and driven. In fact, these practices actually impede the occurrence of professional behaviors and prevent them from being demonstrated.

CRITICAL THOUGHT

Professional delineation and job categories do not mix. In a professional environment job categorization for knowledge work is simply not an adequate delineation of both the requirements and the nature of the work. Position charters and role expectations serve as better tools for defining the accountabilities and obligations of professionals than do job descriptions that focus on tasks and functions.

These identified organizational characteristics have been entrenched in the healthcare system since its onset. Even currently, the long-held system of medical predominance in decision making is supported by a highly vertical, tightly structured organizational construct that has limited the professional growth and development of nursing in significant ways and created particular challenges to the development of a professional frame of reference for nursing practice. Even though contemporary nurses are academically grounded and the profession contains the largest number of bachelor of science in nursing degree and graduate educated women in health care, the traditional challenges to obtaining professional, social, and relational equity commonly achieved by academic parity have eluded nursing. The strongly hierarchical organizational framework for health care and the rigid control of the medical model in clinical decision making has served as a strong impediment to the emergence of the equity necessary to gain and advance comparable professional value for nursing and nurses.

Yet, much has changed over the past 2 decades that has shifted circumstances to create a stronger professional framework for nursing, laying the groundwork for equity, inclusion, and leadership. High levels of success related to advancing the education of nurses, the growth of nurse practitioners and their leadership in primary care, and the expansion of the nursing role in politics and policy development have all converged to create circumstances that have advanced the credibility and status of nurses across a broad range of the public sector. However, in hospitals and healthcare organizations where the majority of nurses work, much of the essential structure driving organized nursing has not fundamentally changed. The introduction of the Magnet program for nursing excellence and the requisites of structural empowerment (shared governance) have done much to recalibrate the professional nurse's role in decisions affecting practice, education, quality of care, and the clinical decision making. Building a professional infrastructure for governing the profession's decision making and relationship to the organization has formed the foundations of a sustainable infrastructure that partners with organizations in a way that advances the interests of quality health care and the integrity and contribution of nursing professionals.

 REFLECTIVE QUESTION

Does the change in the status and role of nursing parallel changes that have occurred as a result of the women's movement over the past 5 or 6 decades, or is the change specifically related to advancing women's education and its impact on nursing?

Personal Obligation for Participating in Governance

One of the basic obligations of members of any discipline is active participation in the life of the profession. Professions depend on the committed, concerted action of individual members who join in the collective enterprise to advance the interests of the profession and to assure the public that the profession is making its best commitment to meet the needs of the public. Professions are not amorphous bodies that do their work in an automatic or mindless manner. Because the profession is a trust held to particular accountability by the public, it must constantly be aware of its obligation to change and adapt to the adjusting needs of the shifting social context. Human existence never remains static. If positive and appreciative work is being undertaken, the human condition advances and improves. Because complexity science teaches us that nothing can stay the same, humans will either advance or they will retreat in their social circumstances. Advancing human interest requires continuous and dynamic proactive effort. This is no less true for the professions than it is for societies in general.

SCENARIO

The nursing staff on the medical unit has noticed that a wide variety of nursing beliefs and practices exist with regard to particular approaches to preventing pressure ulcers in long-term geriatric patients. There is a wide variety of long-held clinical approaches, depending on the learning and experiential background of individual nurses. No uniform standard appears to be used on the unit. The issue has been referred to the unit practice council.

Discussion Questions

1. Does the unit practice counsel have the authority to establish clinical standards and practice for all nurses on the unit?

2. What evidence-based approaches should the unit practice council employ in making decisions about setting a clinical standard?

3. After the clinical standard has been established for the unit, are all nursing staff required to adhere to and implement the standard in their own practice?

4. How does the unit council hold nursing staff members accountable for correctly performing the standard?

5. Should all professional staff expect to serve as members of the practice council, and how is that obligation rotated among staff members?

Nursing has a tradition of difficulty in fully engaging its members to participate in the life of the profession. Because of the long history of job and functional orientation, many, if not most, professional nurses failed to engage the obligations of their profession in a meaningful way to advance its interests, their role, and the practices necessary to meet changing contemporary patient needs. Yet, membership in a profession implies ownership, investment, and engagement. When one becomes a member of the profession, it is a life circumstance, especially within the context of the notion that professional membership also implies social identification of the profession with the person. This "I am" character of professional identification enumerates a kind of personal ownership of the life and work of the profession that is not bound by time, job, organization, or circumstance. One is a member of a profession 24/7/365; there is no respite, escape, or separation of the person from the role. If one seeks only job categorization that can be dropped or forgotten when done or left in the particular workplace, membership in a profession should not be pursued. Professional work can be neither done nor left. It accompanies the professional into every circumstance and activity every day he or she is a member of the profession. For the true professional, every activity he or she pursues represents membership in the profession. Everything the professional is and does is seen by others through the lens of membership in the profession, which therefore demonstrates in that moment whatever they will know of the character of that profession. At every given moment, the public's view of the profession is enumerated by what they see of the individual member and how that person represents the profession in everything he or she does. For that moment, the whole of the profession is on that professional's shoulders, and he or she is, in that moment, the only window others have of what the profession is or is not.

CRITICAL THOUGHT

All professional nurses are members of the professional nursing staff. This means they have a personal obligation to advance the profession of nursing, to fully participate and engage in professional activities that support practice, and to translate the decisions of the profession into personal practice standards in the delivery of individual nursing care.

Participation in the life of the profession for the professional is not an invitation; instead, it is an expectation (Porter-O'Grady & Malloch, 2010). Far too often in organizations and systems where nurses work, they are invited to engage in the life of the profession where they practice. The problem with invitation is it implies the capacity to opt out, to turn down the invitation. Far too often, given the option implied by invitation, nurses readily reject participation. Professions that behave consistently with their character distinguish between the obligations of membership (expectation) and the optional elements of engagement (invitation). For example, it is optional for a professional to engage in social events and gatherings of professional members. At the same time, it is an expectation that they will engage in quality improvement activities that demonstrate the value of their practice.

Professional membership and the structures of governance require the discipline to delineate between expectations of membership and invitational occasions. Members of the nursing profession should be expected to fully participate in decisions affecting practice, quality of care, education and competence, and research and the generation of knowledge. These are the fundamental activities of a profession informing the functional work of the professional. Not participating in these active obligations of members in the nursing profession diminishes the professional character of nursing, limits the performance of its professional work, and presents an image to others of nonengagement, ultimately resulting in task-based, functional, process oriented, employee workgroup behavior.

The Use of Language Characterizing Professional Dialogue

All of these delineations of the professional character of nursing work suggest a critical focus on the appropriateness of language. Language is a more visible characteristic that suggests to both the speaker and the listener a particular kind of interaction (Figure 1-2). Language communication represents a specific kind of dialogue that characterizes both the circumstances and content of the dialogue. Language is important; others hear and perceive in it the character and circumstances of the speaker (Zerbe, Ashkanasy, & Hartel, 2006). For good or for ill, professions have a unique framework for their dialogue that demonstrates specific patterns of communication and interaction that represents the personality of the discipline. Whether the profession is law, architecture, engineering, medicine, or nursing, each has a language that uniquely frames relationships and demonstrates to the world the particular calibration of the discipline.

- Decentralized
- Team based
- Horizontal
- Inclusive
- Engaging
- Accountable
- Point-of-service based

Figure 1-2 Shared decisions

One of the challenges for nursing is the historic language of practice embedded in the traditional job-oriented categorization of organizational work. It is easy to see why the perceptions of nurses and nursing are informed by language that demonstrates the individual's own representations and perceptions of their role and function. When the nurse is heard saying, "I'm just a nurse" or "I'm a floor nurse" or "I'm just doing my job" or "I'm here for the pay," it is not surprising that those listening would assume a more vocational or employee work group orientation of the individual. Such mistakes in identification are not supported when the professional is overheard saying, "my area of practice is" or "our standard for practice is" or "I am Sandra, your professional nurse today" or "let's change our practice plan for this patient." Language frames such as these evidence the content of professional interaction and present the profession to others in a way that creates a perceptive model more closely representing a professional delineation.

For the professional, there are no accidental conversations. Every interaction contains the potential for perceptive reaction. The professional is careful to clearly reflect in her or his personal behavior those images that best demonstrate professional demeanor, interaction, and character.

Personal Presentation of the Professional Self

Along with language, personal behavior plays an important role in representing professional character (Figure 1-3). Personal codes of dress, conversation, action, and expression play a critical role in the representation persons make about themselves to each other and those they relate to (Samovar, Porter, & McDaniel, 2012). Professionals recognize that the codes of conduct defined by the profession and by membership in a profession operate at all times and set the parameters for behavioral and role expectations with self and others. The requisites to respect oneself and all others regardless of personal feelings or differences is an important foundation for the demonstration of collateral and equitable behavior.

- Colleague role with the staff
- Seeks to engage staff decisions
- Provides information for staff decisions
- Open to staff direction and partnership
- Uses good group process
- Models engaging, challenging decisions
- Advocates for staff leadership

Figure 1-3 Personal character of the leader

There is evidence that the perceptual presentation an individual makes during the first 3 minutes of interactions with others sets the perceptual frame of reference that will linger for the longest time in the memory of others (Davidhizar, 2005) (Figure 1-4). There rarely is an opportunity to redo these initial 3 minutes and recalibrate that first perceptual image obtained by others in what is essentially a flash in time. Therefore, it is important for individuals to constantly be aware of how they present themselves to their various publics and what specific image they want others to sustain about them over time.

- Dress
- Grooming
- Eye engagement
- Inclusive
- Confident
- Facial features
- Posture

Figure 1-4 The first 3 minutes last forever

The intention and clarity of the professional person with regard to codes of dress, conduct, communication, competence, relationship, and interaction are critical considerations for both the establishment of professional standards and guidelines for peer behavior. It is important for the professional nurse to remember that at any given moment in time, from the perspective of the patient, whatever image the individual nurse presents to the patient is the one to which the patient will consistently refer in future conversations about the nurse or the nursing profession. If the nurse's demeanor is gruff and uncaring, if an action is brusque and impatient, if the attitudes are egotistical or haughty, if interaction is hurried and dismissive, it will contribute to the observing individual's perception and it will be generalized to the profession as a whole. There are no accidental moments in the interaction between the professional nurse and others. All interaction and communication for the professional is intentional and purposeful and therefore must be carefully considered as the nurse operates within the context of her or his role, knowing that the reflection of these actions will be significant and lingering.

Interactions with Other Disciplines

Perhaps one of the most significant barriers to full professional recognition is the perceptions we create for others with whom we work that influences their view of us (Heuer, Geisler, Kamienski, Langevin, & O'Sullivan Maillet, 2010). If we all remember the basics of our psychiatric clinical studies, we will remember that all behavior has meaning. Also we will recall that in terms of personal identity we are each treated precisely as we expect to be treated and generally no different from that expectation. Although this understanding can be hotly debated, the intent here is to emphasize that how we as individuals clearly enumerate our expectations of self and others in a way that can be fully understood influences what behaviors toward us are expressed and how others generally and consistently relate to us because of those self-expectations.

Behavioral self-expectations need first to be clear to the individual before we can expect to see them in how others treat us. If we are unclear of what those behavioral expectations are within our own role and relationship, it is not surprising that others' perceive mixed messages with regard to what relationships and behaviors are acceptable, marginal, or completely unacceptable to us. Lack of clarity around expectations makes it impossible to determine correct and appropriate patterns of sustainable behavior and responses to each other, facilitating ambiguity and uncertainty that results in confusion and risk in practice and patient care.

On the other hand, in the absence of clearly congruent and well-defined behavioral expectations, others will often respond within the context of what they see regarding our behaviors. If, for example, I am consistently angry and acting out, whether I have defined the expected behaviors from others or not, their reaction to me will be predominantly a reaction to my consistent anger-based behavior. This holds true if I consistently act passively, childishly, aggressively, dependently, subsequently, or if I exhibit behaviors that denote fear, anxiety, uncertainty, lack of confidence, or subordinating, I should expect a direct response to those behaviors, not necessarily the equitable response I want. Without congruence between the behavior I define and the behavior I exhibit, the exhibited behavior will drive the foundation for response to me from others.

Clarity with regard to professional behavior and personal behavior that is congruent with such definitions is critical to ensuring consistent and appropriate interprofessional interaction. Much of my self-perception as a professional depends on having worked through my role and contribution within the profession, issues of equity related to my self-perception and in relationship with other professionals, and how well I demonstrate a clear delineation of expectation that I behave and perform equitably and will expect equitable respect and behavior in return.

Issues of poor self-image within the nursing profession have some notable foundations worth exploration, and they frame further discussion. Indeed, it is important for this discussion to unfold prior to beginning professional practice so that many of the impediments to equitable behavior among the professions can be addressed frankly and critically prior to beginning professional practice. This frank and open discussion between faculty and students should include

SCENARIO

A new drug protocol has emerged for specific cancer patients, requiring a change in the mixture, administration, and evaluation of the drug. A notice has been generated from the pharmacy regarding such changes indicating that there are several changes in both interdisciplinary inter-action and particular discipline-specific clinical actions. There is much reaction to the written directive and some concerns regarding the roles of each of the providers and particular issues impacting clinical administra-tion and evaluation.

Discussion Questions

1. Should there be a regular interdisciplinary meeting or council where critical cross-disciplinary clinical issues are addressed in a common table?

2. What is the nurse clinical leader's role as he or she represents nursing at the interdisciplinary table with regard to participation, decision making, reporting, and implementing decision standards that were arrived at among the disciplines?

3. How do the nursing staff and leadership ensure continuity in collaboration and decision making within the nursing staff and between nursing and other disciplines?

4. Is participation in clinical decision making in a shared governance organization a clinical or a management responsibility? If it is a clinical responsibility, how do we ensure the clinical representa-tive is the most competent person to represent clinical issues at the interdisciplinary table?

conversations related to many, if not all, of the following issues affecting profes-sional equity:

- Overcoming the notion that other disciplines (notably physicians) are better educated and more well informed; have a deeper understanding of patients' needs; are fully knowledgeable regarding the work of others in a way that informs patients' needs; are directly in control of all clinical practice; and are, in the final analysis, the captain of the clinical ship.

- Finding clarity around historic gender equity issues that provide the undercurrent for many interdisciplinary relationships. Exploration needs to include an accurate understanding of the role of women in human history; the unique contribution of women to the human experience; a full understanding of gender differentiation and its role in understanding equity; engaging cultural gender typing, which enumerates subordinating roles for women; the unique values women contribute to knowledge management; and critical thinking, knowledge translation, and decision processing.

- For nursing and nurses it is important to explore traditional and originating role characteristics; the journey from functional to professional delineation; the growing science foundation for nursing practice; the different foundations for clinical judgment and decision making; the centrality of nursing to the coordination, integration, and facilitation of the clinical continuum; and the health script of the nursing role forming its foundations and driving its practice.

- Explore issues related to how nurses present themselves to their peers and their publics. Foundational and practical issues should be explored related to dress, presentation, manner, articulation, clarity, self-acceptance, professional pride, and the dynamics of interdisciplinary interaction. Simulation or practice opportunities that clearly demonstrate appropriate patterns of behavior are critical to establishing a foundation for these behaviors upon which subsequent professional interactions can be built.

- Enumerate sociological, ethnographic, cultural, and economic forces influencing the character of self-perception and the framework for personal expression and interdisciplinary relationships. Include mechanisms that reflect nurses' and physicians' different economic, cultural, and sociological foundations, which underpin self-perception, worldview, relational characteristics, role choices, and relational capacity. Suggest strategies for accommodating such differentiations in the development of behavioral patterns that help the new nurse to adapt equitable behaviors that reflect personal resolution of inequitable circumstances.

Because of the long history of gender and cultural inequity long associated with women in the role of the nurse, it cannot be expected that individuals will automatically or on demand accommodate these prevailing realities and experientially adapt new behaviors to overcome them. A part of the work of nursing as a discipline is grappling with fundamental issues that reflect its history and inform contemporary challenges in building professional practice. This work must be intentional and incorporated into the development of the nurse. Rather than simply identifying courseware within which these contemporary issues will be embodied, it is more important to embed addressing these behaviors inside of the curriculum and clinical practice of the educational and developmental experience of the emerging professional nurse. In addition, faculty and practice leaders must also represent, in their own patterns of behavior, their having addressed and resolved many of these issues for themselves. They must do so in ways that serve to mentor the new nurse and demonstrate the continuing effort to overcome traditional inequities and to better articulate balanced and equitable behaviors inside the role and relationship of professional nurses and their interaction with the world.

CRITICAL THOUGHT

One is always treated precisely as one expects to be treated, and no differently. The real question is, how do you enable or permit others to behave toward you, and how do they closely manifest your own expectations and self-treatment?

The Public and Policy Role of the Profession

All professions work in the public forum. If a profession is to be relevant, contemporary, and share in writing the script for the future, its members must commit to undertaking concerted and informed action in the public sector. Those things that influence a profession to fulfill its social mandate, to achieve the ends of its work, and to make a difference in the lives of the people it serves are important to fully invest in so the profession can advance this effort (Finkelman, 2012).

Because nursing has both been a predominantly employed profession and generally driven by the characteristics of membership in an employee work group, it has been difficult to expand nurses' presence in important roles in the public arena. Physicians and other health professions have recognized the critical value for full participation in the life of the political and policy sector. As a result, this level of engagement has advanced the medical agenda, often created preferred roles and circumstances for physicians that are not always in the best interests of those they serve and society as a whole. Because much of this power and influence has not been equally countered by a fuller, more robust engagement of the public sector on the part of nurses, much of what patients need and nurses require to advance the health of the communities they serve has gone wanting.

Public Policy

Public policy is usually defined as principal action undertaken by governments. It usually involves political decision making and legislative action. Professional involvement in public policy ostensibly represents the profession's interest in advocating for those they serve through influence on government and legislation. Public policy can occur at every level of government in the United States. Indeed, health care generally impacts all levels of government, but localities are more heavily impacted because all health service is essentially local.

Shaping public policy is generally a multifaceted dynamic that usually involves the interaction and concerted contribution of a wide variety of individuals and collective groups that work in their own best interests to advance particular political or policy agendas (Cheung, Mirzaei, & Leeder, 2010). Using a variety of tactics, these individuals and groups seek to influence policy in ways they think is best for themselves or others.

In the policy pursuit advocacy can take many forms and can represent a variety of interests. Advocacy can most easily be defined as the work to influence public policy through educating others, lobbying for specific interests, and working within the political system to make desired or needed change. Advocates suggest that the issues for which they are speaking are critical to the quality of life of those they represent. While it is controversial, many professionals and knowledge workers actively advocate for interests they feel they best represent as they seek to improve the circumstances of those they represent and serve. Questions are often raised, however, as to whether advocates best represent those they serve or if they, in fact, represent their own best interests.

Regardless of the discussion and challenges around advocacy and public policy involvement, it is generally assumed that professionals are interested in the welfare of those they serve. Professionals often link the welfare of the profession with the greater well-being of those the profession serves (Figure 1-5). Although this can be treacherous ground to walk, it is also representative of a strong ethical and moral effort to more clearly articulate the needs of those who are served and better organize public systems to meet those needs in a more effective manner. For good or for ill, policy and political advocates have played a critical role in the establishment of much in health care that has advanced both the quality of health and the quality of life of American citizens. Without such advocates little would change in a democratic society.

Nurses have historically held more advocacy positions than they have actively sought. Although nursing is the single largest health profession in the nation, its per capita representation in the political and legislative arena has not demonstrated the impact that such numbers would suggest. While advocacy for the health interests of the community is central to the role of the nurse, it is difficult to measure that commitment using a numbers count of nursing advocates who are active in the public forum (Jameson, 2009).

- See the welfare of the community
- Link the profession to community
- Have an ethical obligation for health of all
- Ensure the healthcare system meets health needs
- Look for a fit between care and people
- Create a common vision for health

Figure 1-5 Public policy and advocacy

Membership in the profession assumes that a certain percentage of time spent in membership relates to working in the interests of the profession at some level of the public forum. Professionals recognize that policy, political, and legislative action is an important vehicle for advancing improved standards of health, clinical care, and community health. At least some time in the life of each professional should be devoted to addressing issues of public concern. Each professional should demonstrate the fulfillment of his or her personal obligation to make a difference in the life of the broader community and to demonstrate the value of the nursing profession in doing so. There are a number of ways in which the professional can be expected to have an impact on the quality of life of the community:

- Periodically participate in the life of the profession as an active member of a professional organization and potentially as an officer of the organization. Because much of public advocacy is undertaken by professional organizations, participation in the organization strengthens its capacity to speak for the best interests of the population for which it advocates.
- Serving on local boards, committees, and task forces related to health and the quality of life in the community is one of the best ways to demonstrate health advocacy. These roles are generally specific, focused, and time limited, giving the participant an opportunity to

contribute to the local level in a role that can have a broad impact on the quality of health and community.

- Testifying for boards, committees, and commissions regarding specific elements of care and service provides a notable and effective way of having an impact by educating and deepening understanding of specific issues, policies, or changes necessary to advance the health and quality-of-life issues of the community.

REFLECTIVE QUESTION

Does membership in the profession not also imply obligation to the community? Does that not mean that members of the profession have an obligation to demonstrate their commitment by also serving their community in a wide range of public and personal efforts?

- Equally, serving on specific health-related boards, committees, and commissions can expand the option of the nurse to be able to influence policy and strengthen advocacy for particular health causes through the action of collective wisdom in a way that can strongly influence changes in policy, practice, and education.

- Serving in elective office provides a more definitive and specific process in advocating and legislating advancing public policy and law. Full engagement in the political process ensures stronger ownership, direct political accountability, ability to establish law, and the capacity to drive meaningful and sustainable change.

In every level of professional life, from local agency advocacy to representation of broad-based political roles and legislation, nurses have an opportunity to significantly influence the quality of life of the community, the political and social role of the profession, and the passage of law and regulation that can establish firm standards upon which quality, safety, and health can be advanced and assured. Each nurse should be fully aware of the personal obligation the professional has for addressing issues of advocacy and public policy. Making a difference in the life of the community, individual patients, and the profession itself is a fundamental obligation of membership in the professional community (Cowen & Moorhead, 2011). This obligation should not be taken lightly. Each nurse must reflect individually on his or her level of commitment and specific role in addressing personal professional advocacy in a way that advances the interests of those each nurse serves. Such advocacy need not be widely publicized;

instead, it can often be a quiet normative role contribution to making meaningful change in health care. Even the act of writing letters to politicians, participating in the formulation of position papers, gathering data to support advocacy positions, and developing information materials for patients and community members all demonstrate professional participation in public policy. All nurses should see for themselves the extent to which they can participate in such activities, recognizing the essential obligation to have an impact on the public and the health of the community. As Florence Nightingale's life suggests, these are normative obligations for professional nurses and should not be seen as exceptional but, instead, normative functions congruent with the obligations of the profession and representative of its commitment to expanding health in the community it serves.

CRITICAL THOUGHT

For a professional, personal and professional identity act as one. As individuals become members of the profession, they are so identified with the profession that their membership in it cannot be separated from their personal identity. "I am a nurse" is a statement that enumerates who I am, not just what I do.

I Am the Profession

Whatever a profession is or does depends on the contribution and commitment made by its members. How a profession is perceived by others depends on the perception generated by members of the profession who represent its interests to the public it serves. Each person who characterizes him- or herself as a member of the profession has a specific obligation to demonstrate in his or her role the characteristics of what the profession has to offer. Each professional needs to demonstrate the foundations of what constitutes a profession—skills that represent theoretical and evidence-based foundations in knowledge; active participation in the life of the profession in ways that advance the interests of the profession; continuous, lifelong commitment to education and learning; peer-based competency expectations and measurement; meeting the ethical and moral obligations of the profession; demonstrating personal and professional behavior according to the code of ethics for the profession; evidenced by personal disposition, deportment, self-confidence, personal competence, and positive relationship to others, showing the strength and character of the profession. This pattern of professional behavior is exemplified in mentoring, modeling, and contributing to the education and development of peers; and, most importantly, making a difference in the individual and collective lives and health of the community. Each of these demonstrates the characteristics that make up a profession. Collectively they articulate what a profession does and who a professional is. They are the nonnegotiable foundations upon which a profession is built, and they are definitive requisites that form the foundation of professional life. Without them there is no profession. And without the full engagement, ownership, and investment in the activities associated with advancing these characteristics, one cannot claim membership in a professional community. As nursing moves into the adulthood of its professional life, these characteristics become the nonnegotiable characteristics to which each professional member commits in his or her personal behavior, interactions, and clinical performance.

CHAPTER TEST QUESTIONS

www

1. Nursing is a fully mature and adult profession now reflecting all of the particular characteristics of professional delineation. True or false?

2. Professionals act predominently on principle, not simply on their knowledge reflecting a belief that principle drives knowledge. True or false?

3. Evidence-based practice is grounded in good policy and reflects inconsistent standardization and procedures. True or false?

4. The Nurses Code of Ethics serves as a foundation for the exercise of nursing practice. True or false?

5. Shared governance is a voluntary process that invites staff to participate in decisions that affect patient care. True or false?

6. Very few professional decisions are made at the point of service or in the patient environment. Most decisions influencing nursing practice in shared governance should be made away from the patient care setting. True or false?

7. All staff must participate in shared governance activities. True or false?

8. For a professional, the identification of the profession is a part of personal identity such that it is impossible to separate the person from the profession. True or false?

9. Language isn't nearly as important as action is. The way in which a nurse acts is the most important indicator of who the nurse is. True or false?

10. One of the primary roles of the nurse is to coordinate, facilitate, and integrate interdisciplinary interaction around elements of professional practice and patient care in order to ensure synthesis and safety for the patient. True or false?

> **www**
> For a full suite of assignments and additional learning activities, use the access code located in the front of your book to visit the exclusive website: http://go.jblearning.com/leadership. If you do not have an access code, you can obtain one at the site.

References

Allen, D., Calkin, J., & Peterson, M. (1988). Making shared governance work: A conceptual model. *Journal of Nursing Administration, 18*(1), 37–43.

American Nurses Association. (2001). *Code of ethics for nurses with interpretive statements.* Washington, DC: Author.

Becerra-Fernandez, I., & Leidner, D. (2008). Knowledge management: An evolutionary view. In M. E. Armonk (Series Ed.), *Advances in management information systems* (p. 344). Armonk, NY: Sharpe.

Bennet, A., & Bennet, D. (2004). *Organizational survival in the new world: The intelligent complex adaptive system.* Boston, MA: Butterworth-Heinemann.

Bennet, A., & Bennet, D. (2010). Multidimensionality: Building the mind/brain infrastructure for the next generation knowledge worker. *On the Horizon, 18*(3), 240–254.

Cheung, K., Mirzaei, M., & Leeder, S. (2010). Health policy analysis: A tool to evaluate in policy documents the alignment between policy statements and intended outcomes. *Australian Health Review, 34*(4), 405–413.

Cowen, P. S., & Moorhead, S. (2011). *Current issues in nursing.* St. Louis, MO: Mosby Elsevier.

Daly, J. (2005). *Professional nursing: Concepts, issues, and challenges.* New York, NY: Springer.

Davidhizar, R. (2005). Creating a professional image. *Journal of Practical Nursing, 55*(2), 22–24.

Finkelman, A. W. (2012). *Leadership and management for nurses: Core competencies for quality care.* Boston, MA: Pearson.

Hain, L. (2009). Guide to the Code of Ethics for nurses: Interpretation and application. *Nursing Educational Perspectives, 30*(4), 258–259.

Heuer, A., Geisler, S., Kamienski, M., Langevin, D., & O'Sullivan Maillet, J. (2010). Introducing medical students to the interdisciplinary healthcare team: Piloting a case-based approach. *Journal of Allied Health, 39*(2), 76–81.

Jameson, J. (2009). Nursing policy research: Turning evidence-based research and health policy. *Choice, 46*(10), 1973–1974.

Marriner-Tomey, A., & Alligood, M. R. (2002). *Nursing theorists and their work.* St. Louis, MO: Mosby.

McDonald, L. (2010). *Florence Nightingale at first hand.* Waterloo, Ontario: Wilfred Laurier University Press.

Megill, K. A. (2004). *Thinking for a living: The coming age of knowledge work.* München, Germany: K.G. Saur.

Melnyk, B., & Fineout-Overholt, E. (2010). *Evidence-based practice and nursing and healthcare* (2nd ed.). St. Louis, MO: Lippincott Williams & Wilkins.

Porter-O'Grady, T. (2009). *Interdisciplinary shared governance: Integrating practice, transforming healthcare.* Sudbury, MA: Jones and Bartlett.

Porter-O'Grady, T., & Malloch, K. (2010). *Quantum leadership: Advancing innovation, transforming healthcare.* Sudbury, MA: Jones and Bartlett.

Rapp, C., Etzel-Wise, D., Marty, W., Coffman, M., Carlson, L., Asher, D., . . . Whitley, R. (2010). Barriers to evidence-based practice implementation: Results of a qualitative study. *Community Mental Health Journal, 46*(2), 112–118.

Roux, G. M., & Halstead, J. A. (2009). *Issues and trends in nursing: Essential knowledge for today and tomorrow.* Sudbury, MA: Jones and Bartlett.

Samovar, L. A., Porter, R. E., & McDaniel, E. (2012). *Intercultural communication: A reader (13th ed.).* Boston, MA: Wadsworth, Cengage Learning.

Steiger, D., & Steiger, N. (2008). Instant-based cognitive mapping: A process for discovering a knowledge worker's tacit mental model. *Knowledge Management Research and Practice, 6*(4), 312–321.

United States Congress, House Committee on Veterans' Affairs, Subcommittee on Economic Opportunity. (2011). Licensure and certification hearing before the Subcommittee on Economic Opportunity of the Committee on Veterans' Affairs, US House of Representatives, One Hundred Eleventh Congress, second session, July 29, 2010. Washington, DC: Government Printing Office.

Zerbe, W. J., Ashkanasy, N. M., & Hartel, C. (2006). *Individual and organizational perspectives on emotion management and display.* Boston, MA: Elsevier.

Appendix A

Extinguishing Childlike Behaviors in the Professional Nursing Staff

For years the staff have been positioned as the children of the organization. Many of the control mechanisms in the organization were directed to controlling the otherwise undisciplined and misdirected energies of the worker. Because of their relative ignorance and lack of personal discipline and their willingness to escape the demands of work, it was necessary to develop management-derived control mechanisms to provide the frame for acceptable behaviors. Interestingly enough, such mechanisms proved to be a self-fulfilling prophesy for leaders, and the staff ended up behaving exactly as expected. Indeed, such behaviors have now become entrenched within the American workplace on the part of both managers and staff. The staff now exhibit the following patterns of behavior:

- No control over their own work schedules
- No full participation in the assignment of work tasks and responsibilities
- External resolution of personal problems from home or work circumstances
- Nonresolution of relationship conflicts arising out of the work relationship
- Being told what to learn and what is required for personal continuing education
- Parental disciplinary procedures that punish bad behavior and reward good behaviors

Pushing the Children into Adulthood

Leaders must stop the parental patterns of behavior in their tracks if there is to be any meaningful accountability and ownership in the staff. No longer can those parental behaviors be used as a tool of control and staff management. The leader must undertake at least the following if that pattern is to be broken:

- Mama doesn't work here anymore
- Staff must manage themselves and their work schedules
- Staff must be able to problem solve their own issues
- Staff must fully participate in setting work goals and processes
- Evaluation of competence is always a staff process
- Staff must be competent enough to solve their own problems
- Team-based approaches must be used to set direction, undertake work, and evaluate outcomes

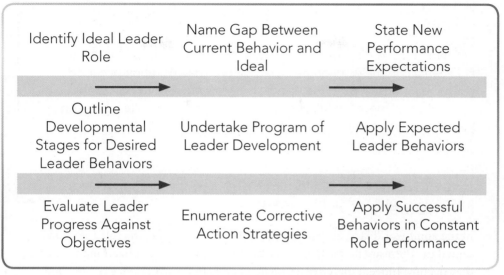

Identify Ideal Leader Role	Name Gap Between Current Behavior and Ideal	State New Performance Expectations
Outline Developmental Stages for Desired Leader Behaviors	Undertake Program of Leader Development	Apply Expected Leader Behaviors
Evaluate Leader Progress Against Objectives	Enumerate Corrective Action Strategies	Apply Successful Behaviors in Constant Role Performance

Leaders of the Profession Extinguish Parental Behaviors

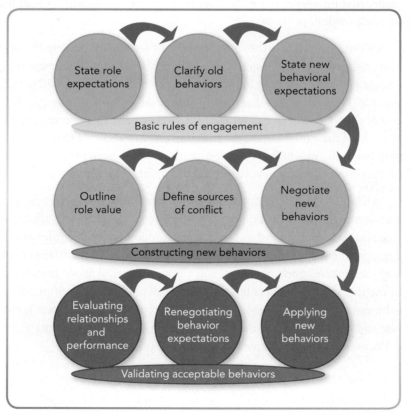

Professionals Get Past Parent-Child Behaviors

> **NOTE**
>
> No one should expect to be invited to the full expression of partnership in the work of the organization. That invitation occurred when one accepted the opportunity to work. Everyone has the right to expect the full engagement of their work colleagues and the commitment necessary to make that successful.

Expectation, Not Invitation (The Professional's Membership Obligation)

In the adult workplace, all participants are expected to play the role they consented to. There are no participants who do not express an obligation to the role they occupy. Indeed, there are no invited guests to the experience of life. One either owns the role played or the role is not occupied. This seems strange at first glance, but on deeper reflection, it is an extremely important tenet of the adult-to-adult workplace.

An invitation to play the full role and partnership in meeting the organization's obligations is not a subset of membership in the work community. One is engaged in work precisely to make a contribution within the skill set defined for the role. It is anticipated that the individual will commit all energies to the exercise of the role without encouragement or coercion. That commitment is a clear element of the expression of the role. Anyone not aware of that expectation as they begin the role isn't going to be expressive of it, even if the person is invited to further commit to the behaviors or expectations for the role.

In the adult-to-adult equation, it is anticipated that all players are equally on board. This notion of equity is a primary centerpiece of the valuing of each role and the expression of its relationship and impact on the roles of others. The aggregated effort of all roles is necessary for the effective interface of energy in a way that ensures good outcomes and work products. Anyone shirking any part of the role will have a clear effect on the work of others and ultimately affect the achievement of good outcomes. In such a circumstance, the effect is a negative one and reduces the net value of the work of all and pulls energy away from the collective effort to add value and produce good outcomes.

Appendix B

The Professional Is a Cocreator

Wise leaders recognize that innovation cannot be unilaterally driven. Ultimately, the creative act is a collective one and requires an ability to excite others and get them on board. No one person is responsible for creating the future, even if the idea was generated out of the thinking and reflecting of an individual. To translate ideas into action requires the concerted effort of a number of committed people in the dynamic act of cocreating—the transformation of an idea into reality.

Creativity Demands Engagement

- Creativity can generate from individuals or teams but must be shared in order to be translated into something of value.

- The leader gathers the creative team together to feed their insight with dialogue, challenge, new thinking, and willingness to explore further.

- The leader can identify in the creative person the unique expression of creativity and make it possible to be nurtured and expressed.

- Creativity within must be regularly nourished by new thinking and exposure to other creative people or it dies.

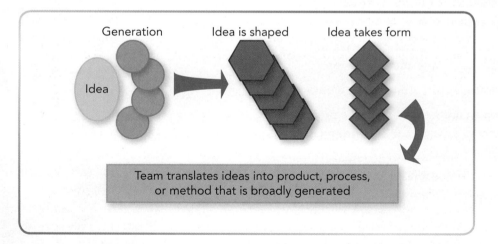

I HAVE AN ALMOST COMPLETE DISREGARD OF PRECEDENT, AND A FAITH IN THE POSSIBILITY OF SOMETHING BETTER. IT IRRITATES ME TO BE TOLD HOW THINGS HAVE ALWAYS BEEN DONE. I DEFY THE TYRANNY OF PRECEDENT. I GO FOR ANYTHING NEW THAT MIGHT IMPROVE THE PAST. —CLARA BARTON

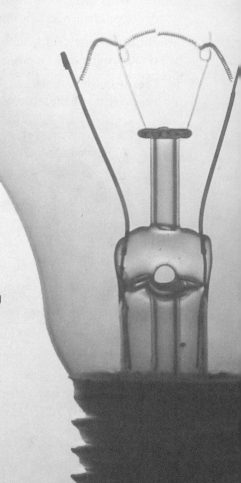

CHAPTER OBJECTIVES

Upon completion of this chapter, the reader will be able to do the following:

» Describe the nature of change and innovation in a complex environment.

» List techniques to assist in the development of change and innovation competence.

» Define the essential competencies and behaviors for effective change and innovation.

» Enumerate specific strategies to embrace change.

» Develop an understanding of the processes for overcoming obstacles to change and innovation.

» Identify the purpose and essential elements of a contemporary business case for advancing quality using change and innovation principles.

Change and Innovation

At some point in time, every nurse realizes that there are better ways to provide patient care, better policies to drive patient care, and better ways to organize and lead a patient care area. These new ideas require change to occur and an understanding of the complex dynamics that often result in chaos, positive or negative events. Improving the processes of patient care to improve outcomes is fundamental to quality patient care and requires skills in change management. What is also important for the clinical leader is to understand the rationale and intended impact for change proposals and processes. Changing without supporting rationale for improvement should be seriously questioned prior to implementation.

In this chapter, the nature of change and innovation along with strategies to embrace new ideas and overcome obstacles are presented. The role of the clinical leader in understanding the dynamics of change and innovation as well as developing skills to challenge assumptions of practice, use innovation techniques, and communicate recommendations for improvements are discussed.

Change and innovation are widely used concepts and the terms are often used interchangeably. Numerous descriptions and definitions of both change and innovation exist and further confound the process of gaining clarity between the two concepts. Innovation, rather than change, is often used to gain attention and infer that something new and special is happening. One of the reasons there are significant variations in the descriptions of change and innovation can be attributed to the various underlying assumptions about the environment and the nature of change.

Many individuals fear change and are reluctant to challenge assumptions and try something different, particularly in the work setting. A smaller number of individuals embrace change as normative and as an opportunity for new and better ways of being. What is important to remember, regardless of one's comfort with change, is that change is ever present and an inevitable attribute of being alive. There is no escaping change—except for death! Thus it makes good and prudent sense to learn as much as one can about the nature of change, how to embrace it, and how to maximize positive changes.

REFLECTIVE QUESTION

Change can be considered a predictable linear process or a complex, highly interrelated process. Are there advantages of each process? Are there times when one approach is more or less useful? Consider a recent change in which a new policy, process, or protocol was implemented. Was the process linear or complex? Describe the areas of success and the areas identified for improvement.

Most individuals and organizations see change and/or innovation as a linear process that can be managed and controlled. This perspective of change as a linear phenomenon guides the processes and decisions of traditional organizations. It is believed that a change in one area will result in a change in another specific area and the change will occur as planned. It is this linear cause and effect assumption that most of our change processes and expectations are built upon.

Project management processes are an example of linear change and focus on predictability, equilibrium, and linear evolution while limiting flexibility, variation, and creativity in order to accomplish the goals of the change project. Deviations from the plan are viewed negatively, and the next steps focus on elimination of variances. While a linear process is helpful in providing order and structure for change processes, it does not recognize the multiple, unanticipated human actions and communications that occur and the dynamic context in which the change is occurring. This linear perspective often becomes rigid, control driven, frustrating, and unsuccessful. While a project may be brought to completion, new issues and challenges emerge quickly. These unanticipated events are often viewed negatively and categorized as project shortcomings when in fact such events are normative and are the evolving results of complex human dynamics.

> ## MYTHS ABOUT CHANGE
>
> - Change can be controlled. False. Change can only be facilitated; it cannot be stopped or harnessed.
>
> - Change is painful. False. Not everyone is reluctant or resistant to change. Some individuals readily embrace change as normative and as a way of living to the fullest.
>
> - Change is always chaotic. False. Change can be planned or unplanned. Planned change focuses on facilitating and managing the process to achieve optional outcomes.
>
> - Strategic planning by a leader will decrease the chaos of change. False. Strategic plans serve as general guidelines that cannot by nature include all of the possible outcomes.
>
> - The environment does not impact a well-thought-out change process. False. The environment is dynamic and continually changing. Necessarily, changes in the environment, such as the economy, the climate, and political decisions, impact strategic plans.
>
> - Change in a digital environment increases the ability of leaders to control processes and outcomes. False. The digital environment provides capacity for increased processing complexity; it does not identify which of the multiple interrelated interactions will occur, nor does a digital resource identify what will occur in the future.

Another perspective from which to view change and innovation is the complexity science perspective (Fonseca, 2002). Complexity science understands the world as a dynamic phenomenon in which movement is continual and unpredictable. The world is in continual motion, and movement occurs in more than linear ways. A change in one area can result in numerous, unanticipated changes in areas not considered. As one individual or a group of individuals interacts with others, numerous actions occur spontaneously as ideas are shared and information is considered. The movement does not cease with the one interaction; it moves on and on and on from one individual to another to another. Interactions in a complexity perspective are characterized by creativity, interdependence, unpredictability, and collective knowledge. Change in the healthcare environment is better understood from a complexity paradigm rather than a linear paradigm because the nature of change is seldom linear and controllable.

CHANGE IS ...

- Something new or different
- To make or become different
- To alter; to make different; to cause to pass from one state to another; as, to change the position, character, or appearance of a thing; to change the countenance
- To alter by substituting something else for, or by giving up for something else; as, to change the clothes; to change one's occupation; to change one's intention
- To give and take reciprocally; to exchange; followed by with; as, to change place, or hats, or money, with another

Source: Webster's Dictionary (1991).

Dynamics of Change and Innovation

These two perspectives provide differing dynamics for change processes; one is linear, the other is highly interrelated and unpredictable. Descriptions of change and innovation are presented in the accompanying box and Figure 2-1.

Change has been described as an alteration of the current state. Innovation is defined as a unique type of change in which there is a novel and dramatic change that fundamentally restructures the deep social and economic value of an organization (Weberg, 2009). Change is considered normative in a complex system. In contrast, change is something to be managed, controlled, and minimized in a linear system.

As clinical nurse leaders embrace change, it is important to establish a common understanding of what is meant by change and innovation among team members and colleagues. The selection of definitions for team members to ensure understanding when change and innovation are discussed serves to decrease confusion and misinterpretation.

INNOVATION DESCRIPTIONS

- Anything that creates new resources, processes, or values or improves a company's existing resources, processes, or values (Christensen, Anthony, & Roth, 2004)

- The power to define the industry; the effort to create purposeful focused changed in an enterprise's economic or social potential (Drucker, 1985)

- The first practical, concrete implementation of an idea done in a way that brings broad-based extrinsic recognition to an individual or organization (Plsek, 1997)

- A slow process of accretion, building small insight upon interesting fact upon tried-and-true process (Dupree & Hessler, 2008)

- A new patterning of our experience of being together, as new meaning emerges from ordinary everyday work conversations; a challenging, exciting process of anticipating with others in the evolution of work (Fonseca, 2002)

- Doing new things that customers ultimately appreciate and value; not only developing new generations of products, service channels, and customer experiences, but also conceiving new business processes and models (Cash, Earl, & Morison, 2008)

Who, Why, When, and How of Change

The dynamics of change and innovation are best understood and advanced when several things are known. These include the key stakeholders of the work to be changed (who), the rationale for the change (why), the content to be changed (what), the timing for change (when), and the techniques to change effectively (how).

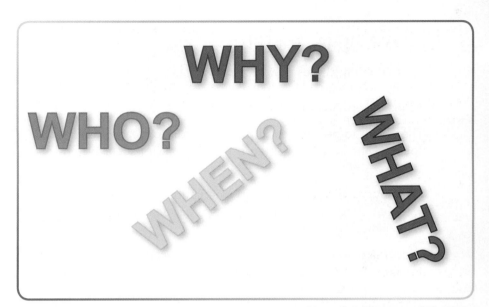

Figure 2-1 Change and Changing

Who Should Change?

Most individuals work to get others to change in hopes of improving processes and outcomes; this work is often futile and frustrating. It is nearly impossible to change or motivate others. While change is best accomplished by engagement of others to support the need and rationale for changing, the process always begins with the individual. Significant effort can be expended to create reminders, guidelines, and checklists for others that do little to advance the desired outcome. The additional work of completing checklists becomes an obstacle to change and decreases the emphasis on the real outcomes desired.

Becoming competent in understanding and thriving in the rapidly changing world requires awareness of personal change abilities first. Individuals need to understand their personal comfort and competence with change. This begins with an assessment of strengths specific to the ability to identify critical issues for change, overcome obstacles, challenge assumptions, recognize areas for growth, provide meaningful feedback, and be resilient. The goal is for each individual to clearly understand him- or herself before attempting to engage with others in advancing change in the areas of knowledge of the change process, personal comfort with change and risk taking, relationships, conflict, and negotiation skills.

When your personal change competence is understood, the next step is to coach others in developing understanding and competence in change and innovation. Most importantly, the change and innovation leader is comfortable with personal limitations and the reality that one cannot possibly know everything there is to know about any one topic and that it is this combined wisdom of the team that creates effective change.

Why Change?

Oftentimes the rationale for change is not clearly identified. When there is not a common consensus and rationale for change among the key stakeholders, the work of change can be resisted through avoidance, benign tolerance, or lack of attention. In our complex healthcare world with limited resources, the rationale for change should be clearly linked to changes that would improve patient care outcomes and the quality of the healthcare experience. Specifically, change should only be considered when patient safety is enhanced, new evidence is available, excellence is advanced, and/or costs are controlled.

Change for Quality Outcomes

Value in health care is measured by the outcomes achieved, not the volume of services delivered. Value is also not measured by the processes of care. Process measures are helpful tactics but do not replace measurement of outcomes and cost. Too often change is made only in selected processes without logical connections to identified outcomes. Improving processes without a clear connection to a change in outcomes is misguided and seldom results in the desired positive change. For example, the limited success of the national quality movement is a product of the linear process change approach. The focus on processes and completion of checklists has not impacted patient value or outcomes and continues to be problematic. Efforts have been made to increase the monitoring and documentation of the integration between process changes and outcomes achieved (Colevas & Rempe, 2011). Also, efforts to tightly link the desired outcomes of providing healthcare information to a patient, documentation of this process, *and* identifying the impact on patient health status as a result of the information are desperately needed and continue to challenge healthcare leaders. Consider the accompanying scenario and identify the needed linkages between processes and outcomes.

SCENARIO

The following five initiatives are identified for all healthcare providers. Consider each of the initiatives and discuss the potential patient outcomes that should occur as a result of these process changes. Discuss strategies to integrate this information into clinical processes to increase engagement of clinicians in monitoring these processes. Discuss alternative strategies to document and measure more meaningful processes to achieve improvements in patient functional health status.

Acute myocardial infarction

- Aspirin prescribed at discharge
- Fibrinolytic therapy within 30 minutes of arrival at hospital
- Primary percutaneous coronary intervention received within 90 minutes of arrival at hospital

Heart failure

- Discharge instructions
- Evaluation of left ventricular systolic function
- ACE inhibitor or ARB for left ventricular systolic function

Pneumonia

- Pneumococcal vaccination
- Blood cultures performed in the emergency department prior to initial antibiotic received in hospital
- Initial antibiotic selection for community-associated pneumonia in an immunocompetent patient
- Influenza vaccination
- Healthcare associated infections
- Prophylactic antibiotic received within 1 hour prior to surgical incision

Surgeries

- Surgery patients on a beta blocker prior to arrival who received a beta blocker during the perioperative period
- Surgery patients with recommended venous thromboembolism prophylaxis ordered

(continues)

Surgeries (*cont.*)

- Surgery patients who received appropriate venous thromboembolism prophylaxis within 24 hours prior to surgery to 24 hours after surgery

Hospital consumer assessment of healthcare providers and systems (HCAHPS)

- Communication with nurses
- Responsiveness of hospital staff
- Pain management
- Communication about medicines
- Cleanliness and quietness of hospital environment
- Discharge information
- Overall rating of hospital

Source: The Federal Register, Vol. 76, No. 9, January 13, 2011.

Change for Evidence

Changing to implement new evidence or to meet newly identified needs of patients is driving much of current healthcare change. When there is a gap between current performance and desired performance in your facility or unit, using an evidence-based practice approach is the most logical. In an evidence-based model, patient care interventions are supported by evidence from a variety of sources and strengths of research support. When there is a gap in the available evidence, patient care needs, and desired interventions, an opportunity can be identified for change and innovation to close that gap. Using the principles of evidence-based practice, linkages between clinical practice and scientific standards, the quest for consistency, minimizing idiosyncrasies, and providing a scientific basis for policy construction are the basic reasons for change in health care. Using an evidence-driven model serves to provide focus and organization of change initiatives; evidence-based practice is the platform for our work. Figure 2-2 provides a diagram of the evidence-based practice process and the emerging gaps that provide a logical impetus for change and innovation (Porter-O'Grady & Malloch, 2010).

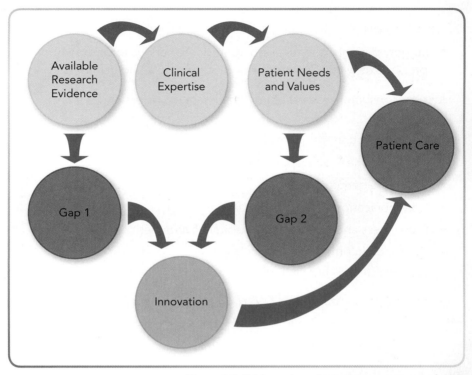

Figure 2-2 Evidence-based practice processes and gaps

ONLINE RESOURCES FOR QUALITY EVALUATION

- Comparative Effectiveness Research (CER) Database: www.npaf.org/images/pdf/NPAFCERDatabase.pdf

- Agency for Healthcare Research and Quality (AHRQ): www.ahrq.gov

- Patient Safety and Quality: An Evidence-Based Handbook for Nurses: www.ahrq.gov/qual/nurseshdbk

- Patient-Centered Outcomes Research Institute (PCORI): www.pcori.org

- National Quality Forum: www.qualityforum.org

- National Patient Safety Foundation (NPSF): www.npsf.org

- National Institutes of Health (NIH): www.nih.gov

- National Patient Advocate Foundation (NPAF): www.npaf.org

CRITICAL THOUGHT

Evidence-based practice is the integration of the best research evidence with clinical expertise and clinical values:

- Best research evidence refers to clinically relevant research, often from the basic health and medical sciences, but especially from patient-centered clinical research.

- Clinical expertise means the ability to use clinical skills and past experience to rapidly identify each patient's unique health state and diagnosis, individual risks and benefits of potential interventions, and personal values and expectations.

- Patient values refers to the unique preferences, concerns, and expectations that each patient brings to a clinical encounter and that must be integrated into clinical decisions if they are to serve the patient.

Source: Sackett, Strauss, Richardson, Rosenberg, & Haynes (2000).

Although there are many reasons for change and innovation, there are also reasons *not* to change, such as a lack of compelling evidence, no specific significant risk to patients and employees, isolated issues that are closely linked with individual performance rather than system performance, and indications that an intervention or change is more likely to be a fad of the moment rather than a solution that is closely linked to a probable outcome improvement. It is important to demonstrate courage to resist moving forward when the change is not appropriate for the conditions and the time.

CRITICAL THOUGHT

- Research is the systematic examination of an idea using rigorous principles of experimentation and measurement.
- **Research utilization** uses knowledge that is typically based on a single study.
- Evidence-based practice applies the relevant research and includes the expertise of the practitioner as well as patient preferences and values.

What to Change?

After a rationale for change, such as new information, patient safety, or increasing value, has been clearly established, the *what* of change can be determined. The what of change begins with the identification of the specific processes and policies that need to be changed, replaced, or created. In addition to specific processes or policies, there are often relational competencies that need to be changed to fully support the transition to new processes. Specifically, individual attitudes toward the change, behaviors to support the change, an understanding of duplicate processes that need to be eliminated, and the potential advancement of technology need to be identified in the desired change measures.

When to Change?

There are several considerations in determining when to change. When to change is best determined with the input of both the specific unit and system needs and resources. Although it has been said that timing is everything, sometimes the options for when to change are limited by the urgency of the situation. Some would ask if there is ever a good time to change or innovate.

CRITICAL THOUGHT

Implementing the second-best idea *now* is a better strategy than doing the best thing a week from now. It is a bigger risk to delay making decisions than to make marginal ones.

The pace and number of changes and new ideas for consideration are often overwhelming. Chaos is normative. It is thus futile to continuously work to eliminate change. It is important not to try to eliminate all change and activity; change is necessary for growth and sustainability of an organization. Most organizations are in the midst of change processes continually—new initiatives, new checklists, new electronic documentation systems, and so on. Learning to support staff with differing types of assignments with degrees of change activity provides a life skill useful in both work and personal settings.

How to Change

Facilitating the change process is much more than identifying what to do and when to do it. Facilitating change and innovation requires very specific competencies to fully engage others and advance the identified processes to achieve outcomes. The following competencies are essential for change effectiveness:

- Personal knowledge and accountability for one's own strengths and limitations specific to change and innovation, including technical capability and computer literacy

- Understanding the essence of change and innovation concepts as well as the tools of innovation

- The ability to collaborate and fully engage team members

- Competence in embracing vulnerability and risk taking

Personal Knowledge

Successful change and innovation agents develop a clear understanding of personal strengths specific to the work of facilitating change and innovation. Previous experiences, abilities to overcome obstacles, engaging with others to elicit meaningful feedback, and courage and stamina to advance new ideas all are important. Knowing that no one can be exceptionally competent in all areas of the change process, but rather comfortable in engaging and empowering team members to contribute their expertise, the clinical leader needs to be comfortable in continuing to forge ahead through obstacles. This work of empowering others is a selfless process in which the work is always the focus and the individual facilitator becomes peripheral to the actual work.

There are several assessment tools to identify communication, relationship, and conflict styles that are quite useful in increasing personal understanding. Myers-Briggs (http://www.myersbriggs.org/), DiSC profiles (http://www .thediscpersonalitytest.com/?view=Assessments_disc&gclid=CMiOyaf_ 4KwCFUhjTAodameDoA) and Kilmann Conflict assessment tools (http:// www.kilmann.com/conflict.html) are some of the available assessment tools that can supplement self-understanding.

Another important tool is peer-to-peer collegial assessment and coaching. Taking time with trusted colleagues to share feedback about communication, relationships, and conflict styles on a regular basis may in fact be more helpful than more formalized assessments.

Asking questions specific to behaviors supportive of change and innovation is vitally important.

Examples of questions include the following:

- Am I open to new ideas?

- Am I able to recognize my own personal limitations and understanding that such limitations are a reflection of reality and not of personal inadequacy?

REFLECTIONS ON PROFESSIONAL NURSING AUTONOMY

- Autonomous practice is a highly evolved clinical attribute.
- Leaders are visible, accessible, and able to communicate effectively with the staff to support decision-making processes.
- Staff leadership is about developing skills of coaching, risk taking, and challenging the status quo.
- Leaders supporting autonomous practice are knowledgeable, strong, visionary risk takers. Their philosophy is clear, well articulated, and guides day-to-day activities.
- A participative management style is pervasive, and staff feedback is not only welcomed but expected by leaders in making decisions about the work of patient care.
- Shared governance is a structure and process that embodies the principles of equity, partnership, accountability, and ownership, which are necessary for autonomy to flourish.
- Competent clinicians, with expertise as autonomous professionals, function most effectively in the context of a team of similarly competent professionals.

- Am I able to clearly identify and share my strengths with others?
- Do I share my wisdom in a kind, caring, and nonthreatening manner?
- Do I trust that the motivations of others are basically good willed?

In contrast, asking colleagues questions specific to barriers that might impact one's ability to relate effectively with others can provide further insight into behaviors. Examples of questions include the following:

- Can you tell me about times when I have displayed an attitude of aloofness or arrogance?
- Are there times when I always need to be right?
- Do I portray serious concern about losing control or that others are more competent than I am?
- Have I expressed fear that others might realize I don't know everything?
- Do my behaviors reflect a belief of personal immunity to anxiety, fatigue, and overwork?

Finally, personal knowledge is about understanding the expectations of a professional. Knowing the accountabilities, expectations, and contributions are important components of each professional and should continue to emerge throughout one's career. As a change and innovation agent, the professional nurse clearly understands that clinical practice autonomy does not imply independence. It is about practicing to the full extent of the nursing scope of practice and licensure in interdependent healthcare teams.

Change and Innovation Knowledge

Specific knowledge about the concepts and theories of change and innovation is an essential tool for those engaged in the change process. Understanding the diversity of descriptions and definitions of change and innovation is helpful in evaluating the understanding of others. Shared understandings of what change is and is not among team members serves to increase consensus and common understanding of the work being done. Finally, an understanding of the course of events in a typical change process further assists leaders in facilitating change (Figure 2-3).

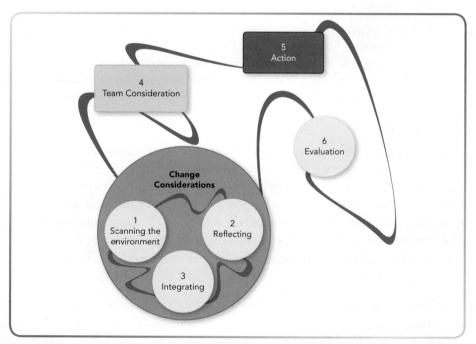

Figure 2-3 The Change Process: Essential considerations for effective change and innovation

In addition to understanding the concepts of change and innovation, basic knowledge of the tools and techniques that support change and innovation advancement is also important. Tools such as **mind mapping**, brainstorming, **directed creativity**, construction of prototypes in innovation spaces, scenario planning, and **deep dive** experiences are helpful in engaging others and increasing the diversity and creativity of dialogue and change effectiveness (Endsley, 2010).

TOOLS TO ADVANCE CHANGE AND INNOVATION

- Deep dive: A particular area is selected for observation in multiple ways. Workflows, photos, interviews, and observations are gathered by a team to analyze current processes and brainstorm new ways of doing the current work processes (Kelly, 2005).

- Directed creativity: A situation is proposed to encourage and advance new ideas. For example, individuals are presented with the following scenario and are directed to respond: "A new unit is being designed for medical surgical patients. If there were no limits on space, technology, resources, staff, or financial resources, how would you design the unit for the future in a way to dramatically improve the cost and quality of the healthcare experience?" (Plsek, 1997).

- Mind mapping: A software tool for collecting, organizing, and synthesizing large amounts of data in layers with complex relationships. A very useful tool for documenting connectivity, interdependencies, and emerging phenomena in health care.

Collaboration

Working together effectively with wide ranges of diverse individuals is another important competency necessary not only with the initiation and implementation of change, but also for sustaining new processes and course correcting when appropriate. Too often, the upfront work of planning, designing, and implementing occur with minimal challenges, and the efforts at fully integrating the new processes into the culture and operations become blurred, minimized, or marginalized. Thus the intended change does not fully occur as planned, nor are the desired outcomes realized.

Collaboration among all team members continues as the problem or goals are clearly identified. In addition, the team identifies processes to be changed, the linkages between this process and other organizational processes, the research evidence to support the change, technology to support the change process, anticipated policy changes needed, clear specification of the evaluation criteria, frequency of evaluation, and processes for course correction.

Embracing Vulnerability and Managing Risk

Oftentimes, change and innovation processes require individuals to take risks and to challenge long-standing status quo work processes and patterns within a strong culture. Taking risks in which the outcome is uncertain requires individuals to be comfortable with the reality that each one of us is indeed vulnerable; no one can be certain of the outcome when challenging the status quo. Despite the uncertainty and the work and challenges encountered in day-to-day work, vulnerability is a positive and enhancing clinical characteristic that is vital for success. Further, the patient safety movement has created a paradoxical situation in health care; standardization has been identified as a characteristic of high reliability processes (Weick & Sutcliff, 2001), and the need to challenge long-standing processes that may not be as safe as previously believed is also a mandate.

CRITICAL THOUGHT

Trust infers that one individual is vulnerable to the actions of another. The greater the trust, the more positive are the expectations that individuals consider others' intentions and actions based on established roles, relationships, experiences, and their interdependencies.

Trust is one individual's willingness to be vulnerable to another based on the belief that the other is competent, open, concerned, and reliable, thus rendering risk taking more rational and realistic.

Taking risks is inherent in healthcare work and requires skills to embrace one's lack of total knowledge and develop rational risk-taking skills. Just as one uncertain situation is embraced and managed, another one appears. The feelings of vulnerability that accompany each risk-taking experience need to be recognized and embraced willingly, rather than avoided. The vulnerable nurse views this work with an openness to new ideas and takes comfort in the reality that not everything works out as intended, no matter how well thought out the plan might be. Taking risks and acknowledging one's vulnerability is not about being irresponsible or incompetent; it is about recognizing the reality of contemporary existence.

Risk can never be eliminated completely; however, it can be minimized. It is important to recognize that there are both rational and irrational risks that need to be differentiated before moving forward.

Risk taking has not been perceived as a positive leadership behavior, nor is it traditionally welcomed and encouraged. Instead, risk taking is viewed negatively and as something that increases the organization's exposure to unforeseen hazards and to loss of net income and reputation. Playing it safe and being a hardworking employee is the more preferred behavior, but the reality is that playing it safe will lead the organization nowhere because the intent is to live in the past and to continue the practices that have been deemed to work yesterday.

Interestingly, there is no better person than the point-of-care clinical leader to identify opportunities for new ways of providing optimal patient care. The clinical leader understands the patient care need, the context in which the care is being provided, and when practices work well and don't work well. Thus, the clinical leader needs to become an expert at identifying opportunities and engaging in rational risk taking as a means to advance knowledge in the system.

Rational risk taking is about taking risks for the right reason. Rational risk taking is more than thrill seeking and experience enhancing; it is focused and consistent with the organization's goals, values, and resources as well as consideration of others involved. The following four categories are considered guidelines for rational risk taking: advancing the organization, developing skills, mandatory reporting, and whistle-blowing.

Advancing the organization, the first category, is about learning to thrive and survive in the organization. Challenges in providing patient care, as well as the external introduction of new ideas, need to be considered carefully and regularly. New clinical interventions, programs, expansion of existing services, selecting equipment, and prioritizing what comes first are common challenges. Choices that are rational and minimize risk are those that are made on the basis of core values of the organization, respect for others, the safety of individuals, strategic goals, and available resources.

In particular, most individuals would benefit from advanced teamwork competencies. Developing skills is the second rational risk category. Regardless of current competence levels, all individuals need to learn new skills to continue to be effective in the ever-changing healthcare environment. Acquiring new knowledge and skills that are rational includes skills specific to the job role and personal preferences to support the role in the most robust way. Considerations should be given to enhancing physical capability, computer skills, public speaking expertise, athletics, art, and personal protection skills. Each of these extend the competence and value of the individual caregiver and leader.

Developing teamwork expertise is vital in times of high risk and uncertainty. The greater the teamwork and support for creativity, the more new ideas that will emerge as the only way to accomplish this challenging and uncertain work. In addition, teamwork competence can be developed by reaching out beyond one's normal network of colleagues to others with related skills. Developing relationships beyond traditional healthcare disciplines can provide new insights and greater depth of understanding. High-functioning team collaboration also includes well-developed professional autonomy and interdependence to maximize each discipline's contribution to patient care.

The third category of rational risk taking is mandatory reporting. Many state licensing agencies require licensees to report the unprofessional conduct of other licensees to the licensing board. The goal is to protect the public from licensees who commit repeated errors, abuse alcohol or drug substances, and are incompetent to do the entrusted work. Proponents of mandatory reporting believe other similarly licensed professionals are best able to identify such issues and thus they must risk speaking up to protect the patient and the profession. According to most state statutes, it is not an option whether or not to speak up, and in fact failing to report known behaviors is considered an act of unprofessional conduct. Examples of unprofessional conduct include repeated medication errors, boundary violations, and theft from patients.

The fourth category of rational risk taking is whistle-blowing. Whistle-blowing is about righting a wrong—a wrong that is believed to be dishonest and that resulted in the mistreatment of others. The need for whistle-blower protection arises when the culture of the organization does not support open communication, honesty, differing opinions, and fairness. When individuals believe they have not been heard on an issue and public interest is compromised, the federal False Claims Act provides a mechanism to report fraud and corruption while protecting those who expose information from wrongful dismissal and loss of security and benefits. Using the protection of this whistle-blower legislation is considered a rational and necessary risk and involves personal and professional risk, regardless of the outcome.

Embracing rational risks requires knowledge, skill, and engagement with the team to best support new ideas and changes. In contrast, avoiding irrational risks is also a learned skill and requires an understanding of the nature of irrational risks. Four categories of irrational risk—a history of failure and oppression, poor judgment, unrealistic expectations, and lack of potential benefit for the action—are discussed in the next section.

CRITICAL THOUGHT

Job security is truly a myth. No job is ever guaranteed forever—or even the next month! Jobs are eliminated as a result of downsizing, the need for new skills, new locations, and different delivery model structures.

The workplace environment changes frequently—new leaders, new colleagues, new work, and so on. The goal for every individual is to always be employable—to always have the skills that are needed in the current and future environment.

Being employed is short-sighted; being employable is futuristic!

When there is a history of failed efforts, it is not prudent to attempt the same change unless there is new energy, new approaches, or new technology to increase the potential for improvement and success. Oftentimes, education programs are provided to increase knowledge or compliance with desired practices, and little improvement occurs. Continuing the same actions is futile without further examination of the situation and consideration of other options.

Poor judgment seems an obvious irrational risk; however, it needs to be recognized. Consider the example of walking out into traffic. The risk of injury to both the pedestrian and those driving is present and probable. This type of irrational risk is similar to the leader who hires individuals without adequate depth and competence for hard-to-fill positions. It is only a matter of time until the inadequate job performance negatively impacts quality and productivity. The organization incurs additional cost and risk. The clinical leader must challenge the assumptions of the position and brainstorm other ways to consider the rational risk approach and assume risk to advance the organization in creating a new role or developing another person's skills to meet the hard-to-fill position. This irrational approach further complicates a situation that is already overly complex and high risk.

Another irrational risk occurs when unrealistic expectations are embraced as the way to do business. Often, there is little potential for success when an organization attempts to implement just one more program or initiative in an environment in which staff are already overwhelmed. It is irrational to believe that such endeavors will be successful, even marginally.

When there is no known benefit for an action, the work can be considered an irrational risk of resources. Examples include planning education programs for which there is no audience, establishing committees for individual attendance when the work can be done electronically, or disciplining employees for outcomes over which they have no control.

In addition to rational and irrational risks, individuals often insert irrational negative fantasies into the discussion and decision-making processes for change and innovation. These negative fantasies can paralyze or hamper individuals from taking action. The irrational fears seem very real to some individuals and need to be challenged. Consider these comments and fill in the blanks:

- My dad will kill me if . . .
- I'll get fired if I say something . . .
- No one will like me if . . .
- The nurses will quit if . . .

Perhaps the most common negative fantasy in health care is the perception that one will be fired for taking risks and speaking up. Individuals worry that speaking up will have a negative impact on their reputation, their ability to communicate openly and honestly with others, and ultimately, the security of their position. The reality is that individuals are seldom involuntarily removed from their jobs for speaking up and taking risks. Involuntary termination is more about incompetence, substance abuse, poor attendance, dishonesty—and *not* speaking up! Identifying and confronting negative fantasies can decrease barriers and resistance to change and innovation (Figure 2-4).

The more risks you take, the more secure your job is . . .

This is true if with every risk, you are growing professionally and learning information that is helpful to both yourself and the organization.

In an organization supportive of creativity and growth, this is certainly true. In a risk-averse organization, this is probably false.

The more risks you take, the greater the probability of being fired . . .

True if taking risks compromises the organization's financial status and reputation when new approaches don't work.

This is true in risk-averse organizations and false when rational risks are taken and the organization is supportive.

The more risks you take, the better the organization will be . . .

True when each new attempt supports a culture dedicated to finding new and better ways to accomplish the work and more efficient ways of doing business that will increase the profitability and sustainability of the organization.

This is false when risk taking overshadows the ability of the organization to accomplish the work at hand. There is a need for balance between operations and stretching the limits of current processes.

Figure 2-4 Taking Risks: True *and* False?

Strategies to Minimize Risk in Change and Innovation Scenarios

Speak Up

The first strategy to minimize risk is to speak up with evidence or a rationale for action. The best safeguard to avoiding poor outcomes is using data, evidence, and a rationale. When there are significant variations in practice patterns, multiple opinions about the best solution, and little use of technology to validate the assumptions, there is a need for focused communication to determine the supporting evidence that is based on standards, experience, and values. To be sure, it is these conditions of uncertainty that precipitate evidence-based practice initiatives and thereby reduce the risks involved in attempting new strategies.

Timing and Tinkering

The second strategy is timing. As previously noted in the section on when to change or innovate, timing is always an important consideration. Not every risk needs to be or must be addressed immediately; sometimes waiting is the prudent approach. Levels of workload, the availability of key participants, and the overall climate of the organization need to be considered prior to taking risks. Classical leadership behavior encompasses strategic planning and the purposeful review of ideas. With the recent advances in information technology, these processes are becoming increasingly ineffective and outdated. The emphasis now includes short-term, incremental strategies similar to the concept of tinkering, introduced by Abramson (2000).

Tinkering becomes the expectation, the status quo—team members seriously challenge assumptions and ask questions, not out of idle curiosity but by looking carefully at current dogma and raising issues that open the door to substantial improvements. The values of tinkering include the following:

- It provides an opportunity to learn how to take risks.
- A little tinkering and a lot of team member experience allow a small group to make changes with big goals in mind and to evaluate the change efficiently.
- Team members' skills are stretched with little risk to the organization; support for constant tinkering minimizes the change that the organization will drift into inertia. Rational risk becomes the norm, change is internalized as essential for survival, and employees gain new experiences and develop new skills.

- Tinkering becomes the expectation, the status quo. Team members seriously challenge assumptions and ask questions, not out of idle curiosity but by looking carefully at current dogma and raising issues that open the door to substantial improvements.

DECREASING FEAR, INCREASING TRUST, AND UPWARD COMMUNICATION CHECKLIST

- Have the right people been involved in making decisions? If not, identify who should be involved and why. Avoid the temptation to complain and mumble, "If they only had asked me."

- Are the goals and values of the organization being respected? If a decision does not seem consistent with the goals and values, take two actions. First, identify what specifically is not consistent with which value. Second, identify what you would like to see done to improve congruence with values.

- Don't get lost in the process. If something is not working, then give it up—even if it means retreating and regrouping. Identify the fact that the work is off course and needs course correction. It is too easy to lose sight of the original goal.

- Identify when work-arounds are created that avoid the real issue. New policies that add work to all employees are often created for isolated, aberrant behaviors. Challenge leaders to address the issue rather than creating another policy.

- When decisions are made on biased or impartial information, offer the additional information. Offer the information not to one-up another, but for the purpose of achieving the best decision with all of the information.

Encourage Upward Communication

The third strategy to minimize the risk of change and innovation is about focused communication; communication that gains the attention and support of decision makers. Top–down communication remains the most common type of communication in an organization. Cultures with shared leadership structures reinforce and support vertical, horizontal, and multidirectional communication more effectively than traditional organizations; however, the need for upward communication remains a great need in organizations. Greater emphasis is needed to assure upward communication to ensure that leaders know what is going in the organization and are able to support the best decisions.

The first step is to realize that leaders cannot and do not know everything; the second step is to learn to share the appropriate information—information that impacts the operations and reputation of the organization. Learning what information to share and when to share it evolves with experience and commitment to core values.

Accelerate Personal Competence

The fourth strategy is to increase one's competence quickly as new equipment, technology, and processes become available. The more one can learn about new approaches, the more competent one is to not only evaluate the innovations, but also to determine if the new approach is right for the organization. Further, this approach reinforces evidence-based principles as the supportive rationale for change. Assuming a posture of risk avoidance and waiting for others to test and critique new approaches decreases the individual's ability to support an organization that is contemporary and able to integrate processes and equipment into the work of patient care.

CRITICAL THOUGHT

- Recognize that mistakes happen!
- Right the wrong as quickly as possible.
- Be sincere and apologize when appropriate.
- Use humor only when appropriate.
- Admit you were wrong—avoid the silent treatment.
- Don't try to rationalize and blame it on someone else.
- Say you are sorry when you are.
- Shake hands and make up!

Further, competence can be developed by reaching out beyond the normal network of colleagues to others with related skills. Developing relationships beyond traditional healthcare disciplines can provide new insights and greater depth of understanding. Embracing environmental psychologists and human factors experts to assist in team collaboration and communication can greatly enrich work processes. Florists and musicians and potters also give new meaning and understanding to the work of healing—and they serve to sustain the focus on healing and avoid the tendency to focus only on technology or publications.

Apologize with a Flair

The fifth strategy to minimize risk is to apologize quickly and appropriately when an error or misstep is recognized. Resiliency is the key. No patient ever expects to be harmed while under the care of a healer; further, no healer ever expects to harm a patient. Yet, unexpected events and deviations encountered in the provision of care do occur and injuries result. All healers will make mistakes no matter how competent one is. The responsibility accepted by a healer is indeed awesome because patients entrust their care to and give caregivers enormous power and authority. It takes considerable spiritual and emotional maturity to accept patient trust, understand that mistakes happen, and modify conditions when needed.

When a misstep occurs, leaders must be resilient and able to regroup and move on when things don't go as anticipated. Recognizing negative situations and acknowledging them with others can be therapeutic. Discussions of unsuccessful events provide an open forum to discuss strategies to avoid repeating similar situations. It is far better to acknowledge the misstep than to ruminate endlessly. This approach avoids leaving others to wonder about your competence and assists you back on the right path (Figure 2-5).

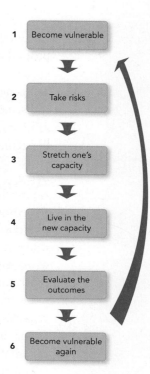

Figure 2-5
The risk-taking cycle

Making Change and Innovation Happen

With a solid foundation of the dynamics of change and innovation, the risks, and risk minimization strategies, the clinical leader is well positioned to move forward. Risk-disposed leaders develop a very high level of self-discipline that allows the processes of change and innovation to evolve. A strong sense of commitment can be more valuable than intelligence, education, luck, or talent. Clinical leaders who are adept at taking risks neither surrender nor overreact to crises or marginally successful efforts; they regroup and return. They take stock of the situation, often pulling back temporarily (but not too long) while they plan the next steps. They realize that sometimes it is best to put aside personal feelings and let bygones be bygones. Finally, they focus on the present and the future, both of which offer perils and possibilities, rather than on the past, about which nothing can be done.

In the complex healthcare world, it is impossible to escape the reality of risk and the associated feelings of vulnerability. The goal for all clinicians is to examine each situation and embrace those risks that are rational and avoid or at least minimize risks that are believed to be irrational. The course of events usually begins with recognizing that one is vulnerable and then recognizes rational risks as a means to stretch one's capacity and ultimately move the work of the organization to greater quality and excellence.

Clinical leaders need to focus across the longer continuum of the change process using reflection, accountability measures, and persistence to ensure full engagement of the change. Appendix A provides specific interventions for the assessment, reflection, and integration phases of the change process. Each phase is discussed in the next section. The change process includes three major phases: assessment of the conditions, reflection with the team specific to the needed work to occur, and integration of information into a plan.

Assessment

Assessment and scanning the environment to determine current practice requires a level of consciousness that allows the leader to take in as much about the environment as possible. Data from multiples sources are involved in the activities of assessment. First and foremost, the leader must become skilled in sensing the environment, listening, and learning from the current activity. *Stilling one's mind* to be open to what is going on in the environment is essential in this process and requires discipline, practice, and commitment. To be sure, there is no template or format in which environmental scanning should occur. Each situation requires different considerations identified by the individual who best knows the organization and situation. The individual scans and assesses the environment based on previous experiences, knowledge of the current environment, and desired outcomes.

Team Reflection

The second phase is discussion with the key stakeholders for the change and innovation work. To begin the discussions, it is important to have the right individuals in the group. Team members should carefully reflect to be sure the needed stakeholders are present so the work can progress. It is equally important to deselect participants who do not add value to the processes of change and innovation.

After the environment is assessed, team members further consider past experiences, the potential impact on current events, and work to avoid negative experiences. Consideration is given to how individuals will react in new circumstances—positively or negatively. This information serves as critical background information in moving forward.

Integration of Ideas into a Plan

The third phase is to integrate the critical information learned in the assessment and reflection processes. The process of integration is the assimilation of the data collected during the assessment and reflection phases, all of the relevant research, values, perceptions, experiences, intuition, and the political, technological, economic, and social data. The ever-present challenge of this phase is developing the skill of which data to include and which data to exclude to effect the best decision. Necessarily, effective integration is not a lone activity; rather full integration of work and efforts of all members of the group is required. To be sure, the preparation for change and innovation is as important as the actual work.

Integrating the data into a business plan template also provides guidance in building and documenting the rationale, plan, and expected outcomes for a change and innovation project.

Caveat: Technology, Change, and the Human Element

Much of the change in health care includes the addition of new devices, software applications for documentation, and communication enhancements to advance the patient care experience. Clinical leaders should regularly ask what value these new technologies provide to improve the patient care outcomes in a way that recognizes that the technology does not drive the work, but rather supports the human work. Bell (2010) reminds us that when everything is digitized and connected, there can neither be stability nor genuine innovation. In particular, decisions still need to be made by humans rather than completely relegated to computer applications. The computer generates the data, and the clinical leader interprets the data within the specific patient care context.

 REFLECTIVE QUESTION

Dare to move to a virtual world. How does one enmesh oneself in the world of technology and still retain the human touch? Moving aggressively to greater levels of technology is about advancing into uncharted territories.

Caveat: Measuring the Impact of Change and Innovation (What Problem Are You Fixing?)

In a world of scarce resources, the goal is to expend resources appropriately with the expectation of success of the desired plan. In spite of the best projections and anticipated risks and benefits, precise and accurate projections of the costs of change and innovation projects are at best estimates—estimates that must be identified as carefully as possible. Creating a business case for innovation can be most helpful in identifying the multiple variables and many of the associated costs. A business case for change and innovation should become a standard practice when resources, efforts, and expertise are expended. Clear and accurate business cases also provide essential information in prioritizing processes for change.

BUSINESS CASE FOR INNOVATION: ESSENTIAL CONSIDERATIONS

1. Clear description of the product or service; work to be done

2. Purpose of the product or service; the goal to be accomplished

3. Projection of costs to begin and manage the project, including staff, equipment, and supplies

4. A list of costs not included and rationale for not including

5. Estimation of benefits and evidence for the anticipated benefits

6. Timeline for development and launching of the project

7. Anticipated profit or loss for the first 2 years

8. Other qualitative benefits anticipated, such as community benefit, reputation, and satisfaction of staff and patients

9. Anticipated risks involved and plans to mediate the risks

10. Summary statement of short-term and long-term value to all stakeholders

Source: Adapted from Malloch (2010).

CRITICAL THOUGHT

The proper unit for measuring value should encompass all services or activities that jointly determine success in meeting a set of patient needs.

Source: Porter (2010).

Another consideration is the challenge of benchmarking innovation work. Phillips (2011) identified the practice from the late 1980s through the 1990s of benchmarking against industry standards as an indication of performance compared to other companies. Interestingly, the relevance, value, and benefit of benchmarking were not determined. Benchmarking innovation methods and processes across the industry may provide insights into practices, as well as differences in practices, which are equally important. Benchmarking specific metrics does not provide similar value and direction.

GUIDELINES FOR SELECTION OF INNOVATION METRICS

- Select metrics to assess innovation progress and costs in advance. Incremental benchmarks are especially important to track and trend progress. Different sets of funding, testing, and performance criteria for incremental, experimental, and potentially disruptive innovations are needed.

- Aim to identify early successes. Major initiatives often require significant time to realize the full benefits. Interim achievements are necessary to demonstrate progress and the likelihood of achieving the full potential of the innovation.

- Get data to back up your gut. Successful innovators begin with the gut feeling and must move quickly to develop the quantifiable, supporting data.

Benchmarking innovations with other organizations is difficult for several reasons. The first is that innovation is closely tied to strategy and vision, which vary widely across organizations and make them difficult to compare. A second reason is that the time in which the innovations were implemented can vary widely, from

90 days to several years. The third reason is specific to the assumptions about the customer or patient. The varying approach to the driving force behind the innovation, namely the company or the customer or patient, provides different perspectives of consumer research and how it is integrated into the innovation work. Some believe that current customers or patients are not able to envision a radically new and better future; thus asking them to participate in the innovation process can vary from organization to organization.

SCENARIO

Oftentimes individuals state they are supportive and want to participate in change or changing; however, the change does not happen. Consider the following underlying assumptions documented by Kegan and Lahey (2001):

- Stated commitment: I want to be a team player.

- I am struggling with making this happen because I don't collaborate enough. I make unilateral decisions too often, and I really don't take people's ideas and input into account.

- Competing commitment: I am committed to being the one who gets the credit and to avoiding the frustration or conflict that comes with collaboration.

- Big underlying assumption: I assume that no one will appreciate me if I am not seen as the source of success; I assume nothing good will come of my being frustrated or in conflict.

Discussion Questions

1. Using your understanding of change and innovation, the process and dynamics, the strategies to manage resistance, and the tools of innovation, how could you and your team address this type of resistance?

2. More importantly, how could the team be proactive in minimizing the chance for this resistance in the planning phase?

Managing Resistance to Change

In spite of the best preparation and planning, resistance to change and innovation occurs. In addition, the results of the anticipated change may not be optimal. In the next section, thoughts on managing resistance and implementing course corrections are discussed.

Resistance to change occurs in many formats from outspoken, verbal reactions to subtle, nonverbal, indirect avoidance of the issue. In general, individuals resist change when there is a perceived threat to their safety and security or position. The culture of an organization or the leadership style can also impede change and innovation (Schein, 2004). Competing commitments have also been identified as a source of resistance. Individuals may want to change; however, there are other deep-seated factors that may become barriers to change. Those involved in change and innovation work are regularly challenged to identify resistance to change as early as possible and begin to work to remove or minimize the resistance.

Course Correction

It is traditional to assign failure to those change and innovation projects that did not result in favorable outcomes. A new perspective that recognizes and values the information gained from less than successful attempts is needed in health care. Embracing these situations as courageous acts that provide new insight and opportunities for further dialogue is congruent with cultures of excellence. When the less than optimal results are identified, the next step is about course correction and remediation. The new knowledge gained from the unsuccessful effort is critical to continuing success; this information serves to inform others of a course of action that should not be repeated.

Documenting this information is essential in advancing change. Further, it is important to avoid individual employee sanctions when the outcomes involve the team and the supporting system. Punishing individuals for outcomes that involved many factors and many individuals is futile and demoralizing. Punishing discourages individuals from future risk taking that could be of great benefit to the organization.

When there is an individual action of concern, remediation is the preferred option. Specifically, remediation is preferred when the potential risk of physical, emotional, or financial harm caused by the incident is low; the event is a singular event with no prior pattern of poor practice; and the individual exhibits a conscientious approach to and accountability for his or her practice and now appears to have the knowledge and skill to practice safely. Punitive actions are reserved for matters of last resort. Punitive actions should be considered only when an individual has repeatedly disregarded advice and directions to modify actions, previous remediation attempts have failed, and there is evidence of incompetence that cannot be rectified.

 ## SCENARIO

When the result is less than optimal, consider the following steps:

- Acknowledge the outcome.
- Correct negative outcomes quickly; ensure personal safety.
- Apologize to those affected by the outcome.
- Review the goal and the selected processes, and identify areas of vulnerability.
- Be sure the goals and work are still the right thing to do.
- Modify the processes to avoid further negative outcomes.
- Never be reluctant to abandon the goal if safe and effective processes cannot be determined.

Consider the scenario in which the goal is for all departments in an organization to use the SBAR (Situation, Background, Action, Recommendation) handoff method for lunch relief and shift change. Several departments, housekeeping, pharmacy, and behavioral health units are now refusing to use the SBAR process because they believe it is cumbersome and not helpful; omissions are still occurring and staff are dissatisfied. What additional information do you need to determine if the SBAR should be continued or discontinued in these areas?

CRITICAL THOUGHT

Innovation leadership is not about being an inventor; it is not about a specific leadership role. It is about envisioning a better future using the following behaviors:

- Having the courage to challenge the status quo
- Being comfortable with risk taking
- Having significant ego strength
- Facilitating and empowering others to be as creative as they can be

Leading and Managing

Clinical leaders need to be able to discern innovations that add value to the work and innovations that serve as obstacles to the work. Creating more work to streamline processes that ultimately decrease productivity and the timely achievement of quality outcomes is not a rational approach.

In times of high risk and uncertainty, the goal is to focus on effective communication through highly skilled teamwork. The greater the teamwork and support for creativity, the more new ideas will emerge as the only way to accomplish this challenging and uncertain work. Encouraging all members of the organization to share and develop their leadership skills requires passion and engagement in the richness of the collective decision-making process.

Looking to the future to support change and innovation requires a clinical leader mind-set that includes a strong personal awareness of one's strengths and vulnerability, openness to other ideas, courage to challenge the status quo, and a highly developed comfort with rational risk taking (Figure 2-6). These behaviors at the point of service are more important now than ever before as new ideas are introduced frequently and the demands for higher quality are emphasized. Shifting from a universal focus on sustaining current practices and being proof driven before attempting new processes that support change and innovation will necessarily require time, persistence, and a different way of thinking.

The clinical leader at the point of care must necessarily continue to look for new role opportunities, improvements in decision-making structures, management of the physical space for patient care, potential partnerships, and equipment and technology needs to support the continual advancement of patient care excellence—and, of course, enjoy this very special journey of advancing healthcare excellence.

Innovation Leadership	Management
• Self-awareness	• Focused on sustaining and strengthening the present
• Courageous, hopeful	• Reactive
• Proactive, future oriented	• Proof driven
• Inquisitive	• Discipline/root cause focused; blame placing
• Optimistic	
• Able to experiment, course correct, remediate	

Figure 2-6 Characteristics of innovation leadership and management

CHAPTER TEST QUESTIONS

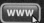

1. Change is (a) always associated with chaos, (b) can be controlled using project management software, (c) an inevitable life process, or (d) is best managed by an individual with expertise in change theory.

2. Innovation and change (a) are similar but distinct concepts, (b) are the same concepts, (c) are based on the same assumptions, or (d) are avoided by health care workers.

3. Timing for change (a) requires assessment and prioritizing of work to be done (b) is best determined by the CEO, (c) is impossible to predict, or (d) requires a multidisciplinary team approach.

4. Resistance to change and innovation (a) increases the chances for creativity, (b) is not uncommon and needs to be mediated, (c) provides a stop gap measure for inappropriate changes, or (d) is limited to individuals with excessive workload requirements.

5. There are certain times when change is not appropriate and should not occur. Change should be avoided when (a) the funding to support the change is not available, (b) the anticipated value is positive, (c) selected team members are resistant or (d) there is no clear rationale or improvement anticipated.

6. Project management templates and processes (a) are ideally suited for complex change and innovation, (b) can remove obstacles to creativity, (c) consider deviations from the plan as negative or (d) accelerate the orderly work of change.

7. Change competencies include (a) common understanding of definitions and descriptions of change, (b) expertise in completing checklists, (c) knowledge of team member abilities to create a business case, or (d) emphasizing the limitations of other team member competencies.

8. Tinkering is about (a) providing input to a complex project management plan, (b) learning how to facilitate team work, (c) using toy models to understand complex processes, or (d) short-term incremental strategies to advance a complex process.

9. Measurement of change (a) is best done with financial metrics, (b) is best done with a single quantitative or qualitative metric, (c) should be distinct from measurement of innovation, or (d) requires consideration of the goals and variables involved in the change.

10. Negative fantasies about change (a) are important considerations in reality checking, (b) encourage creativity and innovation (c) can be serious obstacles to embracing change and innovation or (d) are more prevalent in newer employees.

www

For a full suite of assignments and additional learning activities, use the access code located in the front of your book to visit the exclusive website: http://go.jblearning.com/leadership. If you do not have an access code, you can obtain one at the site.

References

Abramson, E. (2000). Change without pain. *Harvard Business Review, 78*(7), 75–79.

Bell, K. (2010). Will the Internet destroy us? *Harvard Business Review, 88*(11), 138–139.

Cash, J. I., Earl, M. J., & Morison, R. (2008). Teaming up to crack innovation and enterprise integration. *Harvard Business Review, 86*(10), 90–99.

Change. (1991). Retrieved from http://www.merriam-webster.com/dictionary/change

Christensen, C. M., Anthony, S. D., & Roth, E. A. (2004). *Seeing what's next: Using the theories of innovation to predict industry change.* Boston, MA: Harvard Business School Press.

Colevas, A. D., & Rempe, B. (2011). Nurse-sensitive indicators: Integral to the Magnet journey. *American Nurse Today, 6*(1), 39–40.

Drucker, P. (1985). The discipline of innovation. *Harvard Business Review, 63*(3), 67–72.

Dupree, J. R., & Hessler, F. A. (2008). The evolution of measurement. Retrieved from http://www.usatoday.com/money/jobcenter/workplace/kay/story/2011-11-14/show-skills-dont-rely-on-buzzwords/51171274/1

Endsley, S. (2010). Innovation in action: A practical system for getting results. In T. Porter-O'Grady & K. Malloch (Eds.). *Innovation leadership: Creating the landscape of health care,* (pp. 59–86). Sudbury, MA: Jones and Bartlett.

Fonseca, J. (2002). *Complexity and innovation in organizations.* London, England: Routledge.

Kegan, R., & Lahey, L. L. (2001). The real reason people don't change. *Harvard Business Review, 102*(10).

Kelly, T. (2005). *Ten faces of innovation.* New York, NY: Doubleday.

Malloch, K. (2010). Innovation leadership: New perspectives for new work. *Nursing Clinics of North America, 45*(1), 1–10.

Phillips, J. (2011). Why innovation can't be benchmarked. Retrieved from http://www.innovationexcellence.com/blog/2011/07/19/why-innovation-cant-be-benchmarked/

Plsek, P. E. (1997). *Creativity, innovation and quality.* Milwaukee, WI: ASQ Quality Press.

Porter, M. E. (2010). What is value in health care? *New England Journal of Medicine, 363*(26), 2477–2481.

Porter-O'Grady, T., & Malloch, K. (2010). *Innovation leadership: Creating the landscape of health care.* Sudbury, MA: Jones and Bartlett.

Sackett, D. L., Strauss, S. E., Richardson, W. S., Rosenberg, W., & Haynes, R. B. (2000). *Evidence-based medicine: How to practice and teach EBM.* London, England: Churchill Livingstone.

Schein, E. (2004). *Organizational culture and leadership.* San Francisco, CA: Jossey-Bass.

Weberg, D. (2009). Innovation in healthcare: A concept analysis. *Nursing Administration Quarterly, 33*(3), 227–237.

Weick, K., & Sutcliffe, K. (2001). *Managing the unexpected: Assuring high performance in an age of complexity.* San Francisco, CA: Jossey-Bass.

Appendix A

Change Considerations: Scanning, Reflecting, and Integrating

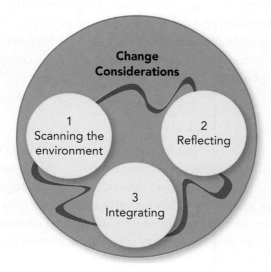

Planning for Change

After an issue is identified, careful analysis is needed to ensure the issue is legitimate and deserving of attention. The depth and range of considerations for a change process include scanning the environment, reflecting on the current and desired state, and integrating critical information into a plan for action.

Note that these steps are deliberately detailed for illustration purposes. When an individual is familiar with these steps, they tend to occur quite quickly and more automatically. However, missing one of the steps can be problematic. A quick move to action without a comprehensive assessment of the situation and reflection with the team can lead to incomplete solutions that will ultimately need to be redone and incur unnecessary costs.

Appendix B

Workgroup Scenarios for Change and Innovation

The following scenarios are designed for small group work in the application of the change and innovation principles, processes, and guidelines. Consider the nature of change or innovation in the project—the who, what, when, and how of the change; plans to manage resistance; measurement of the changes; and a summary business case for each scenario.

Scenario: Span of Control

Given the numbers of people who report to a single individual in a traditional organizational model, as well as the varying degrees of effectiveness of many of the models, create an innovation plan to assess, reflect, and integrate ideas and strategies in a team framework. Given the variations in team sizes and purposes, create guidelines for assessing multiple teams and making recommendations specific to the desired outcomes. Include purposes, goals, variables, competencies, and timelines.

Scenario: Shared Leadership and Decision Making

Implementing an effective shared leadership model requires significant insight, support, employee engagement, regular evaluations, and course corrections to create a sustainable model. Consider the organizational structure, the assumptions of the existing culture, identified core values, and commitment to teamwork as critical for success. Examine your current level of shared leadership behaviors and model (assessment) and create a plan to advance the model to a higher level of performance using change and innovation strategies identified in this chapter. Be sure to include a timeline and evaluation measures.

Scenario: Social Networking

Social networking is a recent innovation and communication trend that has positive and negative connotations. As this innovation continues to emerge, more challenges are appearing specific to personal privacy, Health Insurance Portability and Accountability Act regulations, and reputation management, as well as the potential for using social media in a focused way to connect specific healthcare groups and communities and creatively advance the health status of many community members. What strategies need to be considered in order to maximize the value of social networking and minimize the negative consequences?

NEVER MISTAKE KNOWLEDGE FOR WISDOM. ONE HELPS YOU MAKE A LIVING; THE OTHER HELPS YOU MAKE A LIFE. —SANDRA CAREY

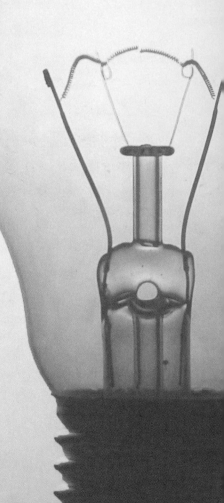

CHAPTER OBJECTIVES

Upon completion of this chapter, the reader will be able to do the following:

» Understand the characteristics and components of personal leadership in a profession.

» Define the role of the professional knowledge worker as a leader in the profession and its impact on the role of members.

» Enumerate the behaviors and practices of the contemporary clinical leader in the skills necessary to exemplify them.

» Outline some of the pitfalls and challenges affecting the role of the leader and sort truth from fiction regarding appropriate leader skills.

» List at least five critical leadership practices that are unique to the leadership role within a knowledge worker frame of reference.

» State your individual personal characteristics and their potential for transformation into the development of your own leadership capacity as a part of a personal leadership development plan.

The Person of the Leader: The Capacity to Lead

Leaders coordinate, integrate, facilitate, and provide a context for the performance of the people of the organization (Maxwell, 2010). This person gives language to the strategic direction of the organization and in that translational capacity he or she gives real life to the work of others. Leaders really do little else than create the context for work in a way that aligns the work to the mission and vision of the organization and ensure that the relationship is continuously played out in the activities of the people of the organization.

Leadership is a capacity all its own. It is a particular skill set. Although it may reflect talents gained from other focuses or activities, its expression is unique to the role. Leadership requires its own time. Cluttering the activities of leadership with responsibilities and tasks of others or assuming the accountabilities that belong to others as a part of the role of leadership both incapacitates the role and impedes its legitimate expression (Watkins, 2004). It is often tragic to see how leaders are subsumed by the activities of others and become overwhelmed with the day-to-day pressures of doing work and getting things done. Although such activities are important, for the leader they are a continuous and constant impediment to the legitimate and full expression of the leadership role.

CRITICAL THOUGHT

Leaders end up in serious trouble when they invest too personally for too long a period of time in busyness, chaos, and the intensity of the day-to-day activities of work. Who will the staff depend on for seeing beyond the day's work and help them find the meaning and sustainability in their work that can come only from rising above it and looking beyond it to discover both purpose and direction?

Leaders can actually lose their legitimacy and the true value of the role by investing too personally for too long a period of time in the busyness, chaos, and continuous intensity of the day-to-day activities of the workplace. Failing to pull away from the ownership of activity and function is perhaps the greatest single impediment to fully engaging the character and function of leadership in a way that will make a difference to the organization and people to which leadership is directed (Zedeck and American Psychological Association, 2011). If the leader is overwhelmed by the intensity of daily activity, the capacity to lead is compromised and the ability of the leader to make a difference in the lives he or she leads will be extinguished.

Self-Knowledge

Over time, leaders are simply unable to hide their true leadership capacity from others. Genuine connection to the real self and the expression of leadership out of the genuine self-expression of the person is a critical centerpiece to the legitimate role of the leader. A refined level of self-knowledge represents a deeper insight into the character, needs, and expression of the person of the leader in a way that represents individual clarity, openness, and vulnerability characterized in the disclosing and humane expression of good leadership. The effective leader represents personal availability to others, to learning, and to change and exhibits the continuous willingness to confront and engage the challenges of life and work head-on with a level of personal enthusiasm and excitement that is palpable to others. One of the real efforts of leadership is the willingness to visibly display struggles and challenges associated with grappling with problems, intractable issues, the challenges of change, and the personal struggles in adapting one's own behaviors when the demands of change call for personal adjustment (Figure 3-1).

Good leaders are many things; they also play many roles. In the 21st century the leader must be:

- A transformer
- A visionary
- A translator of direction
- Communication central
- A pursuer of truth
- A generator of creativity and innovation
- A seeker of the very next thing
- A team expert and role model
- A model of the journey to excellence

Figure 3-1 Who is the leader?

The Continuous Journey of Becoming

Change is a constant. People do not create change, drive change, originate change, or own and control change. Change is, in fact, the condition of existence. Change is a constant more than an activity. It represents the framework of existence and operates as a constant at every level throughout the universe (Hawking, 1988). Furthermore, change is not an event. It does not come and go, it does ebb and flow, but it is consistent and constant, ever present as a part of the condition of living.

As an outflow of this understanding regarding change, personal growth, development, and the engagement of the life experience across the continuum of one's life is the clearest validation of the constancy of change and the demand to continuously engage it in order to find meaning, purpose, and to express value as a member of a dynamic human community. The leader is intimately familiar with this dynamic of change and is able to resonate with this dynamic so he or she is seen as positively disposed and consistently excited about the engagement of the journey of learning and growing as it applies to both the role and function in the system (Werhane, 2007). In fact, this individual so resonates with the reality of change at a personal level that this connection becomes identified with the person. This congruence between the dynamics of change in the person of the leader creates the image of availability, openness, engagement, and embracing the challenges of change as a normative part of the role of leadership. This resonance is so palpable that it represents the person of the leader to others in a way that develops an intensity of relationships where all who represent this interaction share in this level of enthusiasm and equally indicate their connection with the change dynamic and the ability to incorporate it into their own practices and processes.

CRITICAL THOUGHT

The leader creates a context that frames the behavior of the organization in a way that helps the organization achieve its objectives.

It should be evident to the emerging leader at this stage that the personal characteristics and attributes of generative leadership provide the prototype or model for personal leadership (Rondeau, 2007). They present it in a way that generates a community of interest and engagement evidenced by people's ability to seek out, give form to, advance, and create new patterns of response to changing times and circumstances in the organization. This is the power of personal commitment and attachment to the role of leader.

The leader is able to represent within the role a deeper level of understanding of life as a journey, not an event. This simply means that the view of the leader with regard to life experiences is developed from having stood on the balcony of systems, structures, and organizations as a way of better articulating the relationship between the system and the broader context within which it operates. The wise leader is fully aware of the shifts and flows operating at the intersection between the larger social environment and the internal environment of organizations and systems. This leader knows that as those conditions and circumstances adjust and change, the dynamics are altered between the external demands of the environment and the internal response of the system as it shifts in sustainable ways (Guastello, 2002). The leader, understanding the constancy of these shifts, uses a predictive and adaptive capacity to translate that interface into meaningful language related to how these changes will affect the lives and work of the people the leader affects.

Predictive and adaptive capacity demand that the leader is able to quickly shift priorities, conversations, actions, and responses in a way that more tightly fits the circumstances affecting the present. The leader personally understands that what one knows in any given time is not permanently entrenched and doesn't represent a constant value. This leader understands that knowledge is mostly a utility, having value only to the extent that value is current and relevant and represents continuous growth (Wager, Wickham, & Glaser, 2005). The leader is able to surrender attachment to notions, ideas, past practices, rituals and routines—indeed,

WHO AM I AS A LEADER?

Good leaders constantly ask themselves questions that relate to their value and relevance and to the goodness-of-fit between their leadership practices and the changing demands of the organization:

1. Are my leadership practices consistent with the changing goals of the organization?

2. Do I focus my leadership practices on building strong relationships and creating a good fit between people and the work they do?

3. Am I aware of my own continuing developmental needs, always exposing myself to the challenges of changing developments and new learning?

anything that would impede the ability of people and organizations to better adapt to their work and value as the settings (the environment) within which they work shifts. The leader understands that these shifts are driven by what is called the **emergent**. These emergent conditions are driven by new sociopolitical realities, economic changes, technological advances, evidence of best practices, and a host of related shifts that demonstrate that holding onto current practices is an impediment to better engaging work processes in the best interests of those they serve.

The Leadership Mirror

Leaders do not act in isolation. One of the centerpieces of the leader's work is represented in the ability to build and manage meaningful and sustainable relationships with a variety of others. Whether those others are executives, peers, or those who depend on leadership, the leader values and engages in intense relationships, recognizing that it is through this vehicle that effective work and change are accomplished. These relationships are the oil that enables both the organization and its people to continue to work interactively and to achieve effective ends together. Leaders who deeply embrace and can clearly articulate the relational dynamics that drive contemporary network organizations are best able to maximize the energies that result from this knowledge (Mackin, 2007).

CRITICAL THOUGHT

If leaders want to know what kind of leaders they are, they need only look into the mirror of their staff; reflected back will be the quality of their leadership.

Reflected in the person of the leader is a mirror of the continuously emergent realities embedded in social relationships, in the cultural context, and in the business practices involved in the collective work organizations. Increasingly, technology drives much of the functional work in organizations and systems. Technology causes systems to move away from more traditional and outdated manual systems and structures that, in the contemporary world, limit the ability of systems and people to be relevant and viable in a just-in-time, fast-paced technological environment. This new paradigm for work has a number of specific characteristics and elements that directly and radically impact the role of the leader, causing him or her to reflect more deeply on the circumstances that inform effective and legitimate expression of the role (Figure 3-2). Some of these elements to consider might be the following:

- Acknowledgment of and increasing and abiding dependence on both the understanding and valuing of collective wisdom in making decisions and setting priorities.

- Accessing the collective wisdom of diverse work partners helps discern value characteristics of sustainable work. Leaders must now recognize that organizations are systems and networks and these constructs serve as the foundation or context for all work and represent the interconnections that drive decision making and the actions of people in the system.

- The industrial age has long since passed; as a result the world in which the leader leads is no longer mechanistic. It is, instead, a great relationship that is continuously dynamic, interrelated, interdependent, and continuously moving.

- The leader remains servant to the system and its people. The context drives the work of the leader. It is in creating this good fit between the context of work and the content of work that gives the leader's role focus and value. The leader coordinates, integrates, and facilitates this intersection with the intent of creating sufficient and effective convergence between systems and people such that congruence and effective relations work together to sustain both the system and its people.

- Meaning is always informed by purpose. The leader is continually reminded that all people seek meaning in their lives and work and want to see that purpose reflected in the character and quality of the work in a way that represents a contribution of each to advance the sustainability and success of the organization.

- Leaders understand the constancy of change in their own lives. They are able to translate this into the lives of others and into whole systems. Leaders seek the seamless intersection of change events and manage each stage of the change process in a way that ensures engagement of people, their movement in concert and response to meaningful change, and their collective success in advancing their own lives and the organization's interests.

- Leaders make time for self-reflection. If the leader's capacity and confidence in discerning, questioning, and translating change remain stagnant and unrefined, this is reflected in late-stage engagement, reticence, and ineffective response. Furthermore, peers witness this incongruence and are negatively affected with regard to their response to change. The availability to self-reflection, environmental scanning, strategizing, and translating reality is a personal leadership enterprise and contributes to the broader value of the organization and its people only when the leader as an individual has engaged as a personal performance expectation.

- Good leaders are transparent and become exemplars of what is valuable and right. These leaders represent their own personal commitment to engagement and transformation. They recognize that they are constantly being observed, that there are no accidental conversations, moments, or occurrences. Therefore every level of interaction has meaning, value, and impact on others. Good leadership communication is a representation of their commitment, and their connection to change, their willingness to address change, and the effectiveness of how they engage it.

Each of these components of personal leadership briefly describes the expectation of the leader in terms of self-reflection, role expression, and relationship to those to whom the leader relates. Leadership is a role, not a condition. Expressing leadership is intentional work. Leaders make a conscious choice and commitment to the work of leadership. These persons recognize within their own personhood the confluence of characteristics that must converge in a way that demonstrates the character of leadership and the commitment to appropriate and effective leadership behavior.

Conceptual competencies	Interpersonal competencies
Systems thinking	Receptivity and similarity
Acclimation to chaos	Immediacy and equality
Pattern recognition	Integration
Synthesis	Facilitation
Continuous learning	Coordination
	Coaching
	Framing new leadership language
Participation competencies	**Leadership competencies**
Partnership	Vulnerability and openness
Equity	Systems skills
Accountability	Emotional maturity
Ownership	Self-management
Investment	Transformation skills
Involvement	Group process skills
Empowerment	Change management
	Fluidity and mobility

Figure 3-2 Leadership characteristics of the 21st century

Leaders Versus Managers

Leadership and management are two distinct competencies. This textbook focuses on the development of leadership, not on functions of management. Managers have subordinates, leaders have partners. By definition, management is an organizational position and function. Managers require subordinates. Managers generally have a vertical relationship to those they manage. Management is considered a particular position with vested authority given to them by hierarchical organizational management. Traditional employees work for managers and largely do what the managers suggest is appropriate to their work. Management style is largely transactional, such that the manager generally informs employees what the nature of the work is, the direction to which that work is oriented and how it impacts the organization, the functions that are critical to the activities of work, and the training and performance expectations necessary to do the work well (Rippin, 2007).

Leadership has little to do with management. Leaders specifically do not have subordinates or subsequent roles. Leaders tend to influence others by virtue of their relationship skills and advancing the effectiveness of their relationships in a way that supports the collective work of the stakeholders and the effectiveness of their outputs (Gardner, Avolio, & Walumbwa, F. O. (Eds.). 2005). Leaders use well-researched principles of relationship, interaction, behavior, and communication to engage others in mutual commitment that advances the value of all and achieves the purposeful ends of their collective work. Leadership is essentially about the person rather than the work. When focusing on the person of the leader, role expectations relate to group interaction, influential characteristics between leaders and colleagues, innovation and creativity, interactional skills, team dynamics, and personal characteristics that inspire confidence, competence, commitment, engagement, and the support of others. Leadership is generally not fixed in a position; instead it characterizes a role. These role characteristics need to more clearly articulate the leaders' ability to effectively interact, intersect, and engage others, stimulating ownership of their contributions, coaching and develop new insights and skills, and leading others to new insights and understanding about their work system, relationships, and outcomes.

Managers direct from legitimized hierarchical positions, exercising a locus of control enumerated by their formal authority in the system. Leadership can be exercised from any point in the system and, if utilized appropriately, it can change the whole system regardless of where the leader may be located in it. Confidence and capacity are critical elements of the good exercise of leadership, not position. Managers do not necessarily have to be good leaders in order to perform their functions appropriately. However, leaders do not have that same opportunity. Leaders relate by influence, not by control. Northouse distinguished management and leadership in particular ways (2007, p. 10) (Figure 3-3). The distinction between management and leadership is that management is about function; leadership is about movement. The central focus of the manager's role relates specifically to function and activity often enumerated by skill.

Another contemporary differentiation between management and leadership is that management focuses on analysis; leadership focuses on synthesis. **Analysis** is often defined as breaking down the components of a problem or issue into parts or elements (Tilley, 2008). **Synthesis**, on the other hand, works in the opposite direction; synthesis is the act of combining and integrating numerous complex elements or components of the system in order to view it as an integrated whole

(Cowen & Moorhead, 2011). Although synthesis may include analysis as a part of its infrastructure, the ultimate goal is to observe the system acting and interacting as a whole in a way that represents the desired state.

Management produces order and consistency	Leadership produces change and movement
Planning and budgeting	Establishing direction
Establishing agendas	Creating a vision
Setting timetables	Clarifying the big picture
Allocating resources	Setting strategies
Organizing and staffing	Aligning people
Providing structure	Communicating goals
Making job placements	Seeking commitment
Establishing rules and procedures	Building teams and coalitions
Controlling and problem solving	Motivating and inspiring
Developing incentives	Inspiring and energizing
Generating creative solutions	Empowering subordinates
Taking corrective action	Satisfying unmet needs

Figure 3-3 Management versus leadership competencies

CRITICAL THOUGHT

Leadership requires a strong sense of self. It is next to impossible for a tentative leader to influence the lives and choices of others. A context of competence and confidence can sometimes be the only difference between encouragement and failure.

Management tends to look at activities and functions over a short-term, sometimes immediate time frame, and leadership observes longer trajectories of time and deals in broader-framed circumstances related to creating conditions essential for long-term sustainability rather than short-term returns. Management often focuses on efficiency, function, and process emphasis. Leadership, on the other hand, focuses on the relationship, interactions, and confluence of forces that contribute to complexity and how they can be intercepted in order to advance effectiveness or a trajectory of success rather than any moment of success. Leaders tend to embrace risk and experiment with trial and error. Managers tend to eliminate or reduce risk and build on the tried and tested.

The Personal Attributes of Leaders

Although leaders have a wide-ranging number of personalities and personal characteristics, they have a consistent network of attributes that characterize leadership (Leader to Leader Institute, Hesselbein, & Goldsmith, M. (Eds.). 2006). Emerging leaders should ask some basic questions early in their trajectory to leadership to address some of the basic attributes of leadership. Some of those questions might be as follows:

- Do I genuinely like people? My leadership will bring me in contact with many people, and I may have to lead in directions others may not be interested in going at any given time. I will need to be willing to relate to a wide variety of types of personalities, demonstrate sensitivity to their differences, be aware of their needs, and be able to accommodate these differences in my relationships. I genuinely must like doing this work.

- Am I able to live with a high degree of ambiguity and uncertainty? I will be constantly working through a large number of changes. I will need to be an example of willingness, openness, excitement, and engagement of change. I must be able to demonstrate a will to embrace change in my own life and demonstrate my life as a change in motion before I ask others to embrace change.

- How well developed are my communication skills? Communication will be the centerpiece of my leadership expression. I'll be constantly communicating with others at every level of the system. I will need to demonstrate competence and confidence and communicate articulately. I must evidence that I have been informed in my knowledge and expressions. My communication with others must be understandable, and I must be seen as competent and trustworthy.

- Do I have the courage to have crucial conversations and confrontations when required by my leadership? Can I be tough and disciplined regarding decisions and courses of action? Have I have dealt with fear and uncertainty, and am I comfortable with my ability to cope with it and move ahead?

- Am I able to stand alone and encourage support for a position that others are not embracing? I must be able to be firm with regard to a position that is evidence-based, ethical, and appropriate under the circumstances; I must defend it clearly and with firmness. I can address others' concerns and insights and develop my position as it becomes positively informed by others.

- Am I an effective team player? As a leader I see my opportunity to make a contribution to the planning and implementation of critical processes. I can assume leadership in translating necessary decisions to others. I can help others refine their responses to decisions, overcome their concerns, restate their goals, and renew their direction in a way that advances integrity, effectiveness, and sustainability.

Leaders must have the ability to move others in concert. As a person, the leader must be able to connect with both heart and head. The leader helps others find a deeper purpose in their work and to connect that purpose with the collective energy necessary to advance their work and the system to which it is directed. The leader understands the value of emotional and psychodynamic connection to work, to others, and to a cause greater than oneself. Leaders create a culture of ownership and investment in the collective action of work, helping to build a community around the purposes of work and deepening the understanding of the relationship among individual work activities, the collective convergence of that effort, and its power to make a difference (Miner, 2005).

The leader constantly dances with credibility. In order to maintain long-term viability and relationships with others, the leader must be able to reflect values of honesty, transparency, personal integrity, and leadership discipline. These values form the foundation of lasting relationships with others in the workplace. Through the exercise of these values, each person to whom the leader relates develops a special connection to the leader through their own efforts and personal representation of those same values. In the struggle to act consonant with those values, individuals look to the leader as a mentor and validator in a way that keeps them in touch with their own needs and struggles to keep these values at the forefront of their own lives. The leader models these behaviors with personal integrity and values, using them as the vehicle for self-expression and presentation to others. In the case of such values, the leader best communicates them through his or her own personal consistency with personal behavior, generating the understanding that integrity is a way of being, not simply a reaction to a single circumstance or event.

SCENARIO

Many leaders are promoted into a leadership role from staff positions. Often, their selection was a reflection of what good work this individual did as a staff person. In the staff role, this individual became an expert at his or her work. This expertise and effectiveness ultimately led this individual into the role of new leader. The greatest problem with this process relates to the conflict between really great preparation in the work process and the demands of a good leader—often they are not aligned. Leadership skills are unique to the role. Staff expertise may be an indicator of potential competence, but it is no guarantee of transferability into the leader role. The emerging leader must understand this differentiation from the outset. Not doing so skews the new leader's understanding of the role and affects the quality of how the role is applied.

You have been selected to lead the development of the practice counsel in your clinical department. Your manager saw strong leadership potential as evidenced by your commitment to care, your ability to influence your colleagues, and your willingness to help make decisions on the unit. You've never been asked to be the leader before or to organize something as important as a practice council. You are eager to do it well but are a little concerned about your ability to carry it off.

In an effort to get ready for your role, you've gathered some of your colleagues together to help you with some initial questions. How might you respond to the following questions:

Discussion Questions

1. How many and what range of diversity of staff members do you want to gather for the initial council?

2. What are the first personal activities related to your leadership that we need to address before establishing a council meeting time?

3. What specific areas of mentorship would you look for from your manager in guiding you through your initial leadership experiences with the council?

4. What kind of reactions from your colleagues on the staff should you anticipate and plan for as you assume this important role?

5. As you prepare for the first council meeting, what might be some of the first agenda items to establish firm foundations for the council to do its work?

Courage and Leadership

Leadership is not easy work. Invested and committed leaders see themselves as though leadership and their own person are one and the same thing. Leadership is intentional work, and leaders are fully conscious of the implications, meaning, and value of their personal actions (Figure 3-4). Without this awareness of intentionality and the requisite clarity around the impact of the role in the organization and on others, the leader can slip into a sort of passive functionalism that reflects more the characteristics of the management of functions and processes than it does of vision and direction (Kellough, 2008).

Solid self-perception	Strongly self-directed
Ability to relate to others well	
Effective verbal skills	Willingness to interact
Able to clarify issues	Unafraid of ambiguity
Willing to face conflict head-on and early	
Embraces the noise of creativity	
Allows others to be innovative and to break the rules	
Not good at avoiding anything	Lands running
Can live in the reflected glory of others' accomplishments	
Doesn't mind a little chaos	Demonstrates empathy
Loves to celebrate others' successes	

Figure 3-4 Affirming leader competence

Often in nursing leaders are promoted into management roles out of need rather than a clear delineation of skill and capacity. Just as often, individuals promoted into roles of management leadership were often those who were excellent practitioners and were recognized because of the quality of and their passion for patient care. The problem in this process is that clinical work excellence is a poor predictor for management or leadership success (Winkler, 2010). This does not imply that excellent clinical practitioners cannot be good leaders. However, if they are good leaders, it is the result of other circumstances not directly aligned to their excellence in clinical practice. Leadership is a specific set of competencies with unique characteristics and content. The evaluation of the elements and components of leadership suggests different characteristics for success in the role than those who are successful clinical practitioners. Whether an individual is a clinical or management leader, the leadership characteristics and skill sets are precisely the same.

One of those unique ingredients to effective and sustainable leadership is the leader's ability to demonstrate the reasoned and careful judgment related to especially difficult and challenging decisions. The leader's relationship with colleagues is often complicated and involves a myriad of patterns of interaction and communication. Sometimes decisions that are appropriate and correct are not universally acceptable or agreed to. It is at this point where leadership courage becomes especially important. Those times when the current runs counter to the correct or most appropriate decision become the true test of one of the leader's most critical skills. There are a number of elements related to courage that are important to manifest in the personal exercise of the leadership role:

- The courage to initiate and act. Often the leader will need to push the walls of current practices, rituals, and routines of work in favor of implementing new processes, practices, or initiatives. Some of these will not be popular. Yet, the leader must act consistent with the obligation to make sure that clinical action is evidence based and reflects the state of the art. This will often mean challenging colleagues and raising the bar for performance and impact. If the leader has a need for a great number of personal friendships at work, the individual should not seek the role of leadership because it will often call into question personal relationships in the interests of making right decisions.

- The courage to stand up for what is right in others. Occasionally in the work setting, relationships among colleagues may be stressed, stretched, or otherwise subjected to a high level of tension. The leader must be willing to enter the intensity and fray of challenged relationships, and with courage and clarity sort through them in order to identify common ground and to build essential partnerships. The work of the leader focuses on the integrity and effectiveness of the team. In order to ensure that team-based processes and practices remain fluid and consistent, the leader often will need to confront barriers, boundaries, and perceptual relational differences between members of the team. It is here where skill, courage, and the energy necessary to work through differences become critical in the role of the leader. Establishing group norms, clarifying challenges among individuals, building effective relationships, and confronting issues and concerns head-on are acts of personal courage evident in the day-to-day leadership of every system.

- The courage to trust. Often leaders are seen within the context of the capacity to control things. This notion of control is a viable constituent of leadership capacity and is frequently overrated. In fact, the effective leader often is the one who is best able to let go of personal control and to build trust in colleagues that they will act in the best interests of the profession, the organization, and those they serve. Trust is evidence of the quality of the relationship between members of the team. A significant role of the leader is to ensure that expectations, accountability, relationships, and performance are clear enough for team members that each person understands role obligations in terms of an effective work environment and quality practice and patient outcomes. Representing confidence and trust in colleagues and team members best reflects the effectiveness and positive characteristics and the application of the leadership role. Trust reflects effective relationships, clear and understood expectations, consistent and well-articulated accountabilities, and performance results that reveal the aggregation of the best in clinical practice.

- Exhibit a personal connection to leadership courage. Courage is palpable and visible. Others can see courage present in the person of the leader. Through all of the small daily activities of the expression of leadership, the personal courage of the leader becomes evident. How the leader interacts, the voice the leader gives to issues, the leader's personal pattern of behavior, and the critical choices the leader makes in times of challenge or difficulty all represent the expression and character of courage. It is in these small daily events where courage becomes most evident. Some exemplars of daily personal courage are

  - speaking up when one knows his or her voice will not be popular,

  - receiving critical feedback from others regarding personal behavior, positions, or expression,

  - saying no when it is easier and more acceptable to say yes,

  - publicly accepting responsibility for one's own behavior and for the behavior and outcomes of the team,

  - walking away when passions generate childishness, polarization, or lead to unprincipled language or behaviors,

  - speaking with firmness and commitment on issues of principle, best practice, personal rights and integrity, and in the interests of the patient,

  - seeking reflective time when precipitous action may be more expedient or acceptable,

-   defending disadvantaged, discriminated against, aggrieved, or repressed individuals and groups, especially when it is not popular to do so,

-   giving passion and language to vision, innovation, and creativity, especially at points where it is not universally acceptable,

-   admitting error and personal failing with full ownership and accountability,

-   listening deeply when you want to talk and asking when you want to tell,

-   easily giving credit to others, especially when it is easier to take it yourself,

-   finding potential in others and working diligently to develop it.

Courage is generally not reserved for those times of great significance or importance where the gestures of courage can be grand or sweeping. In fact, courage is most often evident in the small and unrecognizable daily acts of integrity, honesty, and commitment to truth. Effective leaders see courage simply as one of the elements present in exercise of the role of leader. Courageous behavior for the effective leader is no big deal, and it is evident in the usual and ordinary behavior of daily leadership. It is the leader who can make courage ordinary and reflect it in every decision and action who best exemplifies the meaning, value, and impact of courage in the act of leading.

Leaders Engage Stakeholders

Good leaders know that they are not the center of the organization nor do they have all of the answers to the myriad questions generated by organizational work. The leader recognizes that he or she is an agent in complex organizational systems (Bergmann & Brough, 2007). While there are many agents in the system, the leader is an unintentional agent located at the intersection of various levels in the system and serves to create opportunities for linkage, interface, and synthesis in the system. This intentional leader is more specifically a capitalist for action rather than the action itself.

The leader as organizational agent recognizes some fundamental elements in the leadership role that are necessary to incorporate in order to best exercise the role of the leader. Some central themes with regard to the role of the leader in the work community are as follows:

- Instead of looking for answers, the leader seeks the right question so that subsequent activity undertaken by organizational members can relate to the most correct issues that best align with the critical requisites of goodness of fit between the organization and its environment.

- Leaders create the circumstances that make it possible to fully engage all relevant and related stakeholders with regard to issues, processes, and problem resolution. The leader does not so much seek the resolution of the problem as he or she seeks to direct the problem to those who have ownership for its solution.

- The leader as agent seeks not to be the locus of control for decisions, processes, or actions. The leader attempts to find the legitimate locus of control for a decision or action in order to ensure that the right stakeholders who have direct ownership for the issue are invested in leading the response to it.

- The leader is always raising the question as to who the stakeholders are that need to be focused on particular issues, concerns, processes, or problem solving. The leader's primary role in this scenario is to set the table with the right players who have ownership and competence in addressing the issue or resolving the problem.

- The leader seeks to ascribe the correct language to a priority, issue, or concern of the organization such that through appropriate dialogue, stakeholders are aligning the right effort to the right issue and devoting the right resources to addressing it.

- The leader serves primarily as a catalyst for issue owners to address and resolve problems, processes, or concerns. The leader makes sure that the right players, tools, processes, and expertise are appropriately aligned to support decision makers in a way that renders the best possible problem solving.

- The leader acts as circuit rider to the deliberation and decisional process, ensuring that the right people, processes, tools, and data are available in a format that best supports arriving at the right solution and undertaking the best action.

Wise leaders are never at the center of the deliberative or decisional activities of stakeholders. Instead, the leaders see that the stakeholders have what they need to exercise full ownership of their issues and to fully invest resources and effort in the appropriate deliberation and decisions related to defining the actions necessary to address particular issues and concerns (Winkler, 2010). In this way, the leader ensures that ownership for the resolution of issues remains in the hands of those upon whom they most impact. Here, the leader ensures that stakeholders develop the right skills, talents, insights, and applications necessary to best address the issues of concern over which they exercise ownership. Although it is easier for the leader to undertake these activities unilaterally and to be the center of problem solving in his or her area of accountability, it is not always wise. Science has shown us that the closer to the point of service a problem is dealt with and resolved by those who have direct ownership for it, the better the process and the better the solution (Barker, 1990). However, it is important to the leader that those who have ownership for problems and issues must themselves undertake the processes directed to addressing them, and they must have the essential tools to do so. It is the leader's obligation to see that needs and resources converge in a meaningful way and that through the application of these resources, issues can be addressed, problems can be solved, and change can be advanced.

The Leader Stays in the Question

Wise leaders know that given any opportunity, the locus of control for an issue or concern will always seek to move from the intensity and volatility of the environment out of which it is generated to a level in the system where volatility, intensity, and anxiety are less concentrated. This basic law of entropy also applies to human dynamics and behavior. Left intentionally unaddressed, most problems will arrive at the manager's desk or in the leader's hands whether they belong there or not.

The leader recognizes that virtually all problems belong where they originated and must seek to return them there if they are to be legitimately and effectively resolved (Figure 3-5). Because the leader does not own them, if he or she attempts to resolve them, resolution becomes symptomatic and iterative. If a permanent solution is to be sought and obtained, the problem must return to its point of origin in order for those who own it to resolve it in a way that permanently addresses the issue they own. It is the leader's obligation to see that the issue returns to its legitimate locus of control and is resolved by those who own it (Malloch, 2010).

Good leaders know that they are not the answer to all the questions that others raise. The leader must recognize that accountability for answers always rests with the questioner. The minute the leader answers the question, a transfer of the locus of control for the answer moves to the leader, essentially absolving the questioner of any ownership of the solution to his or her own questions. This transfer occurs thousands of times every day in the life and role of the leader.

The wise leader recognizes that the accountable answer to any question is the next question. The leader recognizes that ownership of the issue should remain with the person who brings it and that person must be encouraged and enabled to respond and seek the solution that can most be sustained. The leader seeks to have the questioner do the following:

- Retain ownership and control over the issue.
- Identify the resources necessary to pursue a solution.
- Name the barriers impeding a solution.
- Identify the best deliverables related to a sustainable solution.
- Enumerate a mechanism for selecting the best alternative.
- Outline the process steps necessary to address the issue.
- Indicate the impact of the selected approach.
- Evaluate the results of the approach(es) selected.
- Undertake corrective action related to an effective solution.
- Validate the action of the staff.
- Celebrate the success for the staff in resolving their own issues.

Figure 3-5 Leaders engage stakeholders

In order to make sure that a legitimate locus of control is maintained in problem solving, the leader always stays within the question in relationship to issues that belong to others. The leader sees that he or she is not the source of the solution of the problem. Although the leader can access resources, support decision making, provide skill opportunities, and gather the right stakeholders, the leader cannot resolve the problem in any sustainable way on behalf of those who own it. They must resolve it themselves.

In the interests of ensuring this appropriate alignment, the leader stays in the question. This means raising the right issues, engaging appropriate stakeholders, helping others to find the core of the issue or problem, and discerning the right agents for problem resolution and creating the right format and forum for addressing the issue in a way that obtains viable and sustainable solutions. In short, the leader stays focused on the context of problem solving; the staff stays focused on the content of problem solving. This context–content set of parameters helps clarify and distinguish between the elements of the role of the leader and those of the stakeholder. Leaders firmly stay within the context obligations of their role and support stakeholders in addressing their ownership of the content of their issue or concern.

Leaders who stay in the question will find this personal skill set challenging at best. The leader must develop personal attributes that make it comfortable for him or her to refrain from being the centerpiece or the control point for managing, deciding, and directing resolution of issues that belong to the staff. Those who express leadership potential are not often shy, passive, or wilting lily personalities. The unique leadership characteristics evidenced by high energy, strong sense of ownership, creativity and innovation, clear direction, and desire to problem solve often trip up these individuals. Often, they assume that the sometimes much more effective leadership characteristics that remove them as the centerpiece of the action and move them to the side are less meaningful and valuable than being at the "center of the action" (Porter-O'Grady & Malloch, 2010a).

Some self-reflection with regard to leadership capacity is critical to touch base with the intentionality necessary to comprise the leader's role. Understanding motive, leadership role content, and personal attributes are important to the appropriate self-development of the leader in leading a team of equals (knowledge workers/professionals) in ways that best engage them, prevent the transfer of ownership, and create the conditions for effective problem solving. Some of these self-characteristics are as follows:

- Self-confidence and clear awareness of personal ego challenges and reward needs
- A sense of self-direction and the ability to meet one's own needs without depending on the reflected praise of others
- Assertive skills that make it clear to others the locus of control for obligations and accountability
- A strong ability to articulate and clarify issues in a language that can clearly be understood by others, especially those who may own the issues
- A capacity to face the potential for conflict head-on and early enough to help people engage it and translate it into purposeful action

- An ability to embrace the noise of initially chaotic, often creative efforts at aligning stakeholders and undertaking deliberations resulting in creative solutions
- The ability to obtain equal satisfaction and personal reward in the reflected light of the team's accomplishment and in colleagues' recognition of the leader's contribution to creativity or effective solutions
- The capability to celebrate others' success and to make celebration a consistent part of the life of the unit or department in ways that acknowledge successes and other individual contributions toward attaining success

Recognizing Personal Needs for Self-Development

Effective leaders value being effective leaders. These leaders believe that through the development of their effective leadership skills, they will themselves become better leaders. Leaders also believe that they can develop and through personal self-development can grow and become more effective. Leaders also know that a good foundation in self-awareness is essential to anchor the foundations of this leadership development (Figure 3-6).

Awareness of some of the common pitfalls that prevent leaders from developing their skills is in the person's own best interest in developing a stronger capacity for leadership. Many simple situations and occurrences contribute to the incapacitating or early destruction of leadership effectiveness. Developing leadership skills is a lifelong process that demands a continuous level of awareness of the leadership journey, its pitfalls and promises, and the individual hooks and traps that impede one's movement along the leadership trajectory. Some of the more common issues related to effective leadership are ones that are most frequently overlooked. Some of these might be the following:

- An early tendency to self-destruct. Sometimes egos are fragile and new leaders can often come to believe in their own sense of self-importance and thereby lose perspective with regard to their leadership role and impact of the organization. It is not uncommon to see leaders begin to believe that they are more important, capable, and valuable than is truly the case. Often this occurs in the event of recognition or praise with regard to a singular accomplishment. The individual gets lost in the praise and begins to lose his or her center and believes his or her own value far beyond legitimate extents. Allowing the personal ego to run rampant and failing to exercise the same discipline on one's own ego as

Every leader, no matter how experienced, must be aware of the need to continually develop and grow in the role. Competence in the role is neither static nor ensured. Each leader must recognize how dynamic change is, constantly shifting the work landscape and calling all who work to continually reflect on the value of their contribution and the currency of their skills. This means participating in an endless assessment of competence and the need to adjust and grow in the role as it responds to new demands:

- Am I able to see the whole picture, not just the part that applies to me?
- Do I work in systems models and not merely reflect a process orientation?
- Am I able to look past the current issues and see where I am?
- Can I envision the journey and reflect on where I am in it?
- Am I good at translating reality and change so that others understand?
- Am I willing to face issues first before others must contend with them?
- Do I anticipate the needs of the system and of others in it?
- Do I explore different ways of seeing things and expand my thinking?
- Will I experiment with and evaluate options to current routines?
- Is there a place in my life for the uncertain and the chaotic?
- Can I find the energy in stress ad use it to good advantage?
- Am I disciplined in my work and my life without being limited by it?
- Can I see the pain and noise in others and respond with empathy?
- Do I push others into their own challenges and support them in it?

Figure 3-6 Self-reflection: Paying attention to leader self-development

the leader does with others create conditions that threaten the value and viability of the role and tend to make the leader as much of a problem as the issues to which he or she directs attention. When the leader's ego runs rampant and is undisciplined, the leader actually tends to stop the very activities that made him or her successful. A humble but balanced recognition of the contribution to creating a positive context for good team relationships, effective problem solving, and advancing creativity is the best counter to an uncontrolled ego and to a misappropriation of one's role in making meaningful change in attaining sustainable success.

- Failure to accommodate and manage inevitable leadership stress. Burnout is the most common occurrence in leaders. Burnout reflects the loss of personal balance, eroding support system, too much emphasis on the role of the leader, and the diminishment of the moral and ethical center to leadership expression. Often these leaders failed to pay attention to their personal and family supports and the development of close friendships. These leaders often lose connection with the good management of time, become overwhelmed with the work, and have an inflated sense of their own value to others. Failure to attain appropriate leadership peer support and mentorship often contributes to growing leadership stress. If these issues are left unaddressed long enough, they lead to a lack of self-awareness that directly increases impending levels of personal burnout.

- Excessive focus on task and function diminishes leadership effectiveness. Because of the pressures to perform and to achieve outcomes, leaders can be overly focused on short-term functions and results at the expense of long-term viability and sustainability. Leadership over the long term isn't simply about achieving short-term goals; it is more about maintaining continuous levels of satisfaction and performance. The task-focused leader descends into the middle of the fray and becomes a part of the problems that ensue. The distance, objectivity, and long-range view expected of the leader diminishes, and the individual fails to maintain the context or environment necessary to advance creativity and to recognize value in others.

CRITICAL THOUGHT

Self-awareness ensures that a leader is able to confront the challenges that lie within and adjust for the conflicts and challenges that move the individual to grow and develop in a way that takes the person beyond limitation and into the arena of true innovation and creativity. Today most organizations are hungry for just such people.

- Treating everyone the same can lead to problems for the leader. **Equity** does not mean **equality**—one is a measure of value; the other is a measure of condition. Everyone should be treated equally; that is beyond question. However, equity indicates that different roles contribute different kinds of value to the organization and each role must be respected within the context of its unique value contribution. By simply treating everyone the same, you belie the uniqueness that each brings, confuse the specific contribution each role makes, and eliminate the value of diversity to the mosaic of contributions necessary to the life and energy of the workplace. Recognizing and honoring role differences and individual contributions also advance the life and vitality of the leader.

- Admitting personal error does not lead to a lack of credibility; in fact, it advances personal credibility. Regularly making mistakes as a leader is indeed a problem and must be addressed as such. However, effective leaders do not generally make frequent and significant errors. When errors or mistakes have been made, the wise leader owns up to his or her part in the error and demonstrates personal transparency with regard to its disclosure. By so doing, disclosure of errors becomes safe and credible and reduces the intensity and pressure often accompanying the presence of errors. Setting the example of self-disclosure creates a safe space for those behaviors and helps eliminate the personal stress of hiding inadequacy, failure, and personal error.

- The desire to be liked and to be a friend to staff can create significant leadership trauma. In the unique exercise of leadership, friendship is not a part of the quotient. Tongue in cheek, one can say "leaders have no friends." Although this is potentially an overstatement, the truth of this principle lies in the fact that leadership is not a constituent of friendship, and friendship is often an impediment to the exercise of good leadership. Leaders need to be honored, respected, even loved for their excellent exercise of leadership. However, this should not be mistaken for personal affection instead of role and performance acknowledgment. Developing particular friendships within the context of the team format is a formula for stress, crisis, inequity, and personal problem generation. The wise leader develops a balanced view with regard to the role requirements of leadership as distinguished from the personal requirements of friendship. Not working through this misalignment and setting clearly enumerated boundaries in this arena creates a volatile mix that results in diminishing leadership effectiveness and leads to considerable personal harm to both leaders and colleagues.

- Leaders need to be available to each other and to their staff. Leaders who isolate themselves or wall themselves off from communication with other leaders and their own staff or colleagues create conditions that facilitate the development of self-harm. Leaders need to be visible and available to each other and to staff in ways that advance communication, dialogue, interaction, and problem solving. This high level of visibility and interaction creates a relational dynamic that improves the strength of the interaction between the leader and staff colleagues. The leader's exposure to other leaders and the constant interaction this person maintains with other leaders helps keep the leader centered, expands the opportunities for new insights, shares new tools and resources for self-development, and provides opportunities for mentorship and role clarification. Leadership isolation creates the exact opposite and diminishes both the support and the effectiveness of the role, increasing stress and limiting its viability.

- Staying out of touch with the personal and professional issues of colleagues and staff can create emotional isolation for the leader. If the leader becomes so enmeshed in his or her own management or functional activities and becomes captured by them, boundaries between the functional activities of the leader and the relational demands of the staff can accelerate into leadership isolation and stress. Becoming overwhelmed with function and activity is a common condition for leaders. Although many leaders use it as a vehicle for identifying with staff concerns, they fail to recognize their part in the staff concerns does not provide the objectivity essential to help staff deal with their concerns. Availability to problem solve with the staff is critical to building effective staff relationships and preventing leadership isolation. However, the gift the leader brings to the staff and colleagues is a balance to problems and issues that often cannot be attained from inside the problems or issues themselves. Staying in touch with the issues and the staff connects the leader to the staff's concerns, while maintaining the objective leader role and insight lends a new perspective from the outside looking in to support the staff's resolution of issues and concerns.

This sample of common pitfalls that impact leadership effectiveness enumerates the critical needs of the leader to understand his or her own personal needs and attributes and to develop a deeper awareness of those boundaries and traps that can limit leadership effectiveness and sound relationships with colleagues. Leadership development builds on a continuous awareness of the needs for individual growth and the range of competencies embedded in the role of each leader (Figure 3-7). Leadership self-development is a lifelong process that becomes deeper and more enriching as the individual leader increasingly commits to and expands self-awareness and continuous need for growth and development. Seeking out mentorship and leadership colleague relationships helps create a trusting and safe space for the leader to explore personal issues of leadership growth and capacity and a provides a place to discuss the angst and struggles associated with personal growth as a leader (Porter-O'Grady & Malloch, 2010b).

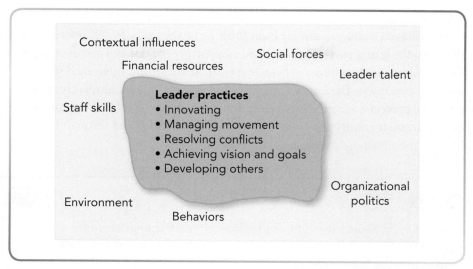

Figure 3-7 Contextual influences

Personal Transparency and Openness

There is nothing more important to the community of people and their relationship to a leader than a real sense of the personal presence of the leader. There is much mythology that swirls around the role of the leader, sometimes even imbued with notions of supernatural or special characteristics. Of course, this is emphatically untrue. Leaders are people who through growth development, role, and position assume important roles in relationship to others. Frequently this role is formal and structured within an organizational frame of reference, but just as frequently it is not. The expression of the role of the leader should be consistent regardless of whether the position is formal or informal. The leader role is differentiated by the context in which it unfolds. Beyond simply being a position title, a leader must not forget her or his personal humanity essentially defines the character of the role, its relationship to others, and, ultimately, its impact on others. At a personal level, the leader must be able to communicate effectively with others in a way that honors their own essential humanity, supporting in others a sense of personal identity that allows colleagues to more fully engage and embrace the leader in a way that supports their own personal work journey (Malloch & Porter-O'Grady, 2009).

In this regard, it is important that the leader represent and express a highly developed level of openness and availability to colleagues in a way that helps the professional community to identify with each other and with the person of the leader. Different from what has been historically held, the leader should never be identified as separate and unique from those he or she leads. In fact, more often than not, the leader should be identified as a partner in the team and exemplify for colleagues the best human characteristics that affirm and value each role and integrated purpose. The leader's openness and availability should represent to everyone present an interfacing connection between members of the team, evidenced by their connection to each other and to the leader, and through it clearly identify their purpose, value, and commitments.

SCENARIO

Leaders must always remember that their primary role is to create a supportive context for the action of change in the organization. This means that the leader recognizes the forces influencing the leader's own expression of encouragement and facilitation of the change process. Understanding the issues of fit between the leader's practices and the conditions that affect them is critical to the good selection of approaches that make change successful. The leader is always aware of this need for good choices and best represents those good choices in his or her own behaviors and practices so that they become a model for the staff and the signpost of how best to respond to the inevitability and engagement of continual organizational change.

Some questions related to the individual leader and his or her commitment to organization goals are as follows:

Discussion Questions

- Do you know the mission, vision, and strategic priorities of the organization and do they influence your actions?
- How do organizational goals get incorporated into departmental priorities and the actions and measures that relate to the department's role in fulfilling them?
- How do you make sure that the staff's personal priorities fit tightly with the organization's goals such that their personal action is an expression of their commitment to fulfilling those goals?

Connection implies support for collective wisdom. Good leaders recognize the value of the whole aggregate of individual insight, knowledge, and experience. This collective wisdom serves as a powerful force for informing the deliberation, effective decision making, and advancing the critical clinical value of the discipline. As mentioned before, good leaders move past the need for control in relating to others and make meaningful decisions and undertake appropriate action. The difficulty, however, is that organizational control was the cornerstone of management and leadership over the course of the 20th century. As systems begin to apply newer and deeper understanding of the complexity and characteristics of organizations, a deeper understanding of how organizations work and change reflects a new set of principles. The impact of complexity thinking and quantum applications in organizations has led to a new understanding of leadership, which emphasizes the shifting understanding of relationships, interactions, and management of life at the intersections of systems and networks. Thinkers in this arena now recognize the importance of network relationships in the synthesis of action (Ang & Yin, 2008). This means that traditional vertical control infrastructures and behaviors are no longer the central capacity driving stability and organizational life in greater work networks. The contemporary leader recognizes the emergent skills related to addressing issues of good fit, functional linkage, relationship and interaction, and convergence and synthesis, all of which are critical elements of human dynamics in complex systems.

Contemporary leaders now recognize that building effective relationships that interface and interact well with one another requires constant attention and continuous reflection on the intersection and interaction of all elements and components in the system, especially those that relate to the human dynamics of that system. Organizational leaders seek now to build a prevailing infrastructure that is predominently relationship grounded. This emphasis on the relationship between people and systems calls for leaders who understand patterns of behavior and are effective in managing the many junctures of organizational networks and can successfully coordinate the linkages necessary to advance and sustain systems. The contemporary leader assures staff that he or she exemplifies essential skill sets that are necessary to lead equitable and value-driven stakeholders collectively and congruently to fulfilling the meaning, purpose, and values of the organization in an ever-changing environment.

CRITICAL THOUGHT

The effective leader always prefers chaos over stability. Stability is a momentary respite in the endless movement and creativity of essential change. Although occasional stability is necessary, stability over time is the enemy of creativity and movement.

The leader's personal attributes and skills work together to ensure that there is consonance between individual purpose and meaning and the organizational value and direction as it fulfills its role and contribution to the broader social network. The leader develops the relationships and interactions necessary to advance, through the work of individuals, the purposes and values of the organization in the larger social environment. In this, at a very personal level, the leader fully engages both self and others in the dynamic interaction that invests everyone in a high level of commitment represented in the convergence of personal talents, capacity, and skills connected to the purposes and value of the larger organization. In this way the leader helps ensure that both personal and collective purpose, meaning, and value are demonstrated in the contribution of each and all and through the collective aggregation of every personal skill and ability and advances the interests and contribution of the organization. This synthesis can be obtained and sustained only through a continuous invitation, gathering, inclusion, contribution, and demonstration of the best and most vital in everyone who participates in the concerted effort to advance the health of those they serve (Ulh-Bien & Marion, 2008). It is to this end that the activities, talents, and the commitment of the leader are directed. The leader's constant and consistent focus on creating an environment of ownership, engagement, investment, and expression creates the milieu necessary to move the caring network in a way that makes a sustainable difference in the health of those it serves. The personal attributes of the leader are what best represents the character of the organization. The clearer the system is regarding those attributes and expectations and the better demonstrated in the person of the leader they are, the clearer and more effective is the role they play in sustaining that contribution.

REFLECTIVE QUESTION

How many times do we hear, "If we could just get to the end of this and know it was done and over with"? Although there is certainly some truth to the incrementalism implied in this statement, there is no truth to its substance. Nothing is ever really done. Everything is always and forever in movement. If the movement of the universe should stop, so would everything in it. We may achieve specific objectives, but if we're seeing them correctly, they are really a small component of a much larger journey— one that never ends. What is your best way of communicating this reality to your colleagues? What story can you tell that reflects its truth to them in a meaningful way?

CHAPTER TEST QUESTIONS

1. It is better to adhere to generally accepted leadership principles than to develop an individual personal leadership plan. True or false?

2. Leadership means providing specific and clear direction to others so that they understand your intention and have a clear idea of your individual leadership vision. True or false?

3. Leadership courage indicates a specific level of self-understanding and personal knowledge about individual motivation, principles, and ethics. True or false?

4. In working with teams, it is important for the leader to let the team know about the decisions they need to make and to provide the team with the appropriate direction necessary to get to the right solution. True or false?

5. One of the differences between the management function and the leadership function is that managers are accountable for staffing, and leaders are more accountable for engaging. True or false?

6. The leader works hard to create trust and does everything to make sure that personal principles of trust are generated to colleagues so they can work in a trusting environment. True or false?

7. Leaders are always interested in finding answers to problems and directing colleagues to seek the most right answers or solutions. True or false?

8. A contemporary differentiation between management and leadership is that management focuses on analysis; leadership focuses on synthesis. True or false?

9. Friendship is not a critical element to leadership. Therefore, the wise leader is reserved about transparency and realizes that self-disclosure can create problems between the leader and those he or she leads. True or false?

10. The leader must set aside time for formal leadership reflection about personal skills and development needs and should develop a strong relationship with the leadership mentor. True or false?

www For a full suite of assignments and additional learning activities, use the access code located in the front of your book to visit the exclusive website: http://go.jblearning.com/leadership. If you do not have an access code, you can obtain one at the site.

References

Ang, Y., & Yin, S. (2008). *Intelligent complex adaptive systems.* Chicago, IL: IGI.

Barker, T. B. (1990). *Engineering quality by design: Interpreting the Taguchi approach.* New York, NY: ASQC Quality Press.

Bergmann, S., & Brough, J. A. (2007). *Lead me, I dare you! Managing resistance to school change.* Larchmont, NY: Eye on Education.

Cowen, P. S., & Moorhead, S. (2011). *Current issues in nursing.* St. Louis, MO: Mosby Elsevier.

Gardner, W. L., Avolio, B. J., & Walumbwa, F. O. (Eds.). (2005). *Authentic leadership theory and practice: Origins, effects and development.* St. Louis, MO: Elsevier.

Guastello, S. J. (2002). *Managing emergent phenomena: Nonlinear dynamics in work organizations.* Mahwah, NJ: Erlbaum.

Hawking, S. (1988). *A brief history of time.* London, England: Bantam.

Kellough, R. D. (2008). *A primer for new principals: Guidelines for success.* Lanham, MD: Rowman & Littlefield Education.

Leader to Leader Institute, Hesselbein, F., & Goldsmith, M. (Eds.). (2006). *The leader of the future 2: Visions, strategies, and practices for the new era.* San Francisco, CA: Jossey-Bass.

Mackin, D. (2007). *The team building tool kit: Tips and tactics for effective workplace teams.* New York, NY: AMACOM.

Malloch, K. (2010). Creating the organizational context for innovation. In T. Porter-O'Grady & K. Malloch (Eds.). *Innovation leadership: Creating the landscape of healthcare* (pp. 33–56). Sudbury, MA: Jones and Bartlett.

Malloch, K., & Porter-O'Grady, T. (2009). *The quantum leader: Applications for the new world of work.* Sudbury, MA: Jones and Bartlett.

Maxwell, J. (2010). *The 21 irrefutable laws of leadership.* Nashville, TN: Thomas Nelson.

Miner, J. B. (2005). *Organizational behavior I. Essential theories of motivation and leadership.* Armonk, NY: Sharpe.

Northouse, P. G. (2007). *Leadership: Theory and practice.* Thousand Oaks, CA: Sage.

Porter-O'Grady, T., & Malloch, K. (Eds.). (2010a). *Innovation leadership: Creating the landscape of healthcare.* Sudbury, MA: Jones and Bartlett.

Porter-O'Grady, T., & Malloch, K. (2010b). Leadership for innovation: From knowledge creation to health transformation. In T. Porter-O'Grady & K. Malloch (Eds.), *Innovation leadership: Creating the landscape of healthcare* (pp. 1–23). Sudbury, MA: Jones and Bartlett.

Rippin, A. (2007). Stitching up the leader: Empirically based reflections on leadership and gender. *Journal of Organizational Change Management, 20*(2), 209–226.

Rondeau, K. (2007). The adoption of high involvement work practices and Canadian nursing homes. *Leadership in Health Services, 20*(1), 16.

Tilley, D. (2008). Competency in nursing: A concept analysis. *The Journal of Continuing Education in Nursing, 39*(2), 58–65.

Ulh-Bien, M., & Marion, R. (2008). *Complexity leadership: Conceptual foundations.* Charlotte, NC: Information Age.

Wager, K., Wickham, F., & Glaser, J. (2005). *Managing healthcare information systems: A practical approach for healthcare executives.* San Francisco, CA: Jossey-Bass.

Watkins, S. (2004). 21st-century corporate governance: The growing pressure on the board toward a corporate solution. In R. P. Gandossy & J. A. Sonnenfeld (Eds.), *Leadership and governance from the inside and out* (pp. 27–36). New York, NY: Wiley.

Werhane, P. H. (2007). *Women in business: The changing face of leadership.* Westport, CT: Praeger.

Winkler, I. (2010). *Contemporary leadership theories: Enhancing the understanding of the complexity, subjectivity and dynamic of leadership.* Berlin, Germany: Physica-Verlag.

Zedeck, S., and American Psychological Association. (2011). *APA handbook of industrial and organizational psychology.* Washington, DC: American Psychological Association.

Appendix A

Old Versus New Leadership Skills

Old		New
Managing people	⟶	Managing mobility
Analyzing processes	⟶	Synthesizing systems
Setting direction	⟶	Reading the signposts of change
Using technology	⟶	Synergizing technology
Motivating others	⟶	Helping others identify their work relevance

Appendix B

Checking Off Basic Leadership Attributes

☐ Do I like people? I will be leading many people, sometimes in directions they may prefer not to go. I must be willing to relate to many types of people and will need a positive sensitivity to the needs of others. I must like this work!

☐ Can I live with a high degree of ambiguity and uncertainty? I will be dealing with a great amount of change. I will have to be an example of excitement and engagement of this change and demonstrate a will to implement it in my own life before I ask anyone else to implement it.

☐ Are my communication skills well developed? I will be communicating with others almost constantly and will need to be informed and articulate in my expressions. Others must understand me and must respect the validity of the information I communicate.

☐ Do I have the courage to handle the discipline issues that my leadership role will demand? Can I make tough decisions and follow through with action when required without fear and uncertainty?

☐ Can I stand alone on an issue when it appears that others are not embracing it? If the position is ethical and appropriate, can I defend it with clarity and firmness, incorporating others' concerns in my own development and positions?

☐ Am I a good team player? I can make a contribution to the planning and implementing processes and then take leadership in translating decisions to others and helping them act in concert with the goals and direction others may have developed for them.

Appendix C

More Leader Core Behaviors

- Leaders reflect flexibility in their approach to all problem solving and in confronting all issues.
- Leaders describe the changes that will affect the staff well in advance of the staff actually experiencing them.
- Leaders translate the goals of the system in a language that others can understand and apply to their own work.
- Leaders represent in their own behavior the patterns and practices they expect to see in others.
- Leaders anticipate the changes that staff will have to make in their work and carefully design approaches to guide staff in accepting and implementing change.
- Leaders recognize the chaos embedded in all change and are not afraid of it, demonstrating engagement of it to others, mentoring acceptance and use of its energy.

Appendix D

What Staff Want from Their Leader

Honesty	Trust
Clarity or role	Opportunity
Open communication	Good problem solving
Personal caring	Engagement
Respect	Meaning in their work

Appendix E

Leadership

Leaders Moving Past the Age of Control

It has been said that control was the cornerstone of organizational leadership in the 20th century. As organizations seek to function in the 21st century, many of the characteristics of change are driven by a different set of principles. Recognizing the impact of complexity thinking and quantum theory, organizations are looking at an emerging significant set of relationships and intersections that require coordination and synthesis. This means that control is no longer the central issue of stability and organization in systems. The good leader recognizes that issues of fit, linkage, interaction, and relationship are the critical elements of all human dynamics.

Leaders recognize that building complex relationships requires constant attention and continual reflection on interaction of all elements in an organization including that of the people who comprise it. Building an infrastructure for relationships calls for leaders to understand linkage and intersections and to provide staff with clarity of meaning and purpose. The leader ensures those who are led that there is value in the work and relationships necessary to advance the purposes and values of the organization. In this, the leader fully engages the participants in an interaction that invests them in the commitment of their work with the purposes of the organization, advancing the meaning and value of their contribution, and to growing and improving their own personal skills and participation. This can be done only through invitation, gathering, inclusion, and encouraging the best and the most vital in all who participate.

Leaders can eliminate the focus on control as follows:

- Help people understand what is happening to them.
- Engage others in defining the content of their own work.
- Reduce hierarchy to its lowest necessary levels.
- Involve stakeholders in setting their own goals.
- Eliminate secrets—disclose whatever is necessary to help others do their work.

> The leader who must control others is expressing a basic insecurity that ultimately results in negative forces and behavior impeding achievement of the organization's goals.

The Leader's Commitment to Learning

The leader cannot expect in others what he or she is not willing to find within. It is important to the consideration of the role of leader to recognize the value of continuing commitment to personal change. The person of the leader represents to others the general commitment to a continuing development that is fundamental to competence and effectiveness. Like all roles, the leader cannot be competent and static at the same time. The leader must demonstrate a willingness and ability to expand the skill set necessary to exercise the role and role model to others.

An endless commitment to learning is fundamental to the role of the leader. Three things are critical:

- A good assessment of leadership skills and needs.
- A good plan with strategies for action and implementation.
- A 360-degree evaluation of the effectiveness of the application of leadership skills.

> Reading the signs of change
> Translating the language of change for others
> Guiding others in adapting to change
> Applying change in the process of work
> Entering into dialogue regarding change impact
> Evaluating the results of change
> Renewing energy for the very next change

A Leader Is Inspired and Is Inspiring

The ability to encourage others and to continue supporting their effort through modeling, motivating, and the leader's own personal commitment is critical to good leadership. The inspiring leader always recognizes that who one is, is as important as what one does. This leader always remembers the following:

- Individuals need to know that their work has meaning and value.
- Individuals hope that their work makes a difference and has a positive effect on the lives of others.

- Everyone wants to know that they are personally valued and have a place as well as play a key role in the world.

- Everyone seeks, at some level, to make a difference and to hear that difference in the words and language of others.

- People want to know that they matter; that their lives have personal value, and that they have an opportunity to express that value in their work and actions.

- The leader always seeks what is good in others, identifies it, and makes other team members aware of the value that an individual brings to their efforts.

- The value of collective wisdom is shared between and among all team members so that their collective impact is recognized by all.

- Nothing is sustained without concerted effort of all stakeholders committed to a common purpose.

- The leader creates the context within which others live and work in a way that encourages engagement, stimulates creativity, and builds commitment.

> The leader's commitment must be such that others can sense it, and from its energy, be encouraged and able to continue their own journey.

IN THE FRANK EXPRESSION OF CONFLICTING OPINIONS LIES THE GREATEST PROMISE OF WISDOM. —LOUIS BRANDEIS

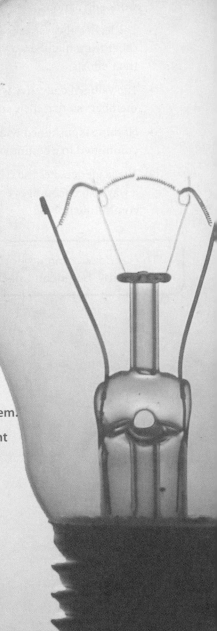

CHAPTER OBJECTIVES

Upon the completion of this chapter, the reader will be able to do the following:

» Understand the fundamental elements that underpin all conflict.

» Define normative conflict and the elements and characteristics of conflict that make it a fundamental part of all human interaction.

» Enumerate the personal characteristics affecting one's own view of conflict and individual relationship to it.

» Outline the effects of unresolved conflict and specific steps that can be taken by the individual to develop personal engagement and skills in addressing it.

» List at least five categories of major conflict, the unique characteristics of each, and key strategies for addressing them.

» State why conflict affinity and skill development is important in the role of the leader and provides one of the critical core functions of leadership expression.

Conflict Skills for Clinical Leaders

First, it is important to state that all conflict is normative (Smokowski & Bacallao, 2011). Conflict is simply a metaphor for difference. Without too much of a stretch, it is observable when one looks around at how unique and different every human being is. Although these differences add to the vitality and wide diversity of human experience, they can also lead to challenges, relational noise, and dispute. Because difference is the predominant condition of most everything in the universe, it best represents what is normative in creation; a vast and unlimited diffusion of diversity and individuality. Within the midst of that prevailing reality, the emergence of conflict is a norm of significant proportions, one that must be recognized as a primary rudiment influencing all human behavior and interaction. Indeed, conflict is more normal than it is exceptional.

Still, there is nothing that can strike more fear and anxiety in the hearts of most people than the potential of being involved in a conflict situation (Rodgers, 2011). Embedded in the fear of conflict are all of the issues of personal security, identity, safety, and relational integrity. The noise and angst associated with the acting out of conflict can range from the incidental to the injurious, resulting in both significant emotional and relational impact as well as the potential for psychological and physiological harm (MacDonald, 2011).

CRITICAL THOUGHT

The leader makes it safe for people to express conflict and to share their experience of it, to develop a language for expression; in short, to make the experience of conflict normal.

The grounds of much human **conflict** are often ideological, identity, personality, psychodynamic, and intellectual differences that display themselves with varying degrees of passion and expression (Blackard & Gibson, 2002). In our contemporary world so many of these religious, identity, sociopolitical, and cultural differences have created such ideological polarization and passionate position taking that polarized positions have moved human behavior into dangerous modes of expression. Because of severely polarized circumstances, the notion of conflict has become increasingly frightening, raising the specter of a wide range of potentials and insights about the dangers of conflict, some of which are life threatening and destructive to the very fabric of society (Tojo & Dilpreet, 2007).

Although there are many significant dangers in broad-based conflict, most conflict operates in a significantly less intense level of interpersonal one on one and small team differences. Well over 90 percent of the conflict that occurs between human beings is local and completely resolvable (LeBaron, 2002). Much of the fear of conflict as it arises in day-to-day relationships and exchanges is unjustified and simply reflects an inadequate understanding of the dynamics of conflict and a lack of competence in its management. Developing basic insights and skills related to addressing elements of interactional and relational conflict more often than not helps take the noise of the conflict dynamic and introduces methodologies and techniques that help people deal with their normative conflicts and move through them to resolution, and it helps build stronger relationships and interactions between individuals and teams.

CRITICAL THOUGHT

The leader listens carefully to people's conversations with or about each other, always looking for the subtext or hidden message that might indicate the presence of the seeds of conflict.

The Early Engagement of Conflict

The most important and best first step in the management of all conflict is the early recognition of its signs and early addressing of its issues (Stahl, 2011). In health care especially, the high-pressure, fast-paced, critically important characteristics of caring work help reduce the conditions and circumstances that can generate the high levels of stress, which are usually always an antecedent to the emergence of conflict. The stress of clinical work provides more than sufficient opportunities for the generation of conflict, a reality that should always put the leader on the lookout for the potential emergence of conflict occurrences (Rodgers, 2011). Often when the individual's perceptions and needs are in conflict with the work and the environment as well as the activity of others, basic stressors are introduced. Many of the stressors are manifested in particular modes of communication, relationships, interactions, or the expression of personal emotions. The leader is always on the lookout for potential conflict emergence. Because conflict is generally the physical manifestation of much of the expressions of individual and group stress, its potential is always present.

Looking for the Signs

At the personal level, there are a number of indicators of stress circumstances that can lead to potential for inevitable conflict. When there is a sense that staff members feel overwhelmed by their work circumstances or situation and feel as though they have few choices or options to do anything about them, the seeds of conflict emerge. Often the first manifestation of early conflict is a situational clash between two individuals that reflects differences in view, opinion, role, relationship, situation, or incidents (Figure 4-1). Sometimes the signs of conflict can be seen or are visible. For example, in an argument between two members of the staff, subsequent negative behaviors can result in exclusion, demeaning the other party, forming cliques, acting out, bad-mouthing, or rivalry. Often a cascade of behaviors occurs over time, resulting in accelerating levels of negative behaviors and circumstances slowly and inevitably cascading out of individual control and creating a broader arc of impact among people, in teams, on units or in departments, and sometimes in the organization as a whole (Lencioni, 2002). Unless these kinds of conflicts are engaged early, they inevitably generate into a broader sphere of influence, and following each cascading extension of the conflict they become increasingly more difficult to resolve. In addition, conflicts left unaddressed do not occupy the same level of intensity, are not fixed, and do not stay local. Conflict, like any other dynamic, has an accelerating pace of its own. It does not stay still; it always grows in intensity over time and becomes increasingly more complicated, difficult, and increasingly irresolvable (Amer & Zou, 2011).

It is for this reason that the simplest and best leadership tool of conflict management is early diagnosis and intervention at the most basic stages of its expression.

- Differences
- Emotions and feelings
- Opposing views
- Acting on or out
- Tension
- Interpersonal
- Disagreeable

Figure 4-1 Sources of conflict

The recognition of early signs that identify conflict require first that the leader be continuously aware that the potential for conflict is always present. The leader's antenna should always be tuned in to departmental dynamics, the character of communication and interaction, differences in individual behavioral norms, and situations and circumstances that reflect elements of controversy or disagreement (Wenger & Möckli, 2003). These early signs of conflict are indicators of the potential for the next stage of conflict, which is often seen in beginning verbalizations, snide remarks, statements of discomfort, cynicism, or outright negative assessments. Each of these views is an early indication of the potential for dissonance, disagreement, and the potential for deeper conflict. Addressing conflict during the symptomatic stage may help alleviate tension related to it and prevent movement into later, more intense stages of conflict expression.

Early identification of conflict helps minimize and even prevent its further development in the clinical setting. The leader should work diligently to gain as much insight with regard to the origin, nature, and character of the conflict and develop appropriate responses that fit the stage of the conflict and help address the parties to the conflict at that time and in that place. Some common personal and systematic responses for framing the early engagement of conflict might be the following:

- Develop an awareness of the norms of conflict in all of the professional peers so they can be coagents in the early identification of the potential for emergent conflict.
- Work with colleagues to organize a unit strategy for normalizing and addressing conflict that includes professional colleagues, interdisciplinary colleagues, associates, and managers.

- Develop specific protocols and processes that automatically click in when a particular conflict is identified and noted by any member of the staff.

- Make sure that there is a portion of the regular staff meeting that addresses a particular challenging issue, circumstance, or event for which there is the potential for conflict or for which signs of conflict already exist.

- Make sure that there are sufficient social and relational outlets that are regularly scheduled for socialization, friendly dialogue, celebration of key events, acknowledgment of successes or accomplishment, or recognition of important life occurrences.

- Regularly undertake feedback, evaluation, problem identification, complaints, or assessment of potential concerns with staff in an emotionally neutral, safe environment that makes such activities a regular part of the way of doing business in the unit or department.

- Establish communication, interaction, and communication norms that represent nonjudgmental, balanced, self-directed communication styles and patterns that eliminate judgment, threats, reactions, or aggression. Make these norms a part of the structure of meetings and of staff and leadership communication styles (Porter-O'Grady & Malloch, 2010).

It is important to recognize that there are common causes of conflict that exist in almost every workplace. Often, ignoring these common causes helps individuals take them for granted and ignore them as significant sources of potential conflict that can generate into increasing levels of stress and inequities at the departmental level. Professional interaction requires an awareness of the simple usual and ordinary issues that exist in the workplace that, if left unaddressed or are found to be inequitable, create the conditions upon which conflict builds. All of these elements require critical and conscious awareness, early engagement, and an organized and systematic mechanism for addressing them if they are not to cause undue influence in the creation of conflict scenarios. Some of these usual and ordinary conflict sources comprising 90 percent of point-of-service conflicts are as follows:

- Personalities: The mix of characters and personal characteristics in a work group is a critical determinant of the areas of concern with regard to communication and interaction in any work group. These personality differences invariably cause impact and fallout regardless of who the people are and where the circumstances within the conflicts may emerge. Recognizing the contribution that diversity makes in the team related to dialogue, decision making, problem solving, and innovation is important to developing a respect for these differences and recognizing how these differences are to be accessed in a positive way. In addition, the challenges that differences in personality create need also to be addressed. When personality challenges emerge in the course of interaction, they must be identified early so the potential to contribute to the dialogue and problem solving can be assessed at the same time as the leader works to limit the potential negative impact or circumstances they may have on group processes.

SCENARIO

Dr. Smith was particularly edgy today and appeared to be taking it out on everyone he met in the operating room. It wasn't as though he was this way often, but staff could never be sure exactly when Dr. Smith would be on the emotional edge. This made it especially hard in the surgical suite when people were already feeling stress about the surgery. Jane, the operating room team leader, was uncertain as to how to handle this situation. She knew that she could not let it go on unaddressed but was uncertain as to what the best approach would be.

Discussion Questions

1. When is the best moment to address Dr. Smith's behavior?
2. Where is the best place that Jane could talk with him?
3. How does Jane deal with her own uncertainty?
4. What might be the best way to open the conversation with Dr. Smith?
5. Should Jane discuss her approach with her peers before beginning?
6. What expectations should Jane have of her conversation with Dr. Smith?

- Personal needs, insights, and requisites: Everyone has a different core set of needs, drives, passions, intentions, and personal values. Each of these converge to create the unique characteristics that an individual brings to his or her profession and work. Sometimes these differences in expression can clash as intently felt motives demonstrate differences in other participant's expressions. Values and purpose are closely aligned with the central integrity of each individual. Giving those a voice, allowing them to be understood by each member of the team, and valuing the array of different value sets that people bring to meaning and purpose help establish a common value theme that can give the work unit a unique identity upon which the team can draw in times of challenge and difficulty. However, in order for this theme to emerge, these values must have a voice, and that voice must be honored, respected, and included in the mosaic that informs the team's integrity and purpose in a way that represents the highest level of meaning.

- Continuously unresolvable issues: Not every circumstance, situation, or condition can be resolved simply because people desire it. Often sociocultural, economic, technological, and regulatory requisites limit the full range of potential responses for problem resolution that people might determine as obvious or clear within their own situation or value set. Sometimes these contextual problems cannot be resolved in a short period of time or resolved in isolation in a manner that would have them cease their perceived negative impact. To the fullest extent possible, and where likely, problems that affect culture and relationship should be addressed and resolved early on. In those cases where regulatory influences cannot be changed, there should be opportunities to discuss them, react to them, and suggest local mechanisms for influencing their application. Participants might even develop new standards that perform in a way that represents a higher measure of performance or behavior than the regulations do. These can all be mechanisms that help participants to accommodate the intractable issues beyond their control or, in some ways, adapt or adjust to them.

- Issues of workload, work distribution, and workload intensity: These are invariably issues that will constantly and continually arise in the workplace. One of the universal conditions of work is that there is always more work than there are resources to address it. Indeed, over the generations the notion that increasing resource use to meet demand is always the preferable solution to address that demand. Supply chain science demonstrates, however, that such solutions are often simplistic and nonsustainable (King, 2011). Still, the perception and demands related to it frequently persist. Discussions and dialogue related specifically to issues of workload, work intensity, and role expectations need a forum and a regular opportunity for expression. The challenges that exist in matching demand to available resources need expression if conflict about them is to be allayed. This means having a regular opportunity in unit or department meetings to discuss issues of workload, resource management, changing demands, and the mechanisms that create balance in the efficiencies among these elements. Giving these issues a voice and a regular opportunity to express that voice and to respond to the issues that are raised in an equitable and efficient manner helps reduce stresses related to them. Giving a voice to these concerns provides opportunity for innovative or creative solutions for making adjustments in them, and provides a forum for discussing modifying resources. Finally, dialogue provides an opportunity for review and evaluation of existing workload strategies, resource issues, financial and budgetary concerns, and a potential for innovative solution seeking (Aiken, Clarke, Silber, & Sloane, 2003).

Personal Comfort with Conflict

Before the leader can engage conflict and others, the leader must be comfortable with his or her own sense of person in the presence of conflict. The effective leader always works to create an environment where colleagues can be comfortable with their own feelings and with the ability to express them. This assumes, of course, that the individual is comfortable in the self-expression of feelings, personal insights, and challenges to prevailing views and circumstances. This leader, of course, needs an environment that is not constraining or controlling or creates structural barriers that make it fundamentally difficult for any individual to identify or express personal feelings. A good leader embraces his or her own feelings regardless of intensity and in doing so represents a level of comfort that is palpable and visible to others. As a result, the leader becomes comfortable with the expression of personal feelings and does so through the development of particular skills that frankly address and express issues of conflict sensitive to the careful consideration of the context and circumstances out of which these conflicts emerge (Shapiro, 2004). The first thing the leader needs to be able to do is test his or her own openness quotient:

- Am I truly comfortable with my own feelings? Is that comfort visible to others?

- Do I personally feel stress in the presence of impending or real conflict?

- Am I uncomfortable when other people express their own feelings and conflicts?

- Do I make it safe and comfortable for others to express conflicts and uncertainties to me? Am I able to embrace another individual in his or her moment of conflict with all the intensity and emotional expression that accompanies it?

- When there is anger or passion displayed, am I able to receive it and be available to it, or do I draw away from it?

- Am I engaging, embracing, and supportive as others express their emotional concerns related to particular conflict issues?

Each of these questions provides an opportunity for the individual leader to assess particular comfort and self-expression in the presence of conflict or conflict situations. It is difficult to ask others to be comfortable in the presence of conflict if personal behavior exemplifies discomfort with the passion, emotions, noise, and expressions of conflict.

Trust: Creating a Safe Space for Positive Conflict

Everyone wants and needs trust in their lives. The safe ability to build commitment, attachment, and mutuality in relationships significantly influences just how well teams will work together, collaborate, express accountability, and have an impact. For the leader, creating a context of trust is the essential framework for the development of a truly safe space where conflict can be dealt with as easily and effectively as any other function, process, or relationship (Shani & Lau, 2005).

Trust is so important that it has a direct impact on the environment of work and the work itself. If a nontrusting environment exists, the degree of involvement and ownership will be lost and will have a direct affect on quality improvement and working methods and procedures in the clinical workplace. In addition, engagement and interaction are essential to the work. If the accuracy of communicating and reporting issues, incidents, and situations based on truth and openness are absent, they begin to shut down trust in the workplace. As well, the potential for mistakes to be detected early is negatively affected when the openness and honesty necessary to early detection and communication are not present and prevent the open discovery and resolution process from working effectively. If issues of consensus, agreement, collective wisdom, common action, and other professional characteristics related to unfolding practice risks are limited or inhibited by an environment that is not representative of openness, integrity, sincerity, mutuality, commitment, conflict inevitably emerges. In sum, the foundations of accountability are shaken by an environment where there is not trust or openness and there exists a lack of willingness to engage real issues, address early conflicts, resolve real problems in the workplace, and confront relational and interactional problems in a safe and trusting environment.

The Need for a Just Environment

The lack of a sense of justice and fairness in the workplace colors individual practitioners' and team members' belief in the fundamental fairness of their environment (Dekker, 2007). The sense of lack of justice comes from what is considered unfair work conditions, procedures, or relationships that are employed by the workplace and impact the team, clinical action, individual decision making, and good leadership. Members of the clinical team begin to believe that there are inequitable opportunities to provide input and influence and make a difference. Individuals begin to experience what they perceive as biased work processes or procedures diminishing not only their own individual commitment to group action or to full participation but also their attachment to the organization, the team, and their trust in leadership (Figure 4-2).

- Regularly review team work processes and mechanisms for working together and problem solving.
- Use an open-ended questionnaire approach as a way of evaluating work team processes and dynamics.
- Use outside facilitation to drill down to issues of inequity or unfairness with the intent to seek equity or find solutions.

Figure 4-2 Antidote for an environment of injustice

Fully Sharing Information

When every leader and team member shares his or her knowledge, experience value is added to the team's decisions. Leaders and staff have many opportunities to fully cooperate in the sharing of useful and helpful information and experiences with each other. In turn, this cooperation makes it likely that every person can fully support the group's final decision. When trust is absent in the unit or department, there is no commitment to the execution of the group's decisions. The staff will stall implementation efforts and sometimes actually sabotage them. You can always know when you have poor cooperation in fully sharing personal views, insights, or opinions in the following situations:

- You observe people nodding their heads or sitting in silence in response to a statement or question raised. This false sense of consensus signals a generalized fear or lack of consensus in sharing opposite viewpoints, critical insights, or opposition in a healthy engagement and dialogue.

- When you notice people stop questioning or raising issues because they fear being labeled as not being team players and are viewed as obstructive or negative in the presence of legitimate questioning.

- Information is presented by individuals who heavily use jargon, generalized factoids, ethereal or nonspecific language, or the use of complex nonunderstandable, convoluted, or simply obtuse language.

Alienation Between Colleagues Is Allowed to Flourish

Collegial attachment unfolds as team members become more familiar with each other, grow in their sense of membership on the team, and feel positive about the opportunities to work together. However, when alienation is allowed to flourish, individuals never arrive at that unique fellowship and strong sense of professional relationship that is a sign of a committed team. Instead, colleague relations disappear and individuals pursue their own self-interests, often at the expense of the collective good of the team. This predominantly individualistic behavior limits group flexibility, particularly in evaluating good choices, practice standards, and action (Deutsch, Coleman, & Marcus, 2006).

In a professional environment, alienation is often unwittingly encouraged by permitting the reflective work of the profession to be sacrificed by unrelenting work expectations and keeping team members busy without the opportunity to think about what they're doing. Reflective work is essential for professionals to be able to determine value, importance, and priorities and make decisions about best practices and necessary changes in patient care (Figure 4-3). When this level of reflective interaction is sacrificed or seen as something extra by the organization or managers, this lack of support for the reflective component of practice actually contributes to the decline of patient care and increases the security of definitive patient outcomes (Webber & Nathan, 2010). In this set of circumstances, members of the clinical team give up participating, recognize that interaction and reflection are not valued, and begin to behave in a more functional employee work group patterns, ceasing to demonstrate the unique behaviors associated with professional practice.

In the midst of harried busyness and chronic addiction to action, emotional connection between colleagues never solidifies, reducing the opportunity for clinical team members to develop trust and to establish sustainable team-based patterns of work. This fragmentation emphasizes unilateral patterns of behavior, inconsistent standards of performance, and low expectations for performance and impact. The result is an uneven workload, unclear impact, competition, resentment, and challenge to the establishment of common standards of patient care practices.

- Ensure that performance expectations and group membership obligations are clearly and specifically enumerated and that performance evaluation includes these values.
- Establish clearly defined indicators of trust and review at least quarterly.
- Clearly delineate that team relationship, interaction, and communication are directly tied to patient care outcomes. Hold colleagues accountable for fully participating in the reflective components of practice.
- Challenge personal agendas when individual priorities predominate over team expectations and standards.

Figure 4-3 Antidote for alienation

Overcoming Personal Barriers to Engaging Conflict

There are generally five personal barriers that have a dramatic impact on the individual leader's ability to understand, engage, and manage conflict (Figure 4-4). The leader must be intentional about conflict in order to bring it to the forefront of consciousness and prevent simply responding to the emotional reaction inherent in almost every conflict situation. Often, breaking the conflict down in a logical sequence of stages helps make the conflict more objective, less personal, and more amenable to addressing and resolving it.

There must be a willingness to confront conflict. When there is a generalized understanding in the unit or department that conflict is normative and will be incorporated into the usual and ordinary activities of managing relationships and interaction, personal reactions can be more safely confronted. Conflict management is a learned process and develops and refines when one has more opportunity to apply skills and test out approaches. When a safe space exists, it should be possible to objectively discuss approaches to particular kinds of conflicts and sensitivities individuals may have with regard to their relationship to that conflict. Bringing these personal issues into the open, discussing them freely,

Fear	First, confront it
	Take three deep breaths
	Examine what's going on inside you
	Talk to someone else about your fear
	Talk yourself through the experience
Uncertainty	Break the conflict down into parts
	Identify which part has greatest impact
	Stay in touch with feelings and reactions
	Identify conflict as early as possible
	Validate with others your identification skills
Negativity	Recall past experiences with conflict
	Visualize yourself within a conflict
	Observe family conflict dynamics
	Talk with other family members
	Write down and review your feelings
No skills	Read about the conflict management process
	Attend classes on conflict management
	Do a role-play on conflict
	Discuss conflict process with others
	Practice conflict scenarios
Poor experience	Seek opportunities to practice
	Begin mediating small conflicts
	Have experts evaluate your progress
	Build experience slowly
	Evaluate your progress with peers

Figure 4-4 Overcoming personal barriers to engaging conflict

and treating the elements of conflict as a process helps diminish the fear associated with it and provides opportunity for the development of conflict-resolving experience.

The second major issue with regard to addressing conflict is the uncertainty about the capacity to handle the conflict emotionally and personally. All conflict has a personal impact and touches individuals in a unique way. Each individual has his or her own experience with conflict and will automatically react to it in the initial stages of the conflict event. Becoming intentional helps overcome some of these issues but does not eliminate their emotional impact. If an individual can give language to the emotional experience he or she is feeling, that experience can be less obstructive and more objective. Each person will have a different alignment with regard to the conflict experience. Breaking down the emotional response to specific patterns of expression helps take from personal consciousness the sense that the whole conflict experience is necessarily rife with stress and pressure. Likely there are stress elements or components of the conflict experience that generate 90 percent of the emotions that one feels in a conflict event. If the leader can grapple with the particular component that addresses his or her specific emotional response, the rest of the conflict management process reflecting that particular element of stress may be much easier to address, providing more opportunities for effectiveness.

Third, it's important to recognize that most people's attitude toward conflict is a negative one. With all the discussion in the world about the positive influences and forces and normative character of conflict, personal history is generally indicative of a negative mindset or set of experiences. These experiences need to be shared among team members. When they are communicated to others and examined as a part of the dialogue together, much of the fear is diminished, resulting in a more objective assessment of the conflict experience. Sharing fears also helps others identify and personalize their own take on their conflict events. This helps defuse the negative experience, objectifies the elements of the conflict event, and makes it more manageable and useful as a tool for learning.

Conflict management reflects the fourth critical element: lack of skill. Conflict management is a learned skill. That essentially means that the initial attempts at managing conflict are often pretty rough and unrefined. Initial attempts by the staff are often halting, rudimentary, and not very elegant. Like all applied experiences, the first stages are usually rough and unrefined. However, with practice and opportunity, skills become refined, talent begins to grow, and effectiveness becomes a common experience. Individuals must realize that this experiential element of conflict handling is critical to personal development and the growing sense of confidence and competence with regard to the handling of normative conflict. Through learning, application, and experiential opportunities, skills develop, become refined, and the maturing conflict **mediator** becomes a role model and mentor for others who are refining their own conflict skill development (Boulle, Colatrella, & Picchioni, 2008). It must be recognized that some people move through this process more quickly and easily than others, which creates an obligation in them for mentoring and supporting others whose developmental process may be more challenging. In this way, skill development gets refined, common experiences get shared, and conflict becomes less dramatic as an element of shared professional relationships.

CRITICAL THOUGHT

One of the most critical elements of addressing conflict is certainty regarding the feelings and insights of others. The mediator must always be sure that others' real feelings can be properly expressed.

Lack of exposure and experience relates directly to the previous discussion about lack of skills. The more opportunities the leader has for actually managing conflict events, the more opportunity there is for skill development, experience, and technique refinement. The growing leader will seek opportunities first to mediate with more experienced conflict managers, and as the leader becomes more competent and skilled, he or she can undertake conflict activities more independently and ultimately become a mentor and model for handling conflict for other colleagues. As a leader becomes more skilled in handling conflict, he or she becomes a resource to the organization and may have the opportunity to resolve conflicts beyond the unit or department as his or her reputation for effectiveness and success grows and serves as an example of conflict effectiveness for the whole organization.

Handling Conflict

Although whole texts are devoted to the management of issues related to handling conflict, some simple rules provide the emerging leader with a basic tool set that will help guide his or her conflict skills development through the initial stages. The conflict management process is well studied, systematic, logical, and intentional. It guides parties from points of high-level conflict toward finding common ground and establishing more sustainable meaning in relationships (Partridge, 2009).

CRITICAL THOUGHT

The mediator does not own the problem and is not responsible for its resolution. The parties own it and are responsible for resolving it.

Where people are given the opportunity to make choices and to manage their own lives, there is always a potential for conflict. As noted, everyone is unique. The differences embedded in the unique characteristics of a wide variety of personalities making up the human community define us as unique individuals and directly influence the roles we play and the contributions we make. At the same time, however, these same gifts can sometimes serve as fundamental sources of potential conflict where those differences run up against the different expressions of others.

However, when handled creatively and effectively, these fundamental human differences can result in richer and deeper experiences and relationships among people. In order for this to happen, however, these differences must be handled with respect, through positive engagement. At the same time the leader must handle the conflict between personalities assertively so it doesn't become or remain a source of constant contention and discord. Unaddressed or ignored, important personality differences (conflict) can create serious ground for psychological and physiological harm. The presence of the existence of human difference represents an emotional and psychological distance between people that frequently manifests in negative feelings, aggression, oppression, antagonism, and alienation between people. In most cases (about 90 percent of the time) managers often called in mediators to deal with interpersonal conflicts that result from a lack of understanding or misperception of personal patterns of behavior between participants (Kellett & Dalton, 2001). It is in anticipating these conflicts and in handling them early that the leader will spend most of his or her time in managing and mediating conflict activities.

CRITICAL THOUGHT

Unaddressed feelings are the most common cause of lingering conflict. These feelings smolder just below the surface, building energy, igniting fuses, and ultimately resulting in a devastating explosion that is very difficult to recover from—for all parties!

Identifying the Problem

The leader's first task as a mediator for conflict is the ability to get the core issues that lie at the heart of the conflict situation on the table and visible to all participants (Kritek, 2002). These core issues are identified by the involved individuals as the triggers that hooked them and brought forth feelings of personal conflict. Good mediation leadership demonstrates the ability to find the central themes or issues and identify them as the drivers that most often hold people to their negative positions or feelings. Remember, these issues do not have to be right or accurate or even legitimate in the eyes of the mediator or anyone else; they simply must be felt, expressed, and clarified. Sorting through the legitimacy of issues comes later in the processes associated with resolution.

Make Sure Issues Are Expressed

It is important that the leader be able to facilitate the individuals' expression of their conflict in a way that is clear, frank, and understandable with regard to what is driving their sense of the conflict. If the individuals experiencing the conflict do not feel as though they've had the chance to fully express their concerns and feelings, these feelings will continue—indeed, deepen—and will emerge later in the process, causing it to slow the process or stop it entirely. Patience and thoroughness around the issue of clarity by the mediating leader in the earliest stages of the conflict often result in fewer problems in resolving the conflict and takes a shorter period of time in processing it. The challenge for the mediator is to stay out of the way of expression and clarification. The mediator must always remember that he or she does not own the problem and therefore does not own its solution. The urge to intervene, to direct, or to control the resolution must be avoided by the mediator so the resolution that is obtained through the processes that are undertaken can be driven by the owners of the problem and through their effort they can move toward resolution. Remember, the mediator has no other goal than helping the stakeholders resolve their own conflict.

Resolving the Five Kinds of Conflicts

Although there are many themes and shades of conflict among people, most conflicts fall into five general categories: relationship conflicts, information conflicts, interest-based conflicts, organizational conflicts, and values-based conflicts (Lansford, 2008). These five categories of conflicts have their own elements and constituents and require different insights in order to address and resolve them.

Relationship Conflicts

The first most important ingredient for understanding relationship conflicts is being clear with regard to exactly how the individual feels and what he or she perceived about the conflict. The most notable kind of relational conflicts are those that build on inaccurate perceptions, especially related to either what was said or heard. Relationship conflicts are filled with emotional content. A part of the clarification process for relational conflicts is providing a safe space and time for expression for the emotional content that one is feeling about the relational issue. Effective mediators create a safe space that can bring individuals closer to the issues and deepen their relationship to them (Figure 4-5). Relationships are filled with meaning and purpose, and the feelings related to the significance of this meaning must be explored sufficiently in order to help the parties more adequately translate their positions into language that communicates them most effectively. However, dealing with feelings and with issues must be separated at the outset so they are not handled in the same way. Expressing feelings is an important part of helping individuals identify their response to their own perceptions of the conflict. As they get clear about these feelings, they can become clearer about their notion of the real issue and can be more supportive of the systematic assessment of it. Each party must be given sufficient time to express feelings and emotions so the full range of sensitivities related to their perception of the conflict has an expression and an opportunity to be stated and recognized. In relationship conflicts, the greatest failure in the resolution is usually found in inadequate allowances for the expression of feeling and the ability to give that feeling a language that can be understood.

- Move the parties away from each other and the place of conflict.
- Support each person in his or her feelings and emotions.
- Accept each individual's own perceptions of how he or she feels.
- Make sure each person has an opportunity to verbalize feelings.
- Don't attempt to resolve the issue before individuals express feelings.
- Be caring and supportive of each person experiencing the conflict.
- Accept whatever emotions are expressed in an appropriate place for it.

Figure 4-5 Creating a safe space

SCENARIO

Rachel didn't know if she could stand one more negative comment from Michael. Ever since she had arrived on the nursing unit, Michael had virtually nothing positive to say to her. He seemed to track her every clinical move and knew exactly when she was overwhelmed or concerned and even when she was behind in her work. It was then that he seemed to comment about her pace, competence, and organization. Again this morning he started with the comments, even suggesting that she might not be able to keep up with the demands of the clinical work. His constant monitoring of her work and comments about her ability to keep up increased the stress level and made her even more tense in this new clinical situation than she would normally feel. Rachel didn't know what to do. If he didn't stop soon, she would either blow up or just throw up her hands and leave.

Discussion Questions

1. At this point in this scenario, what should Rachel's first step be?

2. What kind of environment needs to be created to facilitate expressing conflict feelings?

3. What kind of a relationship conflict would you define this to be?

4. Who will Rachel need to involve in her effort to resolve this conflict?

There are several elements the leader will need to include in the mediation process and make the parties aware of as they explore relationship issues:

- Mutual respect: No matter how divided the individuals are or how attached they are to their positions, keep reminding them of their common humanity and the value each of them has. Good mediators keep aware of the mutuality of weaknesses, frailties, perceptions, and positions each person brings to the table. The mediator reminds the parties of the respect they want for themselves and ensures that they offer it to each other as fully as possible in the circumstances. The mediation leader tries to direct anger to the issues, not to the person.

- Needs versus wants: The leader must help the participants figure out and differentiate between what they really need and what they perceive they want. The leader wants to help parties deepen their understanding of what they need and relate their wants to that particular need. Indeed, in this case, is something the individual must have as a part of this self-expectation or reason to mediate. Although getting what a person needs is critical, getting what he or she wants may be less so. Helping the parties identify need and obtain satisfaction of that need is a significant part of the mediation dynamic.

- Compassion and empathy: One of the intentions of mediation is to help the parties understand each other and to hear the other party's position clearly and with understanding. The leader creates a context for equity and value and translates that value with a sense of compassion and empathy.

- Staying in the "I": In relationship conflict there is always a temptation to blame and focus on the other. The role of the mediator is to keep the parties focused on their own feelings and insights, avoiding blame, name calling, and the prolific use of "you" statements. The mediator consistently reminds the parties to begin their statements or responses with "I" statements, such as "I feel," "I think," "I need," "I want," and "I see." This keeps all parties focused on their role, communication, interaction, and needs.

CRITICAL THOUGHT

People think they have the right information without ever analyzing its source, the perspective it represents, the content, and the meaning it is attempting to project. A great deal of conflict can be avoided if people really think carefully about the information influencing their actions.

Information Conflicts

People often make judgments that reflect their own perceptions, values, and personal processing of what they know and the kind of information that supports it. Sometimes the information they access is inaccurate or inadequate to support their position. When integrated with the individual's values and perceptions, poor or inadequate information can become a potent mix for potential conflict.

Available information on its own demonstrates no bias. Bias occurs when information goes through the perceptive and values filters of the individual reviewing it. In a conflict resolution process, careful assessment of the adequacy, relevance, and accuracy of the information supporting a particular view is critical to the effectiveness of the resolution at any level of appropriate action in the mediation. Before any action can occur (including drawing conclusions or making judgments), the individuals who are party to the conflict should deal with the following critical questions:

- What is the source of the information?
- Is the information relevant to the issue at hand?
- Does the information correlate well with other sources of related information?
- Is the source of the information credible? Is it complete?
- Is there enough information from which to draw any relevant conclusions?
- What are the prevailing views or perceptions in this mediation related to interpreting the information?
- What else needs to be done to clarify or verify information that is influencing the thinking and dialogue in the mediation?

The leader should encourage parties to the conflict to think about the following:

- Are judgments being made before all of the information is available to support them?
- Is the meaning of the information clear to all parties before conclusions can be drawn from them about what action needs to be taken?
- Are all parties' perceptions appropriately clarified so there is a mutual level of understanding and insight regarding the relevant information?

The challenge for the leader is managing information appropriately. Information that conflicts with an individual's fundamental beliefs or ideas about the problem is often difficult to adjust or change. People hold onto their beliefs and levels of understanding regardless of whether the supporting information validates them or not. Cautiously moving through a recalibration of the personal impact of accurate information and understanding about what people know requires careful consideration of the data, its impact on the individuals, the potential for obtainable levels of mutual understanding about the information, and likely usefulness of the information for subsequent dialogue and decision making.

CRITICAL THOUGHT

Most interest conflicts have tremendous emotional and psychological attachment to the issue in conflict. The good mediator attempts to defuse the emotional and psychological passion in order to ensure the parties can get to a level of discourse that can lead to resolution.

Interest-Based Conflicts

Parties to a conflict come to the table with a stake in the conflict. They have interests that need to be resolved. Much of the conflict is about differentiation of their interests. Specifying and naming particular interests is a critical part of what the leader is attempting to accomplish in the dialogue between conflicting parties.

It is important that clarity with regard to individuals' feelings and sensitivities related to their own concerns be established early as a part of identifying conflicting interests. Frequently, the parties are unaware of the fact that they actually may share interests; there may be common ground with regard to what they originally assumed to be conflict related to interests, or misperceptions about the interest and the conflict that generated. Indeed, the real conflict may have nothing to do with the interest that brought them to the table.

Often in the arena of interest conflict, the challenge is more about different insights and perceptions each has about how they know the issues and how they have come to understand their role in relationship to them rather than the real interests. Often what occurs in these kinds of conflicts is that the legitimate interests they share are hidden behind an expressed interest. The mediator must work to get each party to a place where it can become clear about what the underlying or real interest might be that is truly generating the conflict. Moving beyond the perception of interest to actual interest helps deepen the likelihood of conflict resolution.

Of special concern with interest-based conflict is the fact that the parties may not know what their genuine interests are; they may be actually hiding genuine interests; perceptions may be obstructing the emergence of genuine interests; or they may even be unaware of what the actual interests might be. Here the mediator must often bring them to sensitively but more deeply articulate genuine interest issues so the real interests may be dealt with directly and effectively.

Organizational Conflicts

There are innumerable sources of organizational conflict (Figure 4-6). Although many of the sources of conflict in organizations may be obvious to all parties, most are not. Yet, organizational conflicts drive a wide range of personal conflicts because the organization essentially defines the context within which people relate and work. Organizational conflicts relate to questions of accountability, expectations, and systemic communication. In addition, there are questions related to whether a supportive environment exists that supports point-of-service work of the organization and provides appropriate infrastructure and resource allocation for that work to be owned and done at the point of service (Harvey & Allard, 2002).

CRITICAL THOUGHT

Organizational conflicts are best resolved when everyone in the organization is "singing off of the same song sheet." When individuals and groups play out their own agenda at the expense of others or the whole organization, they create the frame for organizational conflict. To get past this or to ensure this does not happen, leaders must be sure that people see themselves as members of the larger organization and are committed to making it successful.

The issues that drive effectiveness of the organizational culture and its facility for limiting conflict are directly related to how well people work together; how team-based activities have been constructed and sustained; how mismatches between the needs of patient care and the distribution of resources have been addressed; and the congruence between the values of the organization and the values of the people who comprise it. Conflicts in organizations can be looked at as having a series of layers—the overall organizational structure, the configuration of the leadership team, the relationship and interaction between departments and services, interdisciplinary collaboration and interaction at the point of service, and the structure and relationships that operate daily at the organization's point of service. All of these elements comprise a network that represents the character of the organization and indicates the confluence of forces in the organization and how they either constrain or facilitate effectiveness at each and every level.

The clinical leader at the point of service can have a radical impact on the roles, relationships, and effectiveness of work within the unit or department.

Certainly, there should be a goodness of fit between broad organizational goals and a specific unit or departmental goals. If general goals of the system are to be achieved, it will be people at the point of service whose work effort acts to translate those goals into action.

- Conflicting goals
- Conflicts between groups
- Intergroup competition
- Inadequate leadership
- Failure
- Compartmental departments

Figure 4-6 Causes of organizational conflicts

Organizational conflict depends on the insight, awareness, and information level of the leader regarding organizational priorities, parameters, policies, and practices. It is important for this leader to carefully observe the action of individuals and teams for their potential to form purposes, goals, or actions that are not in direct relationship to the purpose, mission, and goals of the larger system. Among professional members of the system there is a tacit agreement that a goodness of fit will exist between the purpose, mission, and goals of the system and personal goals of the members who comprise that system (Boddy, 2011). It is the role of the leader to make sure that there is a goodness of fit between these dynamic forces in order to make sure that good alignment exists between the trajectory of the organization and that of the individual member. Some questions related to clarify these issues might be as follows:

- How clear and precise are the purposes and goals of the organization, and how well does that fit with the work done at the point of service?

- Is everyone in the department or unit aware of the personal role they play in fulfilling the organization's mission and goals?

- Is there mutuality and agreements among professional colleagues, managers, and the organization regarding goals, resources, and specific actions to fulfill the effort to advance the agenda of the organization?

- Are performance measures clear and specific enough to tell the story of the staff's contribution to the organization's mission and goals?

- Do leaders at every level of the organization encourage and facilitate providing the necessary resource support, goal congruence, organizational understanding for the goals, and full engagement of all stakeholders in the right response to organizational goals?

- Are financial challenges, constraints, issues of distribution, and opportunities clearly enumerated to all participants in a way that deepens their understanding, or advances their engagement, and is financial management adjusted when performance information indicates the need for it?

- Do the clinical and management leaders in the organization participate in the system's collective effort to delineate strategy, establish priorities, define direction, construct goals, and evaluate the effectiveness of all work effort related to them?

Each of these questions alone is not sufficient to root out conflicting elements in organizational activity, but when taken together they create an integrated framework that provides a context for organizational clarity, specificity of goals and action, congruence between systems and persons, effectiveness, and goal achievement. It is clear that the more the organizational framework, purpose, direction, and goals inform actions, the less likely there will be conflict between and among any of these characteristics. The role of every effective leader is to address those arenas, components, or elements of the organization and its goals, structures, and processes that are not congruent with the achievement of excellence in practice, process, or patient outcomes. A critical openness in organizations is the foundation for all engaged human action in systems. Varying degrees or levels of compromise in any one or more of these elements accelerates the potential for conflict in the organization and raises challenges to personal and organizational effectiveness.

Values-Based Conflicts

Perhaps the most difficult conflicts to address in the workplace are those that relate to personal values. There are many sources of values conflict (Figure 4-7). Fundamental value differences arise from almost any source significant enough to create specific identity differences between individuals and groups. Values conflicts are difficult to resolve because they generally relate to who people are, what they believe, and how they identify themselves to each other and to the world. Values conflicts relate not so much to what people think than to how people feel about who they are in the world and how that is best represented in their person. It is here where the impact of culture, ethnicity, religious beliefs, ideology, internal values, and politics are fully played out and expressed.

The quality and effectiveness of professional and work relationships over time depend, for the most part, on how well people can clarify, accommodate, and adjust to significant values differences. Here again, it is important that each individual be clear about personal values so that the individual's relationship to values can be self-understood and articulated in a way that helps individuals understand themselves and their place in the world better and creates a foundation or premise for translating that to others. Particular questions that need clarification at the personal level might be as follows:

- What does what you see and feel in the world mean to you at a very personal level?
- How do your culture, religion, belief system, values structure, and personal life practices. inform the way in which you live your life?
- How is the answer to the previous question best demonstrated in the image that you present and the way in which you show others how you live your life?
- What is it that you need others to understand about your personal values system?
- How do you demonstrate adherence to your own values and continue to respect the values differences of others as they live their lives?
- In what areas are your values significantly different from those generally expressed, and how have you accommodated them while honoring others' expression of different values?
- Have you resolved your willingness to respect the diversity of values in your work culture, and are you committed to resolving conflicts between them that may affect both work and relationships?

- Different cultures
- Different ethnic groups
- Different religious beliefs
- Different personal values
- Different political ideology
- Different economic and social status

Figure 4-7 Causes of values conflicts

Exploration of these questions is a critical first step for every professional and is nonnegotiable for the leader. Clarity around issues of personal value and one's relationship to the world from that values position is a foundation upon which relationships with others, the organization, and society can be developed and refined. Common responses to values conflicts often reflect a lack of clarity around serious work done in relation to these questions. Common reactions to values conflicts include proselytizing and position taking (lecturing, not listening); minimizing, denying, accommodating, or avoiding any issues with the potential for values conflict in order to keep the peace; and pretending to agree, defer, discount, or ignore values differences in order to simply avoid having to deal with them at all. On the other hand, participants can genuinely acknowledge particular differences, seek common ground, find a broader accommodation of multiple values positions, develop reasonable compromise, and build strong relationships that reflect the values incorporation as a part of mutual understanding.

CRITICAL THOUGHT

Values conflicts can be resolved only when common ground can be established among the parties. There must be some elements of belief and human experience with which the parties can mutually identify and through that experience find a route to building a stronger relationship upon which subsequent interaction can build.

Values conflicts are indeed difficult to address and resolve, but that does not make them impossible or completely intractable. For the leader, however, a unique set of approaches is needed to address constantly existing value differences among colleagues in the workplace. A number of simple, consistent, yet important contextual and role practices can generally be useful in minimizing the potential for values conflict, isolating and focusing on particular values challenges, or exploring a deeper and broader value of diversity and richness in the human experience, dialogue, and relationships. A few of those critical elements are as follows:

- Make a true and abiding commitment to finding common ground and developing win–win compromises in values adjustments between individuals and groups.

- Expand the vocabulary and language of the workplace to include broader terms, expressions, and definitions that are inclusive and respectful.

- Find the common themes and elements between and among values that can anchor relationships and demonstrate the foundation for the expressions of value.

- Articulate and define as a system in your unit that includes the fundamental elements of dignity and respect, which informs all behavioral expectations among members and colleagues.

- Enumerate the legitimacy of the individual differences, the right to have them, and the appropriate forum within which they can be legitimately expressed. At the same time, define and acknowledge environment, context, and situations where the expression of such differences is not legitimate or appropriate.

- Make sure a specific and well-designed ethics process or committee is in place to deal with significant values challenges or intractable values issues in an effort to establish a common frame for behavioral expectations and expression.

- As with other differences, make values conflicts a normative expectation of the dynamics of a diverse membership group, creating a safe space for exploration, an effective process for dialogue and clarification, and a mechanism for conflict resolution.

Although values conflicts can create significant noise within a social system and within professional relationships, those differences need not impede or imperil the essential professional values represented in the provision of patient care. A consistent and ongoing effort to find common ground and stand on it helps create a strong set of relationships, an effective organization, and the medium for acting out of a clearly established set of common values.

The Norm of Conflict

The wise leader will come in time to acknowledge the universal presence of conflict and the continuing and dynamic necessity for addressing it. Conflict will not diminish, disappear, or dissipate in the human experience. It can only be well managed. In the absence of serious and effective management of conflict, it invariably accelerates, increases its intensity, and moves toward the creation of great harm (Figure 4-8).

The role of the leader first must be exemplified within a defined level of comfort with the reality that conflict is a constant companion of human interaction and relationship. Out of this understanding and comfort with the presence of conflict comes the need to develop methodologies and techniques for positively addressing it, engaging it early enough that its positive value can be experienced and that it can ultimately make a difference in the interests of the professional community and those it serves.

The effective leaders sees signs of conflict constantly fomenting in people and in the organization. The conflicting interests and dynamic differences between people and cultures are always a rich source for conflict to percolate.

Leadership:

- Poor recognition of emerging conflict
- Inadequate conflict skills
- Highly competitive
- Seeks own agenda in spite of organizational goals
- Can't tie personal behavior to organizational expectations
- Actually likes conflict; pitting people against each other

Individuals:

- Problems with work competency
- Difficulty establishing relationships
- Personal anger
- Highly competitive
- Unclear about role expectations and goal requirements
- Unable to become a team player

Groups:

- Group relationship unformed or immature
- Groups aggressive or angry with other groups
- Unhealthy level of organizational competition
- Group goals incongruent with organizational goals
- Internally dysfunctional group dynamics
- Failure of the group to fulfill its obligations or achieve goals

Figure 4-8 Seeing signs of conflict

CHAPTER TEST QUESTIONS

1. People are afraid of conflict because they do not have the essential skills to manage it well. True or false?

2. If you engage conflict too early, there is a chance that it might be misconstrued and sufficient time will not have passed to make sure that all of the elements of the conflict have emerged appropriately. True or false?

3. Emotions must be controlled and separated from the conflict so that the real issues can be addressed more directly. True or false?

4. Conflicting personal needs and issues is just one of many sources of conflict but can be the driving force for other kinds of conflict. True or false?

5. The conflict mediator manages all elements of the conflict and assists parties to the conflict in their personal expression and in determining who needs to get what from the experience. True or false?

6. All conflict is normative in group or team dynamics. The role of the leader is to be able to identify the conflict, take care of it, and quickly move the team past it. True or false?

7. The five personal barriers to conflict resolution and problem solving engagement are fear, uncertainty, negativity, a lack of skills, and poor experience. True or false?

8. It is not the mediator's obligation to focus on the core issues of conflict, rather it is the obligation of the parties to know their core issues and to be willing to negotiate them. True or false?

9. Identity issues are the easiest to resolve because they deal only with values and personal belief, which can be quickly identified. When they are clear, they can help move the parties to early and complete resolution. True or false?

10. All conflict is resolvable if there is a good match between commitment and effort of the parties, use of best methodology, and the clarity and effectiveness of the solutions obtained. True or false?

> **WWW**   For a full suite of assignments and additional learning activities, use the access code located in the front of your book to visit the exclusive website: http://go.jblearning.com/leadership. If you do not have an access code, you can obtain one at the site.

References

Aiken, L., Clarke, S., Silber, J., & Sloane, D. (2003). Hospital nurse staffing, education and patient mortality. *LDI Issue Brief, 2,* 1–4.

Amer, R., & Zou, K. (2011). *Conflict management and dispute settlement in East Asia.* Farnham, Surrey; Burlington, VT: Ashgate.

Blackard, K., & Gibson, J. W. (2002). *Capitalizing on conflict: Strategies and practices for turning conflict into synergy in organizations: A manager's handbook.* Palo Alto, CA: Davies-Black.

Boddy, C. (2011). *Corporate psychopaths: Organisational destroyers.* New York, NY: Palgrave Macmillan.

Boulle, L., Colatrella, M. T., & Picchioni, A. P. (2008). *Mediation: Skills and techniques.* Newark, NJ: LexisNexis Matthew Bender.

Dekker, S. (2007). *Just culture: Balancing safety and accountability.* Aldershot, England; Burlington, VT: Ashgate.

Deutsch, M., Coleman, P. T., & Marcus, E. C. (Eds.). (2006). *The handbook of conflict resolution: Theory and practice* (2nd ed.). San Francisco, CA: Jossey-Bass.

Harvey, C. P., & Allard, M. J. (2002). *Understanding and managing diversity: Readings, cases, and exercises.* Upper Saddle River, NJ: Prentice Hall.

Kellett, P. M., & Dalton, D. G. (2001). *Managing conflict in a negotiated world: A narrative approach to achieving dialogue and change.* Thousand Oaks, CA: Sage.

King, T. F. (2011). *A companion to cultural resource management.* Chichester, West Sussex, UK; Malden, MA: Wiley-Blackwell.

Kritek, P. B. (2002). *Negotiating at an uneven table: Developing moral courage in resolving our conflicts.* San Francisco, CA: Jossey-Bass.

Lansford, T. (2008). *Conflict resolution.* Detroit, MI: Greenhaven.

LeBaron, M. (2002). *Bridging troubled waters: Conflict resolution from the heart.* San Francisco, CA: Jossey-Bass.

Lencioni, P. (2002). *The five dysfunctions of a team: A leadership fable.* San Francisco, CA: Jossey-Bass.

MacDonald, G. (2011). *Building below the waterline: Shoring up the foundations of leadership.* Peabody, MA: Hendrickson.

Partridge, M. V. B. (2009). *Alternative dispute resolution: An essential competency for lawyers.* Oxford, England; New York, NY: Oxford University Press.

Porter-O'Grady, T., & Malloch, K. (2010). *Quantum leadership: Advancing innovation, transforming healthcare.* Sudbury, MA: Jones and Bartlett.

Rodgers, D. T. (2011). *Age of fracture.* Cambridge, MA: Belknap.

Shani, A. B., & Lau, J. B. (2005). *Behavior in organizations: An experiential approach.* New York, NY: McGraw-Hill Irwin.

Shapiro, D. (2004). *Conflict and communication: A guide through the labyrinth of conflict management.* New York, NY: International Debate Education Association.

Smokowski, P. R., & Bacallao, M. (2011). *Becoming bicultural: Risk, resilience, and Latino youth.* New York, NY: New York University Press.

Stahl, P. M. (2011). *Conducting child custody evaluations: From basic to complex issues.* Thousand Oaks, CA: Sage.

Tojo, J., & Dilpreet, C. (2007). *Appreciative inquiry and knowledge management.* Northhampton, UK: Edward Elgar.

Webber, M., & Nathan, J. (2010). *Reflective practice in mental health: Advanced psychosocial practice with children, adolescents and adults.* London, England; Philadelphia, PA: Jessica Kingsley.

Wenger, A., & Möckli, D. (2003). *Conflict prevention: The untapped potential of the business sector.* Boulder, CO: Lynne Rienner.

Appendix A

A BRIEF CONFLICT SKILLS ASSESSMENT

In order for conflict to be properly handled, the leader must have specific skills. This is simply the basic inventory of conflict skills. For each of the points made, select the appropriate answer. The higher your score, the greater your conflict skills value. This assessment should be looked at as a developmental tool, not a test.

1. Almost never

2. Sometimes

3. Often

4. Regularly

I have a good sense of the needs of the team at any given moment.

| 1 | 2 | 3 | 4 |

I work hard not to avoid conflicts.

| 1 | 2 | 3 | 4 |

I make it safe for people to identify and express conflicts at work.

| 1 | 2 | 3 | 4 |

Staff have opportunities to test their mediation and conflict resolution skills.

| 1 | 2 | 3 | 4 |

We have fewer conflict events on our service unit since implementing a conflict resolution process.

| 1 | 2 | 3 | 4 |

The trust level on my unit is consistently high.

We regularly evaluate the conflict process on our unit and make changes to make it more effective.

| 1 | 2 | 3 | 4 |

I can anticipate important changes and alert the team before they directly experience the change.

| 1 | 2 | 3 | 4 |

I undertake at least one developmental opportunity a year to refine conflict skills.

| 1 | 2 | 3 | 4 |

There is a staff-driven conflict resolution process in place on my work unit.

| 1 | 2 | 3 | 4 |

The environment is conducive to anyone expressing feelings of conflict.

| 1 | 2 | 3 | 4 |

There is a mechanism in place for following up on conflict resolution and ensuring it was effective.

| 1 | 2 | 3 | 4 |

Staff are satisfied with the conflict process used on our unit.

Scoring:

1–13	Need much work
14–27	Growing
28–40	Building well
40–52	Effective

PLANNING IS BRINGING THE FUTURE INTO THE PRESENT SO THAT YOU CAN DO SOMETHING ABOUT IT NOW. —ALAN LAIKEN

CHAPTER OBJECTIVES

Upon completion of this chapter, the reader will be able to do the following:

» Develop an understanding of patient care delivery models, patient classification systems, and scheduling and staffing.

» Provide an overview of the complexities and interconnectedness of the components of workforce management systems.

» Understand the importance of evidence-driven processes, integration of research, and their impact on nurse satisfaction, patient quality, and organizational outcomes.

» Describe the current measures of staffing effectiveness.

» Gain an appreciation of the challenges in addressing inadequacies or problems of staffing and scheduling.

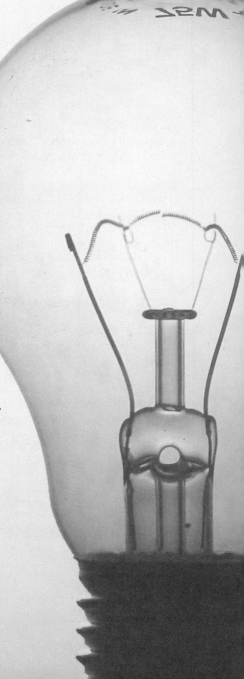

Staffing and Scheduling for Patient Care Excellence and Affordability

Workforce management in health care requires an understanding of the nature and complexities of the dynamics involved in providing the right nurse with the right patient at the right time. Providing the right nurse for the right patient at the right time is more than assigning available nurses to the current list of patients on a unit. It requires an understanding of the critical elements and dynamics of workforce management processes and the translation of these elements into a staffing plan that supports the achievement of the highest-quality outcomes.

In this chapter, the importance of the patient care delivery model, basics of **staffing** and **scheduling**, regulatory, accrediting and research standards for staffing effectiveness, evaluation of the measures of staffing effectiveness, challenges in managing variances in resources, and the role of the clinical leader in ensuring optimal staffing practices are discussed.

Patient workforce management includes five highly interconnected and interrelated components, which include the following (Figure 5-1):

1. Establishment of a patient care delivery model
2. Patient needs and nurse interventions identification
3. Creation of a core staffing schedule to support patient needs
   a. Knowledge of staff competencies and abilities
   b. Integration of staffing and research evidence
   c. Skill mix

       d. Registered Nurse (RN) competencies

       e. Educational levels

4. Daily staffing process to match available staff with identified patient care needs

       a. Interpreting and managing the adequacy of the staffing

       b. Variance between actual staffing and patient care needs

       c. Staffing adequacy indicators/effectiveness

       d. Capacity determination

Workforce management includes distinct processes with special characteristics, processes, and goals.

Caveat: Continuing to attempt to amalgamate patient classification, scheduling, staffing, retention, and recruitment into one process serves only to decrease system validity and frustrate workers with additional unproductive tasks.

Patient Care Delivery Model	→	Describes the infrastructure, roles, accountabilities, and processes for patient care
Patient Classification	→	Patient care needs are identified using a valid and reliable system
Core Scheduling	→	Medical/surgical 12-1 patient/nurse ratio/2 LPN/1 CNA Tele 4-1 RN ICU 2-1 RN Women's & Infants 2 RN PER UNIT MINIMUM (L&D AP/PP, Nursery)
Staffing Assignments	→	Daily adjustments based on actual patient care needs, activity from last shift, and anticipation of Admissions, Discharges, & Transfers for next shift
Evaluate Staffing Effectiveness	→	Assess the relationship between staffing and outcomes and make appropriate adjustments

Figure 5-1 Workforce management

5. Evaluation of value and outcomes

    a. Assess qualitative and quantitative patient, caregiver, and organization outcomes

    b. Nurse retention, satisfaction, and turnover

    c. Productivity monitoring

    d. Financial performance

    e. Modify or update budget, performance targets for staffing effectiveness

A **workforce management** or staffing plan describes the structure and processes by which responsibilities for patient care are assigned and how the work is coordinated among caregivers. In addition, it describes the mechanism for documenting and reporting staffing concerns. This integrated set of processes begins with the patient care delivery model.

The Foundation: Patient Care Delivery Model

Prior to determining how many nurses are needed for patient care, a clearly thought out model or framework for delivering patient care is needed. A **patient care delivery model** is defined as the method or system of organizing and delivering nursing care. It includes the manner in which nursing care is organized in order to deliver the care necessary to meet the needs of the patients. The delivery system encompasses work delegation, resource utilization, communication methodologies, clinical decision-making processes, and management structure (Hall, 2005).

It is important to note that the patient care model emerges from the organizational mission, vision, values, and structure, which include desired outcomes, decision-making authority, and span of control. Thus, the model has a direct and significant impact on the number and levels of nurse caregivers. Patient care delivery models are necessarily dynamic because of the continually changing healthcare environment, needs of the patients, and available technology. The mission, vision, and values remain the stabilizing and focusing forces for the patient care delivery model. Further, the adequacy and effectiveness of the patient care delivery model are essential in supporting a positive practice environment for nurses (Drenkard & Swartwout, 2011).

An effective care delivery system is designed so that the needs of patients are matched to competent caregivers, the caregiver roles are clearly delineated, the quality care provided contributes to the outcomes, and documentation is created to reflect the care provided and outcomes obtained. Specifically, the delivery model is designed to ensure that the right caregiver is with the right patient at the right time and is necessarily linked to the next phase of a workforce management system, a valid and reliable **patient classification system** that is essential in the planning and evaluation of the patient care delivery model. Assumptions from the American Organization of Nurse Executives are included in Figure 5-2.

Numerous patient care delivery models have been implemented with varying levels of success and include functional (work is assigned by tasks), primary (a nurse is assigned as the lead caregiver to plan and coordinate care), team (similar to functional nursing in which a team provides care based on tasks and skills levels and competence), modular (a two-person team providing care to groups of patients), and case management nursing (a nurse coordinates care using clinical pathways and quality criteria) (Sportsman, 2011; Sullivan & Decker, 2009). More recently, interdisciplinary models of care have emerged and include practice partnerships, patient-centered care, and primary care partnerships.

- A systems approach is needed with all disciplines.
- Emerging accountable care organizations will define healthcare reform provisions and impact differing delivery venues.
- Patient safety, experience improvement, and quality outcomes will remain a public, payer, and regulatory focus driving work flow process as demanded by the increasingly informed public.
- Healthcare funding will focus on achieving desired outcomes of improved quality, efficiency, and transparency.
- Interdisciplinary education of health professionals will become the norm, promoting shared knowledge that enables safer patient care and funding for advanced practice nurse (APN) residencies and related clinical education.

Source: American Organization of Nurse Executives (http://www.aone. org/resources/PDFs/AONE_GP_Future_Patient_Care_Delivery_2010.pdf)

Figure 5-2 Patient care delivery assumptions

In each of these models, caregivers are assigned to work from a task perspective, a process or teamwork perspective, and/or an interdisciplinary perspective. Recently, it has become apparent that more considerations are needed for a delivery model to be effective. As the environment for care and clinical work becomes more specialized, a need for additional skills to integrate the specialization or division of labor with the expectations for a continuum of care that integrates all disciplines involved in providing services has been identified. Necessarily, facilitating knowledge work has become an important work process as information generation and communications technology steadily increase and are essential components of a contemporary delivery model. According to Malone, Laubacher, and Johns (2011), there are four areas of focus necessary to get work done in a complex, digital world; how to best divide knowledge work into discrete, assignable tasks; recruitment of specialized workers in terms of their contribution; assurance of work quality; and integration of the work pieces. The situation is similar for healthcare workers—a very complex and dynamic system that requires clear delineation and **assignment** of work based on skills, licensure and competence, recruitment and retention of competent caregivers, assurance of value-based outcomes, and integration of the work of all caregivers into a whole that meets the needs of patients. Indeed, this provides a new lens for the patient care delivery model expectations.

The optimal delivery model for the future is one that is driven by principles and assumptions and ensures coordination of efforts and the achievement of value-based outcomes. How that work is organized and assigned requires a team focus with each caregiver clear as to their work, contributions, and value to the outcome.

Identifying Patient Care Needs

After the patient care delivery model is established, the next step is to identify the needs of the patients being cared for and the required nurse interventions to meet these needs. Time standards and levels of caregivers are then derived from the types of interventions that are performed for patients. The overall goal is to quantify the needs of the patient and family as well as the nurse interventions required to meet the needs. Knowing what the needs and interventions are can then be translated into hours of work for RN, licensed practical nurse (LPN)/licensed vocational nurse (LVN), technician, and certified nursing assistant (CAN) caregivers.

Many healthcare organizations have considered some type of work measurement technique in determining the number and type of staff for patient care units. A variety of approaches are used in health care, including historical usage, staffing grids, legislated staffing ratios, and/or patient classification systems. Many organizations use a combination of approaches. Most of these processes have been manual or at best documented in a spreadsheet. Recent technology advances have resulted in automated systems for calculation and documentation of patient care needs.

The selected technique is then either customized by the facility with a manual or a computerized patient classification system. Some organizations do not use traditional workload measurement systems and rely primarily on ratio or grid staffing. Historically, staffing for patient care has been based on what was actually used for staffing in the previous year rather than from an analysis of current patient care needs and projections from these data. The assumption is that patient care needs remain relatively stable over time. For many organizations, the more staff that were used, the more staff that were budgeted for the next year. These allocations were then used to create a graduated staffing grid identifying how many nurses would be allocated based on the number of patients (Figure 5-3).

Census	RN	Tech	Support	Clerk
24	5	2	2	1
22	5	2	2	1
20	4	2	2	1
18	4	1	2	1
16	4	1	2	1
14	3	1	1	1
10	3	1	0	0.5
8	2	1	0	0.5
< 8	2	1	0	0.5

Figure 5-3 Staffing grid

The underlying assumption of a staffing grid or ratio-based staffing is that all patients are similar in needs. The grid is directly linked to the budgeted staffing. In contrast, legislated staffing ratios identified nurse-to-patient ratios based on experiences and perceptions of nurses and are not directly linked to budgeted staffing. New research is emerging specific to recommended nurse-to-patient ratios. Several advantages and disadvantages of nurse-to-patient ratios are identified in Figure 5-4.

Advantages

- Considers the historical average patient acuity
- Provides incentives for nurses to return to the bedside
- Uses simple to regulate numbers
- Increases nurse satisfaction because nurses traditionally support equal numbers of patients
- Alleviates nurse stress
- Is marginally supported by evidence
- Provides a short-term solution for a complex problem

Disadvantages

- Does not fix the problems in the workplace environment
- Does not consider evidence for effective staffing
- May become maximum staffing levels rather than intended minimum staffing levels
- Does not consider the variation in patient care needs, complexity of care, unit geography, and available equipment
- Does not consider the variations in staff competence and experience
- Assumes that nurses are available to meet the legislated ratios
- Will force closure of some hospitals
- Devalues the role of nurse critical thinking and judgment
- Assumes a manufacturing model is appropriate for patient care
- Shifts staffing accountability from the organization to the government

Figure 5-4 Regulated nurse-to-patient staffing ratios

In addition to recent healthcare reform legislation (Affordable Health Care for America Act), the emphasis has shifted from an event-based model to a continuum accountability model that integrates all settings in which patient care is provided (Day, 2010). Patient care metrics and payment are now based on the provision of integrated care processes and communication across the continuum of care for each patient.

The creation and use of patient classification systems as a tool to improve the clarity and objective identification of patient care needs emerged in the 1960s along with the passage of the **diagnosis-related group (DRG)** payment system.

DRG SYSTEM

The DRG system was developed by a group of researchers at Yale University in the late 1960s as a tool to help clinicians and hospitals monitor quality of care and utilization of services and has been used by Medicare in the United States to pay hospitals.

This system categorizes the types of patients a hospital treats based on diagnoses, procedures, age, sex, and the presence of complications or comorbidities. Briefly, DRGs work by taking more than 10,000 ICD-9-CM codes and grouping them into a more manageable number of meaningful patient categories. Patients within each category are similar clinically in terms of resource usage.

Multiple models for classifying and measuring patient care needs were introduced that included the International Classification of Diseases (ICD), DRG, case mix index, ambulatory payment classification (APC), resource utilization groups (RUGs), Outcome and Assessment Information Set (OASIS), and home health resource groups (HHRGs) (Dunham-Taylor & Pinczuk, 2006; Shi & Singh, 2004). These models identified procedures primarily for billing purposes.

Patient classification systems for nursing care also emerged because the previously mentioned systems did not address a significant portion of nurse work, namely patient education, family support, and interdisciplinary collaboration, that are necessary to support procedural work. Patient care needs are best identified using a framework specific to patient needs that can be translated into nursing work. Nursing Interventions Classification (NIC), Nursing Outcomes Classification (NOC), and North American Nursing Diagnosis Association-International (NANDA-I) are common classifications used to delineate nursing work. Examples of patient care need categories include the following (Malloch & Conovoloff, 1999):

- Cognitive needs: Patient level of consciousness, decision-making capacity
- Self-care needs: Support for activities of daily living—bathing, ambulating, eating, skin care, safety
- Emotional, social, and spiritual needs: Support for stress, anxiety, depression, relationships, and spiritual status
- Pain and comfort needs: Support for varying levels of discomfort from acute to chronic, intractable pain levels

- Family information and support needs: Intentions to assist family and support members with knowledge, information to assist the patient

- Treatments and interventions: Assessments, procedures, medications, fluids, and monitoring through patient care

- Interdisciplinary collaboration needs (includes documentation), patient information needs: Multidisciplinary communication and collaboration among team members to ensure optimal coordination of care

- Transition needs: Support for the transfer of the patient from one level of care to a higher or lower level of care across multiple settings

CRITICAL THOUGHT

Why we need a patient classification system:

- To understand the relationship among patient care needs, interventions, desired outcomes, and the skill level of caregivers as a prerequisite to determine the appropriate type and number of caregivers and support staff needed to provide safe and effective patient care

- To define the amount of staff needed for a particular situation

- To create a valid and reliable system that defines and defends the work of professionals, increases visibility of the role of professional healthcare practice, protects patients from complications, and decreases the vulnerability of professional caregiver staff to budget cuts

These eight categories include the majority of nurse interventions for all clinical patient types, including acute inpatient, intensive care, women's and infants, pediatrics, rehabilitation, behavioral health, and outpatient. The goal of a patient classification system is to provide the most valid and reliable information specific to work that needs to be done for patients. The nature of valid and reliable systems is straightforward; however, it is difficult to achieve in a human work system. A basic understanding of the techniques and challenges in measuring human work is helpful in supporting the processes to achieve the highest degree of validity and reliability.

KEY CONCEPTS

Classification: The ordering of entities into groups or classes on the basis of their similarity, minimizing within-group variance and maximizing between-group variance (Gordon, 1998).

Patient acuity: The level of need or dependency of an individual patient.

Patient classification: A process of grouping patients into homogeneous, mutually exclusive groups to determine their dependency on caregivers or to determine patient acuity (Dunn et al., 1995; Finkler, 2001).

Scheduling: The long-range plan that combines your organization's goals, legislation, regulation, and accreditation requirements and planned patient demand.

Staffing: The real-time adjustment of the schedule based on census, acuity, and the mix of available resources.

Workforce management: The comprehensive system that includes patient classification, scheduling, staffing, and budgeting systems.

Measuring Human Work

Measuring human work, particularly in health care, to determine what is done and how long it takes is a complex process and requires a basic understanding of the techniques available to determine work quantity. There are several techniques to quantify the time associated with tasks performed by workers, and there are at least 25 techniques that assist in the study and measurement of work (Myers & Stewart, 2002). These techniques are used to understand the nature and true cost of work processes and to address the ongoing challenges of reducing costs, effort, and improving the work environment.

Five of the more common techniques often used in health care are provided to better understand the strengths and limitations of each technique as they relate to measuring healthcare work. Motion and time study, work sampling, self-reporting, standard data setting, and expert opinion are each discussed briefly.

The first technique, *motion and time studies*, involves continuous timed observations of a single person during a typical time period or shift of work (Burke et al., 2000). An observer measures primary task occurrences and the length of time to perform the task. Motion study is for cost reduction; time study is for cost control. Motion studies focus on design, whereas time studies focus on measurement.

NURSING WORKFORCE MANAGEMENT SYSTEM: VALIDITY AND RELIABILITY

Validity can be defined as the extent to which a workforce management system measures what it is designed to measure, that is, the ability to quantify and/or predict patient needs for nursing care.

Reliability refers to the extent to which data are reproducible. There are three major types of reliability: stability, homogeneity, and equivalence. The most important for workforce management systems is equivalence or interrater reliability. Equivalence refers to the extent to which different nurses use the same workforce system to measure the same individual, at the same time, to derive consistent results (Alward, 1983; Giovannetti, 1979; Hernandez & O'Brien, 1996a, 1996b).

A motion study is designed to determine the best way to complete a repetitive job. Examples of techniques to study motion include process charts, flow diagrams, multiactivity charts, operation charts, workstation design, motion economy, and predetermined time standards systems. Workload measurement using motion and time studies has been applied to a number of military and industrial problems. Interestingly, while time and motion are often referred to by healthcare professionals, this technique is not often used in health care to identify time standards.

A time study measures the length of time it takes an average worker to complete a task at a normal pace and includes predetermined time standards systems, stopwatch time studies, standard data formula time standards, work sampling time standards, expert opinions, and historical data time standards. In health care, using worked hours per patient day (HPPD) or procedures per year to budget or staff for the next year would be consistent with the standard data set approach. These techniques are problematic for healthcare work in that while many tasks are repeated, such as medication administration, bathing, teaching and so on, each task is unique for the individual patient and the context in which the care is provided.

The second technique, *work sampling*, samples work activities at systematic or random intervals. It involves the process of randomly observing people working to determine how they spend their time. The type and percentage of observations are assumed to represent the typical workload at any given point in time. They do not, however, determine the duration of a particular activity.

In health care, work sampling has been the foundation for some computerized patient classification systems. The caregiver's work is examined for the entire shift or event of care for a selected number of times to achieve a representative range of services. After representative data are collected, the percentage of time spent on specific activities (such as taking and recording vital signs, performing assessments, administering medications, procedures, and discharge planning) is determined. These amounts then create the time standards for determining future **patient acuity** on a daily or shift basis.

Self-reporting is another technique used to determine time associated with activities. Generally, the individual is asked to log the work performed using a data collection tool with start and stop times of each activity recorded. Self-reporting is subjective, but it has been shown to have high face validity (Burke et al., 2000).

Standard data setting, a fourth technique, uses time standards developed from past experiences. It is a common term given to a collection of time values and includes a catalog of basic time standards developed from a database collected over years of motion and time study. It is important to note that these time standards are specific to the individual environment and not readily transferable to another environment without further validation. Standard data are typically the most accurate and least costly to determine for manufacturing settings.

Expert opinion or expert panel is the fifth technique used to determine time standards. A panel of experts or individuals with experience identifies time requirements for certain work. This consensus approach uses professional judgment to determine staff required and provides a flexible approach that focuses on a critical review of nursing practice (Dunn et al., 1995).

Patient care or service work and one-of-a-kind tasks tend to make setting time standards with the more traditional techniques cost prohibitive. Some workers never do the same thing twice, but goals are needed. An expert is needed to estimate every job and to maintain a log of estimates. The best estimation technique is a low-cost, fast, and initially acceptable way of quantifying information using estimation and self-reporting techniques. The expert opinion technique attempts to remedy the criticism of the inability of the work sampling technique to capture professional judgment required in health care (Dunn et al., 1995). Because it can easily become biased and not always reflect current conditions, the expert opinion is reliable only if the results obtained approximate those results generated by experts, and the estimates are valid and reliable.

Many of these techniques are difficult to use in health care where both the worker and the work to be done are highly variable. Health care is very different from the manufacturing assembly line model where the majority of variation lies within the activities of the worker and the machine is stable. The time required to determine specific time standards for the range of patient care profiles and combinations of needs in health care is overwhelming and cost prohibitive to determine using motion, time, and standard data techniques.

Most recently, the expert panel approach has been used to create a comprehensive unit of service as the foundational nursing workload unit of measure for patient care (Malloch & Conovaloff, 1999). Experienced nurses develop workload standards from a comprehensive or shift perspective of the work performed; expert nurses compile the nurse interventions provided to a patient for an entire shift or event; and they identify the time required to provide this care as a unit rather than as a summation of individual tasks. This approach is useful because it integrates the multitasking nature of caregiver work and caregiver interruptions and minimizes the risk of double counting tasks. Typically, an expert panel consists of nurses who practice in clinical, educational, research, and administrative roles, such as experienced staff nurses, clinical nurse specialists, nurse managers, and associate nurse executives. The expert panel then collaborates using a specific nursing intervention framework to estimate the amount of time and level of caregiver required to provide the total care in the comprehensive unit of service.

Patient Classification Systems: Limitations and Challenges

In addition to the challenges of measuring human work, patient classification systems are limited for other reasons. Skepticism about patient classification systems has existed since their introduction. With the variety of patient classification systems available and the years of testing new and innovative ways of capturing time estimation, the nursing profession still struggles with the lack of credible workforce management system.

Five common reasons for the current mistrust of a patient classification system include low validity, misuse of the tool, difficulty in projecting future staff needs, failure to use the data generated, and lack of tool simplicity. Each is discussed briefly.

Low Validity

Failing to account for the full scope of nursing practice, specifically the relational work of nursing, is common in task-based patient classification systems. The absence of the relational work of professional nursing care practices, such as patient education, interdisciplinary collaboration, family support, and delegation and supervision of other caregivers, decreases the validity of the system. Because much of nursing is mind work rather than hand work, it is not surprising that the task-based methods of some systems are quickly manipulated and declared invalid.

At present, there is no single agreed-on patient classification system that adequately represents the full range of nursing interventions. Because there is no agreed-on system, there are few, if any, empirical data sets to describe nursing practice across clinical settings and client populations. The lack of standardized clinical language that makes it difficult to know with any degree of accuracy which type of patient classification system provides the most valid and reliable data for workload management decisions further marginalizes system validity.

One solution for improving the validity and reliability of caregiver work measurement is the attachment of time and skill mix standards to clinical interventions in an electronic documentation system. With documentation driving the calculations for patient needs, the issues of reliability would be decreased significantly.

Misuse of the Tool

The lack of trust between administration and caregivers stems in part from the belief that patient classification systems are a vehicle to increase or decrease staffing levels inappropriately. This lack of trust has serious implications for the ability of hospitals and other healthcare organizations to make the fundamental changes essential to providing safer patient care (Page, 2004). Coupled with low validity, poor reputation, and expectations for the patient classification to do more than identify patient care needs, trust in general is minimal in many organizations. The phenomenon of acuity creep, identified by Shaha (1995), is present when the reported patient acuity increases slowly over time but the actual care does not change. In other words, acuity levels creep to higher and higher levels to justify higher resources use. Creep becomes a problem because it assumes there is an ever-increasing need for patient care resources and labor in an industry where financial resources continue to decrease (Shaha, 1995). Further, the use of a system with low validity makes it difficult to distinguish inappropriate acuity creep from real changes in patient care. Thus the validity and reliability of the patient classification used by an organization is a critical attribute for effective use of resources.

Difficulty in Projecting Future Staff Needs

Projecting patient care needs for the next shift or time period is highly desirable in ensuring staffing adequacy. However, the amount of staff and skill mix has been nearly impossible to determine without an acceptable error range without using a computerized solution. Computerized applications are becoming increasingly useful in assessing current nursing work and projecting from a point in time; however, regardless of the sophistication and accuracy of the calculations of current work, it is still nearly impossible to accurately predict patient condition changes, new admissions, and discharges. Experts continue to work on complex mathematical forecasting models to project patient activities and associated caregiver support into the future. Fitzpatrick and Brooks (2010) analyzed the challenges of predicting patient volumes, needs, and resources and identified the role of clinical leader as logistician. This approach integrates the science of logistics management, including systems theory, mathematical optimization modeling, and human capital planning, and results in significant improvement in outcomes. The value of reconceptualizing the planning and deployment of staff as a logistics problem becomes evident as the staff preferences are maximized, coverage is adequate, skill mix is appropriate, regulations are met, and staffing costs are minimized. Indeed this approach presents opportunities for all staffing offices.

Patient classification system data are useful for both retrospective information of what actually occurred and for projection for next shift staffing. Attempts have been made to classify patients based on the care provided for the current shift or based on what the current caregiver believes the care needs will be for the next shift. Planning for the next shift requires not only information about the patient needs, but also information about the oncoming staff competencies; the previous similar shift staffing (yesterday's afternoon shift compared to the upcoming afternoon shift); facility support for housekeeping, pharmacy, transportation, and teaching staff; and anticipated admissions, discharges, and transfers.

The severity of patient illness, need for specialized equipment and technology, intensity of nursing interventions required, and complexity of clinical nursing judgment needed to design, implement, and evaluate the patient's nursing plan are often not predictable. However, when nurse interventions are reframed to patient care needs, the degree of accuracy increases with clear descriptions of the patient needs.

It is important to note that despite the name implying a measurement of severity of illness or patient acuity, patient classification is in truth more concerned with determining the time required for care; the patient acuity level is secondary information. There is indeed some correlation between acuity and amount of care required, but the correlation is not absolute. A chronic ventilator-dependent paraplegic may score high in severity of illness but not require a large number of care hours because of condition stability and established plans of care.

Failure to Use the Data Generated

Too often the data generated from a patient classification system is not used in staffing allocation, particularly if the projections call for more staff hours. The lack of trust in the process and data generated is often not addressed, and the generated projections are disregarded in favor of the grid or ratio allocations. Unfortunately, if there is a real and valid need for additional staff hours, the need is disregarded by both nurses and support leaders. The basic trustworthiness of the system is questioned by nonnursing hospital leaders, and the system is merely tolerated or ignored.

Lack of Tool Simplicity

To address the credibility gap, and in the expectation of increasing validity, clinical experts worked to develop all-inclusive, objective lists of interventions to create a more valid system. Some systems require the user to review and select from 100 or more items for each patient. Classification systems that try to list every possible intervention become overwhelming, time consuming, and quickly abandoned. Systems that are easily misused, mismanaged, or generate inaccurate data cannot be used by managers to defend their staffing decisions.

CRITICAL THOUGHT

The imposition of mandatory hospital nurse staffing ratios is among the more visible public policy initiatives affecting the nursing profession. Although the practice is intended to address problems in hospital nurse staffing and quality of patient care, it can be argued that staffing ratios will lead to negative consequences for nurses involving the equity, efficiency, and costs of producing nursing care in hospitals (Buerhaus, 2009).

Whenever possible, direct care or interventions specific to patient care that can be directly attributed to the patient, as well as supportive daily planning and documentation, should be included in the patient classification system. Patient care work should include work that is directly attributed to the patient, whether it is at the bedside, in family conferences, or in shift reports supporting the planning process. After patient needs are determined and validated, the department director can then determine the core staffing hours and skill levels necessary to meet patient care needs. The next step in workforce management is creating the core schedule.

Core Schedule

Core schedules represent an aggregated average number and skill mix required for patient care. A core schedule template for each unit includes caregivers, shift length, and calendar days. Based on the identified historical patient care needs for the unit, patient projection volume is used to create the core schedule. The following considerations are important in constructing the basic core schedule: anticipated patient needs volume, caregiver categories, shift length, licensure requirements, experience, education, regulatory minimum level requirements, contextual factors, and available research evidence for staffing effectiveness.

Considerations in Creating the Core Schedule

Projected volume is obtained from historical trend data and budget projections and can be categorized by season, day of the week, and time or hour of the day. Adjustments for fluctuations in patient care volumes resulting from vacations, seasonal variations, and time of day can be forecasted and modeled similar to the work done by Hollabaugh and Kendrick (1998). A five-level pyramid that identified five differing levels of activities and seasons, a hiring plan by varying by census, a more equitable cancellation policy, and active staff involvement resulted in increased continuity of care, increased job satisfaction, fewer patient and physician complaints, and cost savings.

Caregiver Categories

Caregiver categories include advanced practice nurse providers, direct care workers or knowledge workers, preceptors, technical staff, support staff, and clerical staff. Roles can also include a person who is in charge or serves as a resource person during a shift. This person provides leadership, makes assignments, and deals with unusual incidents or difficult situations. This person supports the leadership on issues as they occur during a shift or for a specified length of time.

Staff categorization is often identified as direct, administrative, or indirect. These concepts are defined in each organization and categorize direct patient care hours, unit support hours, or hours away from the unit, such as education, vacation, or sick hours, for cost analysis and payment purposes. The core schedule focuses on identifying those caregivers available to provide care for a specified time period.

Nursing Staff Skill Mix

The skill mix, or numbers of licensed and nonlicensed staff, is determined based on the work that needs to be done, specifically the patient care needs. The specific interventions that are needed by patients are categorized based on which level of caregiver can meet the needs, such as RNs being required for work authorized by the state nurse practice act and the organization, and so on. One anecdotal advantage noted with high RN levels is that less time was needed to communicate with less skilled workers. Determining the ideal skill mix is challenging in light of the multifaceted nature of patients and caregivers.

Advanced Practice Nurse Providers and Clinical Experts

In some delivery models, a nurse practitioner or hospitalist is a member of the team. These providers write orders and provide general patient care oversight. Other practice experts include clinical nurse specialists, clinical nurse leaders, and nurse educators. These nurses provide care and assist staff in the care of more complex patients using the latest evidence in a cost-effective approach.

Direct Caregivers or Knowledge Workers: Registered Nurses

The work of the RN will continue to be the foundational and primary role in the healthcare system. Optimizing the role of the RN requires continually advancing the role to that of knowledge worker at the point of care. An overview of the practice of nursing from a national perspective is provided in the accompanying box.

In addition to the practice of nursing from a national perspective, information specific to the evolving role of the RN as knowledge worker is identified in the accompanying box. Understanding and integrating these values and behaviors into the practice of nursing serve to encourage and support the full scope of RN practice.

THE PRACTICE OF NURSING: NCSBN MODEL PRACTICE ACT

Nursing is a scientific process founded on a professional body of knowledge; it is a learned profession based on an understanding of the human condition across the lifespan and the relationship of a client with others and within the environment; and it is an art dedicated to caring for others. The practice of nursing means assisting clients to attain or maintain optimal health, implementing a strategy of care to accomplish defined goals within the context of a client centered health care plan and evaluating responses to nursing care and treatment. Nursing is a dynamic discipline that increasingly involves more sophisticated knowledge, technologies and client care activities.

Practice as an RN means the full scope of nursing, with or without compensation or personal profit, that incorporates caring for all clients in all settings, is guided by the scope of practice authorized in this section, through nursing standards established or recognized by the BON and includes, but is not limited to:

- Providing comprehensive nursing assessment of the health status of clients.

- Comprehensive nursing assessment is an extensive data collection (initial and ongoing) used for individuals, families, groups and communities in addressing anticipated changes in client conditions as well as emergent changes in a client's health status; recognizing alterations to previous client conditions; synthesizing the biological, psychological, spiritual and social aspects of the client's condition; evaluating the impact of nursing care; and using this broad and complete analysis to make independent decisions and nursing diagnoses, plan nursing interventions, evaluate the need for different interventions, and assess the need to communicate and consult with other health team members.

- Collaborating with health care team to develop an integrated client-centered health care plan.

- Developing a strategy of nursing care to be integrated within the client-centered health care plan that establishes nursing diagnoses; sets goals to meet identified health care needs; prescribes nursing interventions; and implements nursing care through the execution of independent nursing strategies and regimens requested, ordered or prescribed by authorized health care providers.
- Delegating and assigning nursing interventions to implement the plan of care.
- Providing for the maintenance of safe and effective nursing care rendered directly or indirectly.
- Promoting a safe and therapeutic environment.
- Advocating the best interest of clients.
- Evaluating responses to interventions and the effectiveness of the plan of care.
- Communicating and collaborating with other health care providers in the management of health care and the implementation of the total health care regimen within and across care settings.
- Acquiring and applying critical new knowledge and technologies to the practice domain.
- Managing, supervising and evaluating the practice of nursing.
- Teaching the theory and practice of nursing.
- Participating in development of policies, procedures and systems to support the client.

Source: Courtesy of the National Council of State Boards of Nursing.

LPN/LVN

The LPN/VN continues to be an important role in care delivery; however, the role is more commonly used in more stable environments such as long-term care than in acute care settings. The challenges of delegation and communication between the RN and the LPN have been particularly challenging for new nurses. The LPN/LVN role is beneficial in highly functioning teams where the scope of practice of each role is clearly understood.

THE KNOWLEDGE WORKER

The contemporary clinical knowledge worker focuses on a new level of accountability for moving forward to informed, evidence-based decisions. No longer does the clinical knowledge worker rely on past practices, individual experiences, and tradition. The work of the knowledge worker emphasizes conceptual synthesis of knowledge and experiences for practice. Reliance is on principles and values rather than on processing policies and procedures. The focus is on the product (not the processes) of work and the value produced. Responsibility is about how well the work is done and is based on knowledge, evidence, competence, and efficiency. It is about doing the work well and doing it right. Knowledge workers own the tools and capacities necessary to do patient care work and the responsibility *and* accountability for this work. Knowledge workers cannot transfer the locus of control for their patient care work accountability to institutions, organizations, or supervisors.

Unlicensed Assistive Personnel (UAP)

UAP assist the RN with carrying out professional activities. Healthcare organizations use these workers in a variety of roles, some that are more focused on supporting the patient care environment rather than the patients themselves. The goal in using assistive personnel is to provide the highest quality patient care at the lowest cost. Thus, if support personnel can safely provide certain aspects of patient care under the supervision of an RN, then integration of these roles into the team is the prudent approach.

UAPs have been used in a variety of roles, in addition to the traditional primary support functions at the bedside; some perform simple housekeeping or secretarial tasks, and others perform higher level clinical or technical tasks, such as electrocardiograms and phlebotomy. Because there is no one accrediting body common to all types of UAPs and because state laws vary regarding their use, hospitals have been relatively free to experiment with different care models under the guidance of their internal nursing leadership (McClung, 2000).

Shift Length

The variations in shift length are much easier to manage with the availability of computerized scheduling and mathematical calculation of the impact of ranges from 2-hour shifts to 12-hours shifts. The selection of traditional 8-hour or 12-hour shifts must necessarily be done within the context of the type of patient care provided, specifically care for a short time interval or a longer interval. Continuity of care and consistency in caregivers in settings where care is provided for several hours or less can accommodate more flexible shift time lengths. The hand-off process and change of shift is less complicated with short-interval patient care. In areas where care is provided over several days, the challenges of care continuity and hand-offs increase in complexity because of the nature of the patient illness. Regardless of the shift length, the selection is best made first on the patient care needs and second on the preferences of the caregivers.

Licensure Requirements

Each state jurisdiction maintains a nurse practice act that identifies the duties and responsibilities of the RN. While similar in most respects, there are differences that the nurse must be aware of when moving to new practice settings. In general, the Model Practice Act clearly identifies the expectations of the role and practice of nursing.

Education

The significance of educational preparation and continuing development is documented in several of the research studies noted in Appendix A of this chapter. The importance of at least a baccalaureate degree in nursing is recognized as required entry-level competence for contemporary patient care situations.

Goode and colleagues (2001) described the BSN RN as having greater critical thinking skills, less task orientation, more professionalism, stronger leadership skills, more focus on continuity of care and outcomes, greater focus on psychosocial components, better communication skills, and greater focus on patient teaching.

Experience/Competence

In creating a core schedule, a balance of experienced and less experienced or learning nurses is desirable. A mixture is necessary to support the highest quality care and provide opportunities for new nurses to learn complex patient care processes. Mentoring new nurses is a critical role of the professional nurse.

Regulatory Minimum Requirements

In several cases, minimum staffing levels are defined by state, national, and professional agencies. The minimum number of staff that are needed to ensure safety and caregiver vigilance apply to most patient care units and in particular those areas where unstable patient conditions are the norm. The core schedule identifies the minimum regulatory requirements. In addition, regulations specific to overtime must also be honored. Given that regulations change regularly at the state level, it is important for nurses to be aware of both state and national requirements.

Contextual Factors

Staffing effectiveness is influenced by an extensive list of contextual factors, such as facility leadership, nurse–physician relationships, available technology and supplies, and numbers of external nursing staff. In addition, Berkow and colleagues (2007) have identified wide fluctuations in patient volume, percentages of protocol-driven care, geographic locations, and teaching status of the facility as significant influences in workforce staffing.

Staffing Effectiveness Research

Significant research is emerging in which the role of the RN is correlated to patient outcomes and cost. Appendix A of this chapter includes a summary of selected research evidence specific to RN levels and hours of work per day and per week. In general, the outcomes research in selected studies indicates that a higher RN number results in lower length of stay, fewer complications, lower mortality, lower costs, increased nurse satisfaction, and increased patient satisfaction. While there is increasing evidence supporting a positive relationship and impact of the role of the nurse on patient outcomes, the results are not generalizable nationally. Also, while specific numbers of nurse-to-patient ratios are identified, this number is also not generalizable across the country. Numerous other variables need to be considered to achieve an optimal nurse assignment.

Daily Staffing Process

Matching patient care needs to scheduled core staff on the day in which care is to be provided is the next step. The amount of patient care staff, skill mix, and necessary support staff needed to assist in providing the care is compared to the identified patient needs. Daily staffing is driven by informed decision makers who consider multiple factors (Douglas & Kerfoot, 2011).

Optimized staffing processes are achieved from approaches that are centralized, decentralized, or a combination of both. Most recently, a combination or hybrid staffing model is preferred to support unit involvement and decision making and central records management. A hybrid model also allows for consideration to both the unit and organizational needs. Situations of over- and understaffing are addressed to ensure a balanced staffing plan that meets patient needs, minimizes premium labor costs, and supports staff satisfaction (Crist-Grundman & Mulrooney, 2011).

AMERICAN NURSES ASSOCIATION PRINCIPLES FOR NURSE STAFFING

The American Nurses Association (ANA) supports regular and evidence-driven dialogue about staffing effectiveness. In particular, ANA emphasizes the importance of recognizing the complexity of effective nurse staffing and the solution is not simple. In addition, several considerations are also recommended:

- The needs of the patient drive staffing allocations.
- In addition to patient needs, the skills of the nurse and the influences of the environment must also be considered.
- Registered nurse input into the staffing processes is always necessary.
- Interprofessional and ancillary support is necessary to optimize patient care outcomes.
- A culture of safety is reinforced.
- Evaluation of staffing effectiveness is logical and includes multiple variables impacting staffing.

Source: Adapted from American Nurses Association. (2011). Principles for nurse staffing (draft). http://www.nursingworld.org/DocumentVault/CNPE/Draft-Principles-for-Nurse-Staffing.aspx

Variance management is an essential component of daily staffing. One of the most often missed processes in workload management is the identification of and management of the variance between needed staff and actual staff hours. Figure 5-5 presents an example of essential data for variance analysis. Managing the difference between actual hours of staff and required hours of care requires analysis of individual caregiver variances as well as total variance hours. The figure includes a variance analysis data form that displays the actual hours, required hours, and variances. Once a significant variance is determined, variance actions are considered, implemented, and documented. These data provide valuable trend information for nurse leaders as they continually work to create effective workload management systems.

CRITICAL THOUGHT

Expecting caregivers to "do one's best" in an impossible situation continues to fuel the flames of caregiver dissatisfaction and ultimately leads to premature exit from the workforce.

Addressing variances is a routine activity of nurse leaders that requires an examination of the required staff needed for care and the actual staff. What is not routine is the systematic documentation of the difference between required and actual hours and the interventions to address and mediate the variance or gap. Both positive and negative variances need to be addressed and documented.

WILLING TO WALK: A NEW APPROACH TO FLOATING

To address the challenges of nurse floating, the team at Aultman Hospital created a "Willing to Walk" program to minimize stress and create a positive experience for both the receiving unit and the nurse who is floating or *willing to walk*.

The Aultman program is proactive in that nurses are asked to sign up for the program to be considered for floating to selected areas within their realm of competence. Nurses meet the requirements for each of the units they agree to work. In addition, nurses are asked each time there is a need for floating. The program has resulted in increased autonomy, satisfaction, and lower turnover rates over a 7-year period (Good & Bishop, 2011).

Examples of both short-term and long-term interventions to address the variance or gap between needs and actual staffing include the following:

- Reevaluating patient acuity ratings
- Postponing admissions
- Calling additional staff
- Postponing nonemergent patient care
- Floating existing staff to the unit in need

- Sending staff home early
- Eliminating non-value-added work

The challenge of managing increasing workloads requires new strategies beyond working faster (Storfjell, Ohlson, Omoike, Fitzpatrick, & Wetasin, 2009). Rather than changing the speed of work, examining work to determine what work is not adding value to the outcome and eliminating this work becomes a more realistic option and strategy to manage the variance between required work and available staff. Wasteful, non-value-added work is often subtle and difficult to identity. Decreasing the waste in required work becomes a potential pathway to increased productivity and quality care.

Evaluation of Workforce Management

Evaluation of staffing, scheduling, and patient classification systems considers the infrastructure, the processes, and the outcomes of the integrated workload management system. Assessment of these three areas includes evaluation of the presence of factors identified within each area.

Infrastructure for Excellence Assessment

1. There is a clearly defined patient care delivery system that includes support for nursing participation in decision making at the point of service, expectation for professionalism, and shared decision making.

2. A valid and reliable system to determine patient care needs drives the staffing process. Specific consideration is given to the following:

   - Number of patients
   - Acuity of patients
   - Length of stay/intensity factor
   - Unit geography
   - Skills and experience of caregivers
   - Appropriate skill mix

3. Scheduling and staffing systems are developed collaboratively by leaders, managers, and direct caregivers/knowledge workers.

4. Consideration for unit functions that support the delivery of patient care is included in staffing hours (indirect time).

5. Staff clinical competencies are identified for differing patient populations.

6. Expert resources are available to support less-experienced staff.

Process Excellence Assessment

1. Collaborative scheduling is the norm. Historical trend data, patient care needs, and staff preferences (in that order) serve as the basis for scheduling. Patient care needs are always the first priority.

2. Mandatory overtime is not used.

3. The fatigue factor is recognized; long stretches of 12-hour shifts are not considered safe practice. Nurses do not work more than three 12-hour shifts in a row.

4. Leaders and staff work together to manage variances (staff shortages) between available staff and patient care needs.

5. Experienced clinical experts are available to assist less-experienced staff in organizing and providing patient care.

Evaluation Excellence Assessment

1. Multiple indicators are used to evaluate staffing effectiveness. Indicators include patient outcomes, staff satisfaction, and organizational cost. Performance indicators do not focus solely on hours per patient day (HPPD).

2. The analysis includes individual patient care as well as aggregate analysis. Ranges as well as averages are evaluated.

3. The analysis includes both census averages and outliers (ranges).

4. Indicators that are sensitive to nursing scheduling and staffing are examined at least monthly. These include but are not limited to the following:

    - Patient satisfaction with response to call lights

    - Patient increased knowledge of clinical condition

    - Patient/family's increased ability to manage their own care

    - Absence of adverse outcomes (e.g., dermal ulcers, nosocomial pneumonia, patient falls, and medication errors)

Leading Versus Managing in Staffing and Scheduling: Concluding Thoughts

The complexity and dynamics of nurse scheduling cannot be understated. The initial work of the nurse is to understand the components of this complex system and process. The next step is for the professional RN to analyze and interpret the effectiveness of the workforce plan specific to his or her ability to provide patient care effectively. Immediate feedback to address quality concerns with proactive recommendations is critical for system success and effectiveness. Managing and adjusting current situations with a strong rationale necessarily supports improvement of patient care and the system. To be sure, it is simple to identify what is not working. It is professional and courageous to figure out what needs to be done for improvement and to build a case that is so powerful that everyone agrees with the recommendations for more effective staffing.

CHAPTER TEST QUESTIONS

www

1. Staffing adequacy (a) is determined by multiple factors including nurse competence and patient care needs, (b) does not vary by shift, (c) can be assured with good planning of nurses work schedules, or (d) requires experienced nurses and supportive managers.

2. Equitable nurse patient assignments (a) require experienced nurses to create nurse assignments, (b) are positively related to nurse satisfaction, (c) are nearly impossible in complex patient care settings, or (d) are typically limited to core staff.

3. Core schedules (a) are based on budgeted hours, (b) should be adjusted at least quarterly, (c) are based on trended patient care needs over time, or (d) are inconsistent with ratio staffing models.

4. Ratio staffing (a) is strongly correlated to positive patient outcomes, (b) is strongly correlated to nursing satisfaction, (c) requires specific state legislation to implement, or (d) does not consider the variations in patient care needs.

5. Non-value added work (a) will continue due to patient expectations, (b) should be identified and eliminated whenever possible, (c) can be identified easily during unit focus groups, or (d) is not an area of significant concern for nurses.

6. Measuring staffing adequacy (a) requires knowledge of recent research evidence, (b) is essential for Medicare certification, (c) is a quarterly evaluation of evidence for nurse staffing, physician availability and reimbursement, or (d) is an ongoing evaluation of matching patient care needs with appropriate nurse staffing and outcomes achieved.

7. Evidence for staffing specific to nurse fatigue (a) is unique for each team of nurses on a particular unit, (b) is inconclusive for healthcare workers, (c) identifies work practices that can be performed safely, or (d) includes information specific to shift

hours worked, weekly hours worked, and number of days worked in a row.

8. Reliability of patient classification systems (a) requires the use of a standardized nursing language, (b) is high when the ratings by system users are identical, (c) requires use of the system for at least 12 months, or (d) does not exist if the inter-rater reliability is below 85%.

9. Validity of patient classification systems (a) is about the accuracy of the system to measure the work of patient care, (b) requires a minimum amount of clinical intervention categories, (c) does not change over time, or (d) is only essential when the data is used for patient billing.

10. Patient care delivery models (a) are most commonly based on the team model, (b) are best used in academic medical centers, (c) are required for Medicare reimbursement, or (d) form the foundation for workforce management goals.

References

Alward, R. (1983). Patient classification systems: The ideal vs. reality. *Journal of Nursing Administration, 13*(2), 14-18.

Berkow, S., Jaggi, T., Fogelson, R., Katz, S., & Hirschoff, A. (2007). Fourteen unit attributes to guide staffing. *Journal of Nursing Administration, 37*(3), 150–155.

Buerhaus, P. I. (2009). Avoiding mandatory hospital nurse staffing ratios: An economic commentary. *Nursing Outlook, 57*, 107–112.

Burke, T., McKee, J., Wilson, H., Donahue, R. M., Batenhorst, A., & Pathak, D. (2000). A comparison of time-and-motion and self reporting methods of work measurement. *Journal of Nursing Administration, 30*(3), 118–125.

Crist-Grundman, D., & Mulrooney, G. (2011). Effective workforce management starts with leveraging technology while staffing optimization requires true collaboration. *Nursing Economic$, 29*(4), 195–200.

Day, J. (2010). Affordable Care Act (ACA) summary and updates. Published May 28, 2010. Retreived from http://www.wid.org/affordable-care-act-aca-summary-and-updates

Douglas, K., & Kerfoot, K. M. (2011). Forging the future of staffing based on evidence. *Nursing Economics$, 29*(4), 161, 167.

Drenkard, K., & Swartwout, E. (2011). A commitment to optimal practice environments. *Journal of Nursing Administration, 41*(7/8), 52–53.

Dunham-Taylor, J., & Pinczuk, J. (2006). *Health care financial management for nurse managers: Applications from hospitals, long-term care, home care, and ambulatory care*. Sudbury, MA: Jones and Bartlett.

Dunn, M., Norby, R., Cournoyer, P., Hudec, S., O'Donnell, J., & Snider, M. (1995). Expert panel method for nurse staffing and resource management. *Journal of Nursing Administration, 25*(10), 61–67.

Finkler, S. (2001). Budgeting concepts for nurse managers. (3rd ed.). Philadelphia: Saunders.

Fitzpatrick, T. A., & Brooks, B. A. (2010). The nurse leader as logistician: Optimizing human capital. *Journal of Nursing Administration, 40*(2), 69–74.

Giovanetti, P. (1979). Understanding patient classification systems. *Journal of Nursing Administration, 9*(2), 4–9.

Good, E., & Bishop, P. (2011). Willing to walk: A creative strategy to minimize stress related to floating. *Journal of Nursing Administration, 41*(5), 231–234.

Goode, C., Pinderton, S., McCausland, M., Southard, P., Graham, R., & Krsek, C. (2001). Documenting chief nursing officers' preference for BSN-prepared nurses. *Journal of Nursing Administration, 31*(2), 55–59.

Gordon, M. (2001). Nursing nomenclature and classification system development. Online Journal of Issues in Nursing. Retrieved from www.nursingworld.org/ojin/tpc77_1.htm

Hall, L. M. (2005). Quality work environments for nurse and patient safety. Sudbury, MA: Jones and Bartlett.

Hernandez, C., & O'Brien, P. (1996a). Validity and reliability of nursing workload measurement systems: Review of validity and reliability theory. Part 1. *Canadian Journal of Nursing Administration, 9*(3), 16–25.

Hernandez, C., & O'Brien, P. (1996b). Validity and reliability of nursing workload measurement systems: Review of validity and reliability theory. Part 2. *Canadian Journal of Nursing Administration, 10*(3), 16–23.

Hollabaugh, S., & Kendrick, S. (1998). Staffing: The five-level pyramid. *Nursing Management, 29*(2), 34–36.

Malloch, K., & Conovaloff, A. (1999). Patient classification systems, Part 1: The third generation. *Journal of Nursing Administration, 29*(7), 49–56.

Malone, T. W., Laubacher, R. J., & Johns, T. (2011). The age of hyper-specialization. *Harvard Business Review*. July/August, *89*(7), 56–65.

McClung, T. (2000). Assessing the reported financial benefits of unlicensed assistive personnel in nursing. *Journal of Nursing Administration, 30*(11), 530–534.

Myers, F., & Stewart, J. (2002). *Motion and time study for lean manufacturing* (3rd ed.). Upper Saddle River, NJ: Prentice Hall.

Page, A. (2004). *Keeping patients safe: Transforming the work environment of nurses.* Quality Chasm series. Washington, DC: National Academy Press.

Shaha, S. (1995). Acuity systems and control charting. *Quality Management in Health Care, 3*(3), 22–30.

Shi, L., & Singh, D. (2004). *Delivering health care in America: A systems approach* (3rd ed.). Boston, MA: Jones and Bartlett.

Sportsman, S. (2011). In P. S. Yoder-Wise (Ed.), *Leading and managing in nursing* (5th ed.) St. Louis, MO: Elsevier Mosby.

Storfjell, J. L., Ohlson, S., Omoike, O., Fitzpatrick, T., & Wetasin, K. (2009). Non-value-added time: The million dollar nursing opportunity. *Journal of Nursing Administration, 39*(1), 38–45.

Sullivan, E. J., & Decker, P. J. (2009). *Effective leadership and management in nursing.* Upper Saddle River, NJ: Pearson Prentice Hall.

Appendix A

Selected Staffing Effectiveness Research Evidence

Significant progress is being made in identifying the relationship between the role of the nurse and patient, provider, organization, and cost outcomes. This appendix lists the specific areas of impact and supporting references. The increasingly broad range of evidence provides support for effective staffing plans and adjustments to daily staffing assignments. Specific relationships between patient outcomes, nurse characteristics, and nurse schedules are illustrated. Reference numbers are listed with the identified variables.

Patient outcomes:

- Patient mortality/failure to rescue: Pneumonia, postoperative DVT/ pulmonary embolism: 1, 2, 3, 7, 8, 9, 13, 15, 16

- Patient adverse outcomes: Pneumonia, postoperative infections, urinary tract infections, acute myocardial infarction, congestive heart failure, patient falls, medication errors, pressure ulcers: 2, 10, 13, 14, 15, 16

- Smoking cessation counseling rates: 12

- Pneumococcal vaccinations rates: 12

- Length of stay: 7, 17

- Patient satisfaction: 6, 14

- Patient experience of care: 14

- Physician satisfaction: 14

- Readmission: 8

- Cost of care: 8, 17

Nurse characteristics:

- Clinical nurse leader role: 4, 14

- Education level: 2, 3

- Percentage of RN staffing: 1, 7, 10, 13

- Experience at the shift level: 10

- Shift hours: 3, 8, 9, 10, 11

- Number of days worked in row: 13, 15

- Number of hours worked in a week: 13, 15

- Unit admission, discharge, and transfer activity: 9
- Nurse turnover: 14
- Nurse fatigue and sleep cycles: 12

Environment of care:

- Foundations for quality of care: 3, 5
- Nurse manager ability, leadership, and support: 3, 5
- Collegial nurse/physician relationships: 3, 5

References

1. Aiken, L. H., Clark, S. P., Sloan, D. M., Sochalski, J., & Silber, J. H. (2002). Hospital nurse staffing and patient mortality, nurse burnout, and job dissatisfaction. *Journal of the American Medical Association, 288*(16), 1987–1993.
2. Aiken, L., Clarke, S., Cheung, R., Sloane, D., & Silber, J. (2003). Educational levels of hospital nurses and surgical patient mortality. *Journal of the American Medical Association, 290*, 1617–1623.
3. Aiken, L. H., Clarke, S. P., Sloane, D., Lake, E. T., & Cheney, T. (2008). Effects of hospital care environment on patient mortality and nurse outcomes. *Journal of Nursing Administration, 38*(5), 223–229.
4. Alward, R. (1983). Patient classification systems: The ideal vs. reality. *Journal of Nursing Administration, 13*(2), 14–26.
5. Finkler, S. A. (2001). Measuring the costs of quality. In A. Kovner & D. Neuhauser (Eds.), Health services management readings and commentary (7th ed., pp. 114–121). Chicago, IL: AUPHA Press/Health Administration Press.
6. Gabuat, J., Hilton, N., Kinnaird, L. S., & Sherman, R. O. (2008). Implementing the clinical nurse leader role in a for-profit environment. *Journal of Nursing Administration, 38*(6), 302–307.
7. Gordon, M. (1998). Nursing Nomenclature and Classification System Development. *Online Journal of Issues in Nursing, 3*(2), 1, Available at www.nursingworld.org/MainMenuCategories/ANAMarketplace/ANAPeriodicals/OJIN/TableofContents/Vol31998/No2Sept1998/NomenclatureandClassification.aspx
8. Institute of Medicine. (2004). *Keeping patients safe: Transforming the work environment of nurses.* Washington, DC: National Academies Press.
9. Kutney-Lee, A., McHugh, M. D., Sloane, D. M., Cimiotti, J. P., Flynn, L., Felber Neff, D., & Aiken, L. H. (2009). Nursing: A key to patient satisfaction. *Health Affairs, 28*(4), 669–677.
10. Kane, R. L., Shamilyan, T., Mueller, C., Duval, S., & Wilt, T. J. (2007). *Nurse staffing and quality of patient care* (Publication 07-E005). Agency for Healthcare Research and Quality.
11. Kohlbrenner, J., Whitelaw, G., & Cannaday, D. (2011). Nurses critical to quality, safety and now financial performance. *Journal of Nursing Administration, 41*(3), 122–128.

12. Needleman, J., Buerhaus, P., Pankratz, V. S., Leibson, C. L., Stevens, S. R., & Harris, M. (2011). Nurse staffing and inpatient hospital mortality. *New England Journal of Medicine, 364*(11), 1037–1045.

13. Patrician, P., Loan, L., McCarthy, M., Fridman, M., Donaldson, N., Bingham, M., & Brosch, L. The association of shift-level nurse staffing with adverse patient events. *Journal of Nursing Administration, 41*(2), 64–70.

14. Rogers, A. E., Hwany, W., Scott, L. D., Aiken, L. H., & Dinges, D. F. (2004). The working hours of hospital staff nurses and patient safety. *Health Affairs, 23*(4), 202–212.

15. Shaha, S. H. (2010, June). Nursing makes a significant difference: A multihospital correlational study. *Nurse Leader*, 36–39.

16. Sochalski, J. (2004). Is more better? The relationship between hospital staffing and the quality of nursing care in hospitals. *Medical Care, 42*(Suppl. 2), 1167–1173.

17. Stanley, J. M., Gannon, J., Gabuat, J., Hartsranfi, S., Adams, N., Mayes, C., . . . Burch, D. (2008). The clinical nurse leader: A catalyst for improving quality and patient safety. *Journal of Nursing Management, 16*(5), 614–622.

18. Trinkoff, A. M., Johantgen, M., Storr, C., Gurses, A. P., Liang, V., & Han, K. (2011). Nurses work schedule characteristics, nurse staffing and patient mortality. *Nursing Research, 60*(1), 1–8.

19. Trinkoff, A. M., Johantgen, M., Storr, C., Gurses, A. P., Liang, V., & Han, K. (2011). Linking nursing work environment and patient outcomes. *Journal of Nursing Regulation, 2*(1), 10–16.

20. Unruh, L. (2003). Licensed nurse staffing and adverse events in hospitals. *Medical Care, 41*(1), 142–152.

Appendix B

Case Study: The Flaw of Averages

The flaw of this averaging process for health care is that the average situation may never occur. According to Savage (2002), the averaging process distorts accounts, undermines forecasts, and dooms apparently well thought-out projects to disappointing results. In healthcare staffing, average caregiver needs are often used to create monthly schedules. Although this process is efficient, it may create more challenges in the long run. Consider the situation in which the average number of staff per shift is five and the range for each day of the week is three to nine on the basis of patient activity. No shift requires five staff persons, yet every day is staffed with five persons.

Using the specific number within the range of relevant numbers, in this case a number between 3 and 7, rather than the average of 5 for each shift results in more accurate staffing. The wide range of time required for similar—but different—patient situations is often significant.

1. Examine two to three 4-week schedules and compare the projected core schedules with the actual numbers of staff worked.

2. What are the differences between scheduled and worked, including percentages over and under the core scheduled numbers?

3. What is the range (from the lowest to the highest) of differences?

4. What are the implications of examining both averages and ranges?

5. List three strategies to decrease the differences.

Reference

Savage, S. (2002). The flaw of averages. *Harvard Business Review, 79*(11), 20–21.

Appendix C

Perfect Staffing

Perfect staffing is about having the optimal (not too much, not too little) staff resources to support the right number of qualified caregivers to do their work effectively and timely in an organizational setting that is affordable and available.

While the achievement of perfect staffing seems impossible, nevertheless, this must be the goal of all caregiver teams. It is a journey that begins anew every day with the recognition that health care is complex and uncertain. It is also important to recognize that technology has increased opportunities for more efficient work and course corrections. As the caregiver team works toward perfect staffing, evidence is now our beacon for making things better, and it is readily available with the digital resources that are being introduced every day.

Perfect staffing goals include the following:

- Zero never events

- 100 percent quality compliance

- 100 percent patient, physician, and nurse satisfaction

- 100 percent working and available equipment

There are four key steps in creating a plan for perfect staffing:

1. Create the ideal story for a patient population.
2. Select data elements (focus on 15 or fewer).
3. Analyze the results.
4. Intervene at points of deficiency.

Consider the following scenario or story for a medical cardiac patient care unit and begin with one clinical condition for analysis. (Note: Groups of patients can also be considered.) Outcome indicators for current performance are identified and compared to the team-developed perfect staffing metrics on the accompanying table.

In addition, nurse expectations for perfect staffing include the following:

- 12-hour patient care assignment that includes:
  - Five patients with acuity requirements for 11.5 hours of care
  - Effective hand-off from previous shift
  - An ergonomically safe environment
  - Good communication/collaboration with team members
  - Safe medication administration principles
  - Available supplies for patient care
  - Effective interactions with patients/family, including education

Given these guidelines for creating the conditions for perfect staffing, develop a plan to implement a perfect staffing plan in a selected patient care area. The plan should include the following:

1. The type of patient population
2. Current and expected performance metrics
3. A plan for analysis of data that includes the rationale for targets
4. Number and types of caregivers required
5. Assumptions about the patient population needs

Develop an implementation plan that includes key stakeholders, timelines, plans to address resistance, and communication of results. Include the next steps to achieve perfect staffing on a regular basis.

	Perfect Staffing	Actual Staffing	Variance
HPPD	6.0	5.9	0.1
% RN	40%	42%	2%
% New Graduates	50%	30%	20%
Average Years of Experience	3.0	4.5	1.5
LOS	4.5	4.4	0.1
Cost/Case	$4,000	$3,800	$200
Re-admissions	0	0	0
Call Light Response Satisfaction	5.0/5.0	4.8/5.0	0.2
Pain Management Satisfaction	5.0/5.0	4.8/5.0	0.2
Medication Errors	0	1	1
Patient Falls with Injury	0	0	0
Overall Satisfaction	5.0/5.0	4.9/5.0	0.1
Nurse-Physician Satisfaction	5.0/5.0	4.7/5.0	0.3
Overall Employee Satisfaction	5.0/5.0	4.9/5.0	0.1
Turnover Rate	<5%	3%	2%

Enjoy the challenge of this important journey for optimal outcomes!

Appendix D

Eliminating Non-Value-Added Work

Eight common areas have been identified as sources of non-value-added work and result in wasted time (Storfjell, Ohlson, Omoike, Fitzpatrick, & Wetasin, 2009):

- Admission, discharge, transfer activity
- Shift report
- Supplies/equipment
- Pharmaceuticals
- Diagnostics
- Documentation
- Communication
- Staffing

Within each of these areas are opportunities to eliminate wasteful work. Examples of wasteful work include inefficient hand-offs in which information is incomplete, searching for information or reports, waiting for others to complete their work, fixing equipment, and repeating calls to fill requests. Select two areas from the previous list and brainstorm with a colleague to address these issues or questions.

1. In examining a recent experience, what areas of waste can I identify? How much time is involved?

2. Develop a plan to share this information with members of the team and create a specific plan to decrease the wasted time for this particular event. Be sure to include a specific timeline to complete this work.

3. List the challenges in gaining support from the team and in documenting the value of this work to the team and to the patients.

4. Develop a plan to communicate the challenges in addressing basic waste at the point-of-patient care and the importance of continuing to address nurse work from a positive perspective.

Reference

Storfjell, J. L., Ohlson, S., Omoike, O., Fitzpatrick, T., & Wetasin, K. (2009). Non-value-added time: The million dollar nursing opportunity. *Journal of Nursing Administration, 39*(1), 38–45.

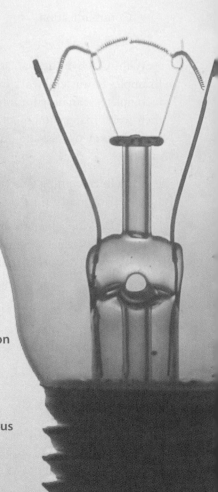

EVEN THE MOST RATIONAL APPROACH TO ETHICS IS DEFENSELESS IF THERE ISN'T THE WILL TO DO WHAT IS RIGHT.
—ALEXANDER SOLZHENITSYN

INTEGRITY WITHOUT KNOWLEDGE IS WEAK AND USELESS, AND KNOWLEDGE WITHOUT INTEGRITY IS DANGEROUS AND DREADFUL.
—SAMUEL JOHNSON

CHAPTER OBJECTIVES

Upon completion of this chapter, the reader will be able to do the following:

» Describe the key concepts and related concepts of healthcare ethics.

» Identify the risks and consequences frequently experienced when personal values and organizational values are different.

» Identify the challenges for nurses in addressing common ethical dilemmas.

» Describe strategies to address ethical dilemmas related to patient, nurse, and organizational issues.

» Delineate strategies to develop competence in ethical decision making.

» Analyze the potential ethical risks in using technology applications specific to patient privacy and confidentiality.

» Gain an appreciation of the personal risks in taking courageous ethical actions.

Principles of Ethical Decision Making

Doing the right thing is not always straightforward. In a complex world, especially health care, ideas, influences, motivations, principles, and individuals contribute to interactions that are far from simple. Making the best decisions in each and every situation in light of these influences is seldom straightforward or found in a reference book. Oftentimes, differences become evident among patient values, nurses' values, and the organization's values, creating conflicts known as ethical dilemmas. In spite of the challenges of making those quality decisions from an ethical perspective, there is an incredible amount of information available to guide individuals in not only being proactive about ethical challenges, but also in course correcting when better decisions are identified. In this chapter, the basic concepts of healthcare ethics are discussed along with the challenges of making appropriate decisions and strategies to support the best ethical work. It is important to note that the information presented in this chapter provides an overview of ethical concepts and challenges and beginning strategies for nurses to identify and address common ethical issues as well as to seek further information to better understand the complexities of such situations. In no way should this chapter be considered a comprehensive presentation of ethical issues in nursing. Every ethical situation is unique based on the environment, the individuals, and the values involved. Much like the inevitable nature of change, so too are ethical issues.

The Basics

The science of ethics and ethical decision making has a language of its own. Knowledge of these basic concepts provides a foundation for nurses when exploring and discussing ethical issues in a professional manner. The following definitions, key concepts, and related concepts are described and expanded to provide the greatest understanding for nurses providing patient care and faced with ethical dilemmas.

Definitions, Key Concepts, and Related Concepts

Autonomy—The right to self-determination; being one's own person without constraints by another's actions or psychological and physical limitations (Dahnke & Dreher as cited in Lachman, 2006); the capacity of a rational individual to make an informed, uncoerced decision. In moral and political philosophy, autonomy is often used as the basis for determining moral responsibility for one's actions (Autonomy, n.d.). Autonomy means that individuals are respected and allowed to make their own decisions about issues that affect them. It means we do not interfere if a person genuinely has the capacity to decide.

Beneficence—The duty to do good. The term refers to actions that promote the well-being of others. In the medical context, this means taking actions that serve the best interests of patients (Medical ethics: Beneficence, n.d.).

Betrayal—A person's words or actions that indicate he or she lacks good intentions toward another; the breaking or violation of a presumptive contract, trust, or confidence that produces moral and psychological conflict within a relationship between individuals, between organizations, or between individuals and organizations. Often betrayal is the act of supporting a rival group, or it is a complete break from previously decided upon or presumed norms by one party from the others.

Bioethics—A subdiscipline of applied ethics that studies questions surrounding biology, medicine, and the health professions. Issues explored in bioethics include questions of research ethics, the use of patients in clinical drug trials, stem cell research, human cloning, etc. (Dahnke & Dreher as cited in Lachman, 2006).

Boundary crossing—Brief excursions from an established boundary for a therapeutic purpose, for example, disclosure of bits of personal information or small gifts. The crossing is brief with a return to the established limits of the professional relationship. Crossings are made based on what is best for the needs of the client (Arizona State Board of Nursing, 1997).

Boundary violation—A deviation from the established boundary in the healthcare provider and client relationship where the healthcare provider's needs and the client's needs are confused. Boundary violations are characterized by role reversal, secrecy, and sometimes the creation of a dual relationship with the client (Arizona State Board of Nursing, 1997). Favors, self-disclosure, and/or physical contact in a professional relationship are examples of boundary violations. Performing favors such as providing lunch, transportation, or running errands are outside of the therapeutic relationship. Disclosing information about one's personal relationships, financial status, or health status are also boundary violations. Touching or hugging a patient without permission is considered an unwelcome violation of one's physical space and should be avoided.

Code of ethics—Guidelines for behavior specific to a moral framework for professional practice. Many codes look to the four basic principles of medical ethics: autonomy, beneficence, nonmaleficence, and justice (Ethical code, n.d.).

Collective ethical wisdom—The sum total of individual and collective experience, knowledge, and good sense; know-how in which the individual and collective knowledge, experience, and good sense result in sound ethical decisions and judgment everywhere and every day; the sum of experience, knowledge, and good sense, which provides subtle signals that alert us to the possibility that something is wrong and worth checking on, and which is driven more by intuition than by an assembly of facts (Gilbert, 2007).

Ethical dilemma—A problem that confronts one, with a choice of solutions that seem or are equally unfavorable (Dahnke & Dreher as cited in Lachman, 2006); a complex situation that often involves an apparent mental conflict of moral imperatives, in which to obey one would result in transgressing another (Ethical dilemma, n.d.). An ethical dilemma ensues when one value is placed against another value. For example, one person may believe that health care should be available to everyone. Others may believe that because of inadequate funding for health care, only those between certain ages and with certain health statuses should be provided healthcare services.

Ethical erosion—The subtle, even unnoticed, slippage of ethical standards; a pervasive, subtle negative dynamic resulting from a decreased focus on values in small and often unnoticed slippages; slight deviations from the normal course of events (Gilbert, 2007).

Ethical fading—A process that obscures the ethical dimensions of a decision (Curtin, 2011).

Ethics—The philosophical study of right action and wrong action; also known as morality, ethics delineates the highest moral standards of behavior (Dahnke & Dreher as cited in Lachman, 2006); a discipline in which one applies certain principles so as to determine the right thing to do in a given situation (Curtin, 2011).

Ethics of care—A recently developed moral theory based on the insights of Gilligan that rejects the traditional male-centered ethics that focused on rationality, individuality, and abstract principles in favor of emotion, caring relationships, and concrete situations (Dahnke & Dreher as cited in Lachman, 2006).

Fidelity—Duty to keep one's promise; the quality of being faithful.

Health advocacy—Supports and promotes patients' healthcare rights and enhances community health and policy initiatives that focus on the availability, safety, and quality of care (Advocacy, n.d.).

Justice—The elimination of arbitrary distinctions and the establishment of a structure of practice with a proper share, balance, or equilibrium among competing claims (Rawls, 2001); a concept of moral rightness based on ethics, rationality, law, natural law, religion, or equity, along with the punishment of the breach of said ethics. The act of being just and/or fair (Justice, n.d.). Justice is about treating individuals fairly and equally.

THREE CAUSES OF MORAL DISTRESS

- Poor-quality and futile care
- Unsuccessful advocacy
- Raising unrealistic hope

Source: Schluter, J., Winch, S., Holzhauser, K., & Henderson, A. (2008). Nurses' moral sensitivity and hospital ethical climate: A literature review. *Nursing Ethics, 15*(3), 304–321.

Medical futility—Care at the end of life for which there is little hope of benefit (Trossman, 2011); the belief that in cases where there is no hope for improvement of an incapacitating condition that no course of treatment is called for. Withholding futile medical care does not encourage or speed the natural onset of death. One could say that it is impossible to reach a firm definition of futile medical care because this would depend on universal agreement about the point at which there is no further benefit to intervention, and different involved parties may always disagree about the amount and type of benefit under discussion (Futile medical care, n.d.).

Moral reasoning—The process in which an individual tries to determine the difference between what is right and what is wrong in a personal situation by using logic (Moral reasoning, n.d.).

Morality—Designates the conventional beliefs of a particular society (Dahnke & Dreher as cited in Lachman, 2006); the degree of congruence between what one perceives as right and one's actual behavior (Curtin, 2011); the differentiation among intentions, decisions, and actions between those that are good (or right) and bad (or wrong). The adjective *moral* is synonymous with *good* or *right* (Morality, n.d.).

Nonmaleficence—Duty to do no harm. The concept of nonmaleficence is embodied by the phrase *first, do no harm*, or the Latin *primum non nocere*. Many believe the primary consideration (*primum*) is that it is more important to not harm your patients than to do them good (Medical ethics: Beneficence, n.d.).

Organizational integrity—The means of producing stronger, sustainable performance through ethical pathways consistent with the vision, mission, and values of the organization (Gilbert, 2007).

Personal integrity—A state of wholeness and peace experienced when our goals, actions, and decisions are consistent with our most cherished values (Gilbert, 2007).

Pragmatism—An American school of philosophy that rejects the esoteric metaphysics of traditional European academic philosophy in favor of more down-to-earth, concrete questions and answers. According to Dewey, the scientific method is used to solve moral problems from this perspective. Proposed by Kant, a moral action is distinguished from an immoral action in that the person acts from a sense of duty, not from inclinations or feelings (Dahnke & Dreher as cited in Lachman, 2006).

Principle—Guideline derived from philosophical perspectives (utilitarian, rights based, duty based, etc.); a law or rule that has to be, or usually is to be followed, or can be desirably followed, or is an inevitable consequence of something, such as the laws observed in nature or the way a system is constructed. The principles of such a system are understood by its users as the essential characteristics of the system, or reflecting the system's designed purpose, and the effective operation or use of which would be impossible if any one of the principles was to be ignored (Principle, n.d.).

Professional boundary—The limits of the professional relationship that allow for a safe therapeutic connection between the healthcare provider and the client.

These include, at a minimum, time, location of patient care, money, exchange, favors or gifts, self-disclosure, and physical contact.

Rationalization—When a person knows what is right and doesn't want to do it (Curtin, 2011); a term used in sociology to refer to a process in which an increasing number of social actions become based on considerations of teleological efficiency or calculation rather than on motivations derived from morality, emotion, custom, or tradition (Rationalization, n.d.).

Right choices—Those choices that conform to ethical norms or principles, and others can know whether or not one has made a right choice.

Trust—The degree to which one can be relied on without surveillance by the observer (Gerck, 1998). Trust has been called the ugly duckling of science, believed to be subjective, imprecise, and unreliable.

Utilitarianism—The principle of utility or the greatest happiness principle; actions are chosen that will produce the greatest amount of happiness for the greatest number of people.

Veracity—Truth telling, or the duty to tell the truth.

Whistle-blowing—Action taken by a person who goes outside the organization for the public's best interest when the organization is unresponsive after the danger is reported through the organization's proper channels (Lachman, 2008); an informant who exposes wrongdoing within an organization in the hope of stopping it (TheFreeDictionary, 2008).

Resources for Ethical Decision Making

In addition to key concepts and definitions, there are several resources, both internal and external to organizations, that are readily available. Internal resources include ethics committees, which typically serve the function of educating employees and providing consultative services. Each organization structures this consultative resource to meet the specific needs of the community and the organization. Whenever possible, nurses should consider attending ethics committee educational meetings and discussions of specific cases. A selected list of additional resources—including textbooks, journals, and online information—to supplement understanding of the ethical aspects of health care are listed in Appendix A.

Ethical Issues and Challenges

There are numerous differing values, perspectives, motivations, and levels of understanding among patients and caregivers. These differences often lead to various approaches to issues and conflicting perspectives on how to proceed when there is an ethical dilemma in the provision of patient care services. To be sure, discussion and resolution of these differences is essential to avoid ethical fading or ethical erosion at both the individual and organizational level. The importance of resolution cannot be underestimated as the goal of reconciling personal values and organizational values is advanced.

CRITICAL THOUGHT

Why is it so difficult to develop good, long-lasting relationships? Is it the fear of disclosure, fear of failure, or a lack of accountability for performance? Is it lack of trust? Or is it something completely different? To be sure, trust is a large component of healthy relationships. Healthy relationships in an environment of continual and complex change require not only a high level of self-awareness and shared values, but also that each individual is comfortable not knowing everything and is able to trust that colleagues have the same shared values and will perform to their best ability.

In this section, several of the sources, common issues, and challenges in the provision of healthcare services that could result in ethical dilemmas are discussed. Not surprising, the source of ethical dilemmas is varied and can arise from values, communication, diversity, legislation, nurses, patients, and organizational differences.

The first general category is values, which includes those situations related to trust, timeliness, accountability, and personal appearance features in which individuals differ. Diversity of values and different perspectives on age, gender, location, political views, role, education, culture, and religion are examples of the sources of differences among individuals (Figure 6-1). This multifaceted diversity is frequently the source of misinformation or misunderstanding that can lead to an ethical dilemma. Disrespect for differing values and behaviors among individuals is often subtle and unintentional. When these differences result in obvious conflict situations, it is helpful to use ethical concepts and principles to identify the specific issues and begin to resolve the conflict situation.

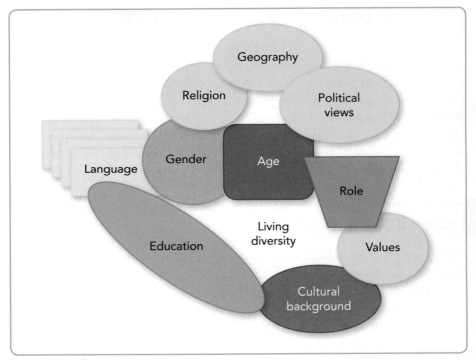

Figure 6-1 Diversity types

Communication style can be a source of conflict that leads to misunderstanding, divergent actions, and ethical dilemmas. Individuals have developed and reinforced communications styles that have worked for them, however offensive or intolerable they may be to others. At times, individuals do not always share complete information, or they share it in a way that is unclear, or, even worse, they remain silent and do not share information that would facilitate and enrich the discussion. Sharing partial treatment information with a patient, such as what to expect in a procedure, may be motivated by the desire to protect the patient from upsetting information; however, partial information discounts the patient's right to know information that is pertinent to his or her care. Motivations for partial truth telling or withholding information are varied and need to be explored when such behaviors are recognized. Ethical issues of autonomy, beneficence, betrayal, boundary crossing, justice, nonmaleficence, and personal integrity could all be involved in inappropriate communication.

Communicating in an aggressive manner can also create ethical concerns when the rights of others are violated. Consider communication behaviors between nurses that reflect horizontal violence or nurse–physician communication that is demeaning and intimidating. Bullying is another concept identified as an unhealthy communication behavior.

When one person asserts physical or emotional power over another person, many ethical issues arise. Ethical issues of autonomy, beneficence, betrayal, code of ethics, justice, nonmaleficence, boundary violations, and personal integrity can all be involved in aggressive and intimidating communications.

Legislation can also be a source of ethical dilemmas when it differs from an individual's values. An ethical dilemma can emerge related to the right to choice for an abortion, which conflicts with the personal values of some individuals who support right to life. While this might seem like a straightforward resolution in favor of the person involved, that is not always the case. It is not only the values of the individual that must be considered, but also the context in which the individual is requesting services. If the organization's values are based on beliefs that differ from the individual's, the organization is not able to provide the desired services and the individual would need to move to a facility that supports abortion services. An ethical dilemma can also arise from the individual nurse caregiver value perspective. Nurses whose values are in conflict with those of the organization have several options. One, of course, is to choose not to work at the organization; another is to frankly discuss the situation with managers and determine how to modify assignments to not be involved in the areas generating the ethical dilemma. What is not appropriate is to ignore the dilemma and work in a conflicted state. Ethical issues of autonomy, boundary violations, code of ethics, pragmatism, rationalization, and personal integrity could be involved in legislative issues.

Nurse–Nurse Ethical Dilemmas

It seems natural and obvious that nurses, given their education, would all have similar values and beliefs about patient care. Given the wide range of diverse values previously discussed, nurse-to-nurse relationships and behaviors encounter the same variations and dilemmas. Nurse-to-nurse ethical dilemmas arise from these multiple sources and impact perceptions and professional role behaviors.

An area of great concern and challenge for nurses is the nurse-to-nurse ethical dilemma in which nurses espouse different standards of practice from one another. The American Nurses Association's Code of Ethics clearly defines standards of practice, yet not all nurses follow these professional standards. Oftentimes, nurses support professional standards in the strictest manner, while other nurses tend to cut corners or ignore some professional standards, resulting in different levels of patient care. Autonomy, beneficence, betrayal, code of ethics, fidelity, nonmaleficence, rationalization, veracity, and personal integrity are all involved in substandard practice.

CRITICAL THOUGHT

Trusting relationships cannot be bought or recruited from the outside; they must develop over time and through experience.

In many states, nurses are required by law to report unprofessional and unsafe practices to the board of nursing as a requirement of their license. The requirement to report nurses who do not follow the professional standards of practice should not be taken lightly. Specific guidelines are available from the American Nurses Association and each state board of nursing. Examples include the following requirements to report nurses to the appropriate state board of nursing:

- Information that a nurse may be mentally or physically unable to safely practice nursing
- Conduct involving practicing beyond the scope of practice of the license, such as giving a medication not authorized by a provider or an unauthorized adjustment of a dosage (boundary violation)
- Conduct that appears to be a contributing factor to high risk or harm to a patient and required medical intervention (nonmaleficence)
- Conduct involving the use of alcohol or chemical substances to the extent that nursing practice may be impaired (nonmaleficence, personal integrity)
- Actual or suspected drug diversion (nonmaleficence, personal integrity)
- Pattern of failure to account for medications or wastage of control drugs (nonmaleficence, personal integrity)
- Pattern of inappropriate judgment or nursing skill (rationalization, nonmaleficence, personal integrity)
- Professional boundary violations, such as sexual conduct with a patient or patient's family member
- Conduct involving theft or exploitation of a patient (boundary violation)
- Practicing without a valid license (code of ethics)

When a nurse identifies or recognizes behaviors believed to be in violation of professional standards and regulations, the issue should be escalated to the next individual in the organizational chain of command or reporting structure to determine how and when to be compliant with the reporting requirements. The reporting of colleagues can be quite unsettling for the individual and can also impact team dynamics. When the issue is not addressed, ethical fading begins and can lead to ethical erosion. Doing the right and ethical thing requires courage and conviction of one's actions.

Substance use disorders are another area of great nurse-to-nurse conflict. Of all the professional issues among nurses, addressing impaired nurse behaviors is probably the most difficult. The number of nurses impaired by substances is of great concern to the profession and the public and represents the most common reason nurses are reported to boards of nursing (Darbro, 2011). As difficult as it is to report a colleague with probable substance abuse issues, the importance of getting assistance is critical in getting impaired nurses into recovery.

Reentry into practice from substance use disorders often presents another dilemma for nurses. Nurses who have successfully completed initial rehabilitation and are engaged in their recovery from substance abuse often have difficulties reentering the practice setting. Practicing nurses are often reluctant to put forth the additional effort to monitor and mentor the returning nurse. One ethical dilemma that arises between nurses who practice safely and the returning nurse pertains to why nurses without substance abuse issues should be expected to oversee and monitor the nurse who violated professional standards. Ethical issues of autonomy, beneficence, fidelity, nonmaleficence, and rationalization are common in these situations.

Nurse–Patient Ethical Dilemmas

The second category of specific types of ethical dilemmas is related to the nurse–patient relationship. During the course of providing patient care, numerous ethical dilemmas can emerge. Issues related to decision-making authority, pain management, the dying process, futile care, patient privacy, and communication among providers are not uncommon dilemmas and require investigation and resolution.

Historically, physicians directed patient care treatments based on the belief that physicians held the best and most reliable information about medical treatments. Patient autonomy was deferred to the physician. More recently, the belief has shifted. It should be recognized that the patient or user of the healthcare system owns his or her decisions about healthcare treatments and has personal autonomy. For example, autonomy can come into conflict with beneficence when a patient disagrees with recommendations that healthcare professionals believe are in the patient's best interest. When the patient's wishes conflict with his or her welfare, the wishes of a mentally competent patient will dominate even if healthcare providers believe the patient's choice is not in his or her best interest. Patient knowledge, culture, religion, or other values can be the source of disagreement with providers.

Patient restraint is another recurring challenge for nurses in ensuring a safe environment. Restraining a patient necessarily decreases patient autonomy in favor of beneficence or nonmaleficence. Similarly, when a patient or family selects palliative care rather than all possible care at the end of life in support of patient autonomy, nurses may in fact disagree that appropriate care is not being provided and harm is being brought upon the patient by withholding antibiotics or tube feedings.

Another nurse–patient ethical dilemma is related to technology, specifically to monitoring alarms. The management of alarms on monitoring equipment has gained attention recently. As the number of monitoring devices increases, the number of associated alarms has also increased, rendering the patient care environment a cacophony of sounds. The noise and false alarms have resulted in alarm fatigue, and nurses often turn off alarms to decrease the noise and interruptions from false alarms (Inglesby, 2011). Several concepts and principles are involved in these types of situations and include rationalization, nonmaleficence, morality, beneficence, and personal integrity.

Nurse–Organization Ethical Dilemmas

The third category of specific types of ethical dilemmas is between the nurse and the organization. Interactions between an employer and employee can lead to ethical dilemmas in several ways. To be sure, it is important to be clear how an organization addresses ethical patient care situations. When there is a lack of congruency among nurse values, individual patient needs, and the demands of the organization, an ethical dilemma emerges. Caregivers become disenfranchised and dissatisfied with their work. For example, if caregivers believe their primary obligation to the patient (health advocacy) is compromised, an ethical dilemma is present. Being able to work in an organization in which difficult patient care problems are discussed and decided so the primary obligation to the patient is honored is essential for caregiver satisfaction and retention. Caregivers are empowered, trusted, and included in the decision-making processes of ethical dilemmas. Examples of nurse–organization ethical dilemmas can be related to error management, staffing adequacy, technology management, and many others.

Another nurse–organization ethical dilemma between nurses and the organization is related to the management of errors. Historically, if a nurse commits an error, he or she was disciplined for poor practice. More recently, the investigation of errors and considerations of a just culture have emerged as important considerations in the management of errors (Benner, Malloch, & Sheets, 2010). Specifically, the recognition that errors are inevitable in a human system, the nature of the interconnectedness of systems, and the morality of treating persons fairly and humanely when an error occurs have dramatically shifted the management of errors in healthcare organizations.

This shift in thinking is the result of error research and the emphasis from systems theory that practice deficiencies can seldom be understood in isolation and individuals are rarely responsible for anything but the most egregious errors (Goeschel, 2011). The new dilemma is now about assigning accountability and administering sanctions with fairness. Specifically, the work is now to determine team accountability and administer sanctions fairly?

Staffing adequacy is also associated with ethical dilemmas. When nurse staffing is less than adequate, patient care can be compromised. Oftentimes nurses are in a position in which a nurse does not report to work and no replacement is available, leaving the nurses on the shift to add additional responsibilities beyond their capabilities. Nurses have accepted this situation in the belief that patient care would be worse if they refused the additional, unreasonable assignment and they were the only ones who could protect the patient. The principles of beneficence, nonmaleficence, ethical fading, fidelity, rationalization, boundaries, and rationalization are all potential explanations for the ethical dilemma.

Documentation technology is another source of ethical dilemmas. The large influx of technology to document and monitor patient care has resulted in increased access to information and challenges in documenting the information in a timely and individual manner. The increased availability of protected and private patient information in an electronic environment has resulted in inappropriate disclosure of confidential patient information. Accessing patient information without a clinical relationship with the patient for care has resulted in both discipline and termination of employment. Principles of beneficence, betrayal, fidelity, nonmaleficence, personal integrity, rationalization, and veracity can all be involved in understanding these types of ethical dilemmas.

These ethical issues provide a general overview of the most common situations faced by nurses. It is hoped that readers of this information will use the key concepts and common dilemmas as foundations for discussion of ethical issues that arise in their own organization. In addition, multiple clinical scenarios are provided in Appendix B for nurses to analyze ethical situations using ethical concepts to gain skill and competence in this important area.

BEHAVIORS OF INDIVIDUALS WITH HIGH SELF-AWARENESS

- Are aware of personal values related to culture, religion, race, gender, etc.
- Able to articulate personal and professional boundaries specific to physical space, thoughts, sense of identity, and relationship with a higher power
- Communicate in an open style and question frequently to gain a greater understanding
- Communicate likes and dislikes
- Able to separate data from opinion in making decisions
- Value multiple perspectives and diversity of ideas
- Recognize the impact of both verbal and nonverbal communication behaviors
- Do not talk down to others; use language that is easily understood
- Strive to be concise in communication and avoid rambling on; do not filibuster or tolerate filibustering
- Know the purpose for the relationship and what is expected of each person

Strategies to Address Ethical Issues

Recognizing moral dilemmas and the associated concepts is just one step in ensuring ethical decisions and behaviors. Strategies to address ethical issues specific to self-knowledge, trust building, organizational team building, practice breakdown management, and managing personal risks are discussed to guide the nurse in becoming competent in this area.

CRITICAL THOUGHT

Can I trust you? Can you trust me?
How do I know if I can trust someone? Certain behaviors reflect trust more than others. Consider the following trust-enhancing and trust busting behaviors as you develop your relationships.

CRITICAL THOUGHT

Numerous healthcare situations call for courage. Examples include breaking bad news regarding a poor prognosis, challenging a colleague who appears incompetent, delivering care to an infectious patient, confronting an angry relative, and raising concerns about unethical practice.

What is common to all of these situations is the fear that may be experienced as the practitioner considers the cost of the action and the consequences of a particular intervention or of getting it wrong. There may be fear of an extreme emotional reaction, violence, contamination, negative reactions from colleagues, or losing one's job.

Self-Knowledge

Self-knowledge specific to ethical concepts, issues, and resolutions is a necessary first step. Understanding the concepts and examples of specific applications begins the development of one's competence. A regular discussion of ethical issues and application of the associated principles is an important practice for nurses. It is important to remember that no two situations are ever the same; however, the principles for assessing and addressing ethical dilemmas are always consistent.

SCENARIO

There continues to be ample evidence that nurses do not always feel they can do the right thing in their everyday practice. In some instances, this may be because they lack virtues—such as moral courage, wisdom, and integrity—that are required to speak up and bring about change. In other instances, however, when organizational cultures are defensive, unsupportive, and potentially punishing, the virtue of courage may not be adequate to change a situation.

Discussion Questions

1. In a small group, share your thoughts on this dilemma.

2. Which ethical principles are involved?

3. What strategies should be considered to address this problem?

Demonstrating moral courage is a competence specific to one's ability to be assertive in addressing ethical issues. When faced with a situation in which a nurse knows the right thing to do, but does not feel able to do the right thing or live his or her professional values, moral courage is needed—courage to confront the situation in a logical, unemotional manner focused on doing the identified right thing. To be sure, there are risks and consequences when one asserts him- or herself to address ethical dilemmas. The reality of speaking up and risking one's position is real and often cannot be avoided. Developing moral courage begins with competence in concepts and scenarios specific to ethical dilemmas. In addition, working within a team setting focused on organizational integrity further assists those faced with ethical dilemmas to confront those situations with moral courage—assertiveness, clarity, timeliness, and beneficence. Managing the personal risks of ethical behaviors requires all of the strategies identified in this section.

Clarity of one's professional role is another strategy for effective ethical dilemma resolution. A clear understanding of the expectations of a professional includes autonomy as a professional nurse, advancement of the science and evidence for healthcare practices, and a focus on results in providing patient care (O'Rourke, 2003) to assist nurses in maintaining the boundaries of the practice of nursing.

Trust Building

Being able to communicate openly and honestly (fidelity, integrity) with colleagues, patients, and families is foundational to ethical behaviors. Caregivers know that health care is fundamentally based on personal, professional, and trusting relationships between individuals seeking care and those who care for them.

Trust infers that one individual is vulnerable to the actions of another. The greater the trust, the more positive the expectations that individuals have about others' intentions and actions based on established roles, relationships, experiences, and their interdependencies. Trust is one individual's willingness to be vulnerable to another based on the belief that the latter party is competent, open, concerned, and reliable. When trust is lost, feelings of betrayal, stress, and vulnerability emerge, often resulting in ethical dilemmas.

BEHAVIORS THAT REFLECT TRUST

1. Sharing relevant information in a timely manner to support the best decisions. Sharing partial information or sharing information after the fact does not engender trust. Rather, hesitancy emerges because one never knows if someone is holding back and for what reason.

2. Revealing concerns even when you are not exactly clear what the concern is. Exploring intuitions with others encourages dialogue and openness.

3. Working to understand others and their perspectives before telling others your plans and goals. Allowing for mutual influence to avoid a sense of personal superiority.

4. Reducing controls to engender trust in the abilities of others and decreasing the need to oversee other individuals.

5. Meeting expectations as promised.

6. Letting others know their work is valued.

7. Recognizing contributions not only by financial reward but also by presence, concern, and support of effective relationships.

8. Sharing information regarding the rationale for changes in order to fully engage others in the change process.

9. Requesting input whenever possible to be sure the best decisions are made on the basis of the collective wisdom of the team.

10. Making eye contact to reflect openness and honesty (note that this does not apply to all cultures).

There are several behaviors that facilitate effective ethical decision making. The following activities should be embraced by all members of the team:

- Support an environment in which a nurse feels comfortable speaking up to any member of the healthcare team.

- Establish rules of engagement for the team specific to ethical issues. The goal is for every member of the team to know and understand key concepts, common dilemmas, and expectations, and for team members to be competent to do the right thing the first time.

TRUSTBUSTER BEHAVIORS

- Jumping to conclusions
- Avoiding discussion about sensitive issues
- Demonstrating insensitivity to the beliefs and values of others
- Interrupting while another is speaking
- Expressing an opinion before a person has an opportunity to share an idea or opinion
- Being too busy for dialogue about controversial topics
- Encouraging competition—winners and losers
- Changing a course of action depending on who is present
- Working in isolation and then presenting ideas to others as complete
- Dishonesty

- Make sure that people hear the real messages that are communicated. This often requires validation of communication and reiteration of expectations.
- Make expectations clear and make sure they are understood. Communicate in several ways: verbally, in writing, and electronically.
- Develop principle-centered policies and practices. Emphasize principles for ethical behaviors and minimize specific rules. For example, the practice to provide a safe environment is a principle; a requirement to always have side rails in the up position is a rule. The principle of providing a safe environment can be met in many ways. In fact, elevating side rails may decrease the safety of the environment if the patient attempts to climb over the rails out of the bed. Other interventions, such as lowering the bed to its lowest position or placing the mattress on the floor, may be consistent with the principle of providing a safe environment.
- Adhere to principles—do not bend them for anyone!
- Discuss areas of disagreement until common ground is found.

- Support an environment of trust and hold people to their words and promises.

- Respect every team member's contributions and build on team values.

- Work out ethical situations quickly and establish new rules as needed.

CRITICAL THOUGHT

Thoughts on trust:

- Trust is that which an observer knows about an entity and can rely upon to some extent (your spouse or coworker).

- Trust is that which can be relied upon without surveillance by the observer.

- Trust is received information that has a degree of belief that is acceptable to an observer.

- Trust depends on the observer; there is never absolute trust. Trust only exists as self-trust; trust of others will always have surprises.

- Mutual trust is a two-way street in which you trust me and I trust you.

Managing Practice Breakdown Errors

As previously noted, errors in health care are now being perceived from a more humanistic perspective. Errors, recently identified as *practice breakdown*, are defined broadly as the disruption or absence of any of the aspects of good practice (Benner et al., 2002). This new conceptualization allows nurses to identify and examine not only the error, but also the category of professional practice error, the role of the system in the error, and the opportunity to prevent other similar breakdown situations. It is important to identify the root cause of the practice breakdown, thereby identifying an area for additional education or training to improve practice and system deficiencies rather than punishment of an individual for an error that is believed to be his or her sole responsibility. The ethical issues of beneficence, justice, integrity, nonmaleficence, and utilitarianism are served with this type of approach rather than disciplining single individuals for errors that often involve team members and system flaws.

The most common sources or rationale for nurse practice breakdowns in 884 cases studied by the Taxonomy of Error Root Cause Analysis and Practice-Responsibility (TERCAP) Committee of the National Council of State Boards of Nursing included lack of professional responsibility, lack of clinical reasoning, and lack of intervention (Zhong & Thomas, 2012). Further, 72 percent of the cases involved unintentional human errors, and 27 percent involved intentional misconduct or criminal behavior. More than 50 percent of the cases did not cause harm to the patient. When system factors were analyzed, 65 percent involved team members as a contributing factor, as well as communication, interdepartmental breakdown or conflict, and inadequate orientation and handoff procedures. These data support a more humane approach to this ethical dilemma of whether to punish an individual or view the incident first as a specific type of nursing practice breakdown that can be studied and improved upon.

MOST COMMON PRACTICE BREAKDOWN ERRORS

- Lack of professional responsibility (77 percent)
- Lack of clinical reasoning (51 percent)
- Lack of intervention (50 percent)
- Documentation error (44 percent)
- Lack of interpretation (40 percent)
- Medication error (32 percent)
- Lack of attentiveness (25 percent)
- Lack of prevention (24 percent)

Note: The percentages exceed 100% because some cases were classified in more than one category.

Source: Zhong, E. H., & Thomas, M. B. (2012). Association between job history and practice: An analysis of disciplinary cases. *Journal of Nursing Regulation, 2*(4), 16–18.

Concluding Thoughts

Creating an ethical environment in an organization requires persistent and ongoing dialogue as well as validation of appropriate behaviors. Recognizing the complexities and multiple variables involved in ethical issues requires nurses to develop and maintain competence so that patient values continue to drive patient care. Addressing ethical issues and dilemmas requires logical, prompt, and principle-based actions. As noted earlier, the complexity of ethical issues cannot be understated.

CHAPTER TEST QUESTIONS

1.   An ethical dilemma arises from (a) inadequate patient assessments, (b) differing values, (c) differing gender, generational, and educational competencies, or (d) unsuccessful or negligent patient care.

2.   Trusting relationships are essential in managing ethical dilemmas. Trust is characterized as (a) complete support of a colleague, (b) an ugly duckling, (c) a relationship in which one individual is vulnerable to another, or (d) nearly impossible to create and sustain.

3.   Ethical erosion is (a) subtle, even unnoticed slippage of ethical standards, (b) a common organizational phenomenon, (c) an increase in sensitivity to diverse values, or (d) the result of poor patient care.

4.   Ethical principles are helpful in (a) determining the specific cause or explanation of an ethical dilemma, (b) assigning blame to the individual violating the principle, (c) forming guidelines for appropriate behavior, or (d) resolving patient care errors.

5.   Promise keeping or fidelity is (a) an agreement in nurse–nurse relationships, (b) the same as nonmaleficence, (c) a foundational ethical principle for resolution of ethical dilemmas, or (d) a difficult principle to validate.

6.   Oftentimes nurses rationalize a situation because (a) it is necessary to fully understand a situation, (b) the right thing is not easy to do, (c) other more appropriate actions might become available, or (d) the pragmatic approach is not effective.

7. Boundaries from an ethical perspective (a) include activities specific to nurse–patient assignments, (b) emphasize boundary violations as inappropriate behaviors, (c) require interpretations from a moral perspective, or (d) delineate the professional limits of a therapeutic relationship.

8. Impaired nursing practice is (a) about substance use disorders impacting safe nursing practice, (b) not common in the nursing profession, (c) readily reported by colleagues who become aware of the impaired practice, or (d) a relatively new issue in health care.

9. Practice breakdown strategies represent ethical issues (a) in identifying the cause of errors, (b) specific to fair and just treatment of nurses, (c) requiring more stringent discipline of those making errors, or (d) supporting rationalization of healthcare errors.

10. Conflict in ethical situations arises from (a) morality, (b) nonmaleficence, (c) value diversity, or (d) financial resources.

> **www** ⌖ For a full suite of assignments and additional learning activities, use the access code located in the front of your book to visit the exclusive website: http://go.jblearning.com/leadership. If you do not have an access code, you can obtain one at the site.

References

Advocacy. (n.d.). In *Wikipedia*. Retrieved from http://en.wikipedia.org/wiki/Advocacy

Arizona State Board of Nursing. (1997). Arizona State Board of Nursing guidelines for sexual misconduct and boundary violation cases. Retrieved from http://www.azbn .gov/documents/Substantive%20Policies/Guidelines%20for%20Sexual%20 Misconduct%20&%20Bondary%20Violation%20Cases.pdf

Autonomy. (n.d.). In *Wikipedia*. Retrieved from http://en.wikipedia.org/wiki/Autonomy

Benner, P., Malloch, K., & Sheets, V. (Eds.). (2010). *Nursing pathways for patient safety: Expert panel on practice breakdown. Overview: NCSBN practice breakdown initiative.* Philadelphia, PA: Elsevier.

Benner, P., Sheets, V., Uris, P., Malloch, K., Schwed, K., & Jamison, D. (2002). Individual, practice and system causes of error in nursing. *Journal of Nursing Administration, 32*(10), 509–523.

Curtin, L. (2011). Quantum ethics: Coming to grips with the dark side. *American Nurse Today, 6*(11), 48.

Darbro, N. (2011). Model guidelines for alternative programs and discipline monitoring programs. *Journal of Nursing Regulation, 2*(1), 42–49.

Ethical code. (n.d.). In *Wikipedia*. Retrieved from http://en.wikipedia.org/wiki/ Code_of_ethics

Ethical dilemma. (n.d.). In *Wikipedia*. Retrieved from http://en.wikipedia.org/wiki/ Ethical_dilemma

Futile medical care. (n.d.). In *Wikipedia*. Retrieved from http://en.wikipedia.org/wiki/ Medical_futility

Gerck, E. (1998). Toward real-world models of trust: Reliance on received information. Retrieved from www.mcg.org

Gilbert, J. A. (2007). *Strengthening ethical wisdom: Tools for transforming your health care organization.* Chicago, IL: AHA Press.

Goeschel, C. (2011). Defining and assigning accountability for quality care and patient safety. *Journal of Nursing Regulation, 2*(1), 28–35.

Inglesby, T. (2011). Being everywhere at once. *Patient Safety and Quality Healthcare, 8*(2), 44.

Justice. (n.d.). In *Wikipedia*. Retrieved from http://en.wikipedia.org/wiki/Justice

Lachman, V. D. (Ed.). (2006). *Applied ethics in nursing.* New York, NY: Springer.

Lachman, V. D. (2008). Whistle blowers: Troublemakers or virtuous nurses? *Medsurg Nursing, 17*(2), 126–128, 134.

Medical ethics: Beneficence. (n.d.). In *Wikipedia.* Retrieved from http://en.wikipedia .org/wiki/Beneficence_(ethics)#Beneficence

Moral reasoning. (n.d.). In *Wikipedia.* Retrieved from http://en.wikipedia.org/wiki/ Moral_reasoning

Morality. (n.d.). In *Wikipedia.* Retrieved from http://en.wikipedia.org/wiki/Moral_ compass

O'Rourke, M. W. (2003). Rebuilding a professional practice model: The return of role-based practice accountability. *Nursing Administration Quarterly, 27*(2), 95–105.

Principle. (n.d.). In *Wikipedia.* Retrieved from http://en.wikipedia.org/wiki/Principle

Rationalization. (n.d.). In *Wikipedia.* Retrieved from http://en.wikipedia.org/wiki/ Rationalization_(sociology)

Rawls, J. (2001). Justice as reciprocity. In S. Freeman (Ed.), *Collected papers* (pp. 190–224). Cambridge, MA: Harvard University Press.

Schluter, J., Winch, S., Holzhauser, K., & Henderson, A. (2008). Nurses' moral sensitivity and hospital ethical climate: A literature review. *Nursing Ethics, 15*(3), 304–321.

TheFreeDictionary. (2008). Whistle-blowing. Retrieved from http://www .thefreedictionary.com/whistle-blowing

Trossman, S. (2011). Issues up close: The practice of ethics. *American Nurse Today, 6*(11), 3233.

Zhong, E. H., & Thomas, M. B. (2012). Association between job history and practice error: An analysis of disciplinary cases. *Journal of Nursing Regulation, 2*(4), 16–18.

Appendix A
Selected Healthcare Ethics Resources

American Medical Association Journal of Ethics. http://virtualmentor.ama-assn.org

American Nurses Association. Code of Ethics for Nurses. http://nursingworld .org/codeofethics

Baillie, H. M., Garrett, R. M., & McGeehan, J. F. (2009). *Health care ethics: Principles and problems* (5th ed.). Upper Saddle River, NJ: Prentice Hall.

Bioethics.net covers information related to health care and biotechnology and includes news articles, editorials, book reviews, and a blog. www.bioethics.net

EthicShare is a research and collaboration website offering reference materials, news items, group discussions, and bioethics information. www.ethicshare.org

Fremgen, B. F. (2012). *Medical law and ethics* (4th ed.). New York, NY: Pearson.

Hastings Center Report. http://www.thehastingscenter.org/Publications/HCR/ Subscriptions.aspx

Health Ethics Trust. http://www.healthethicstrust.com/?gclid=CM3iguDO-qwCFWmhtgodcjjJTA

JONA's healthcare law, ethics, and regulation. http://www.lww.com/webapp/wcs/ stores/servlet/product__11851_-1_9012052_Prod-15209229

National Institutes of Health. Bioethics resources on the web. http://bioethics. od.nih.gov/

Nursing Ethics: An International Journal for Health Care Professionals. http://www .uk.sagepub.com/journals/Journa1201821

Pozgar, G. D. (2009). *Legal aspects of health care administration* (11th ed.). Sudbury, MA: Jones and Bartlett.

Purtilo, R. B., & Doherty, R. (2011). *Ethical dimensions in the health professions* (5th ed.). St. Louis, MO: Elsevier Saunders. http://www.eu.elsevierhealth.com/ Health-Professions/specialty/book/9781437708967/Ethical-Dimensions-in-the-Health-Professions

Santa Clara University's Markkula Center for Applied Ethics offers online articles, end-of-life materials, case studies, and resources on medical decision making. www.scu.edu/ethics/practicing/focusareas/medical

Yale Journal of Health Policy, Law, and Ethics. http://www.yale.edu/yjhple/

Appendix B

Ethics Discussion Scenarios

When faced with an ethical dilemma, it is helpful to approach the situation as logically as possible. These scenarios are posed for discussion to broaden your understanding of ethical issues and potential solutions. For each scenario, consider the following seven questions. Issues specific to autonomy, beneficence, betrayal, boundaries, fidelity, justice, integrity, nonmaleficence, rationalization, trust, and utilitarianism should be considered for each scenario. Additional comments are also included in selected scenarios to assist in furthering the discussion after the ethical aspects of the scenario are discussed.

1. What is the background of the situation?

2. What are the facts that can be verified?

3. What is the ethical dilemma? Which ethical principles or concepts are involved?

4. What are the options for resolution?

5. What activities or resources are necessary for resolution?

6. What will be required to implement the decision?

7. What are the anticipated consequences of the decision?

Scenario 1: Nurse–Organization–Professional Role. The organization discourages nurses from becoming members of professional nursing organizations because of the commitment to collective bargaining. Nurses want to join because they believe the association sets the standards for nursing practice and believe their participation on organizational committees is a professional obligation.

Comments: Nurses are hired by organizations on the basis of their nursing skill and knowledge that is based on their profession's principles and standards. Participation in and commitment to one's profession is a hallmark of professional practice. While the bargaining arm of some organizations may be problematic to many human resource directors, it is important to determine other purposes of the professional organization, such as standards setting, education, and mentoring. Each nurse should work to educate those in the organization who resist professional membership with information that clearly describes the essence of the American Nurses Association. Failure to resolve this issue may require the nurse to seek a more supportive employer.

Scenario 2: Nurse–Organization–Professional Role. Several of the nurses on your unit are reluctant to participate in unit activities, discussion of patient outcome data, or nurse–physician relationships.

Scenario 3: Nurse–Organization. The organization emphasizes the need for continuing education and excellence as core values. However, in light of the limited resources and cutbacks in reimbursement, recognition and reward programs are limited to a standard annual pay rate increase for all employees, occasional movie tickets, and pizza.

Scenario 4: Nurse–Nurse. One nurse on your team is chronically late to work, complains about assignments, and seldom assists others even when asked. No one, including the manager, has given feedback to the nurse that this is unprofessional behavior and negatively impacts the team and patient care. The nurse is a relative of a prominent physician and regularly talks about their relationship and frequent interactions.

Scenario 5: Nurse–Patient End of Life. A dying patient's family is not ready for their mother to die in spite of the poor prognosis and demands that everything be done, including antibiotics, ventilator care, and tube feedings. There is a 24-hour waiting list for intensive care unit (ICU) beds, and this patient is in an ICU bed and therefore preventing an admission. Several nurses reduce the ventilator settings and delay tube feedings because they believe it would be a better use of resources if the patient was allowed to die.

Scenario 6: Nurse–Patient Pain Management. The elderly mother of a local physician in a rural setting is admitted to the hospital with pneumonia for the third time in one year. The patient is somewhat confused and receiving oxygen. The physician son orders morphine to be given every two hours around the clock to keep her comfortable. When a nursing instructor is working with students, she questions the order because the patient is not responsive and experiencing increasing difficulty breathing. She wonders if euthanasia is being practiced.

Scenario 7: Nurse–Organization–Staffing Adequacy. The organization is experiencing declining revenues and requesting increased efforts to control expenses. The nursing manager believes she should decrease staffing to contribute to the cost reductions in spite of increasing patient acuity and nurse dissatisfaction. Nurses are frustrated and not able to complete the expected patient care.

Scenario 8: Nurse–Nurse–Team. The chief nursing officer (CNO) has supported the implementation of a shared governance model and states that nurses' decisions must be respected. Nurses have become concerned because the CNO has begun to override decisions of the council and change the priorities of the council.

Comment: The adage of *walking the talk* in this situation can be the ultimate challenge for leaders. Learning to transition to the role of coach, mentor, and guide is difficult for even the most committed leader. The appropriate approach is a direct one because discussing the problem without the CNO would be counter-productive. Clear identification of the overriding of council decisions to the CNO and asking for guidance on how to manage the situation are the first steps. If the CNO rationalizes that this approach is necessary, further discussion is warranted to determine what shared leadership means to the CNO and how such situations should be managed.

Scenario 9: Nurse–Organization–Non-Value-Added Work. All nurse managers are required to attend the safety committee in person on a monthly basis. The managers do not believe their presence is necessary because their input or opinions are never requested. They believe this meeting is a waste of their time. Nurse managers have requested to attend via conference call and/or be accountable for reviewing minutes.

Comment: Meetings that consist of only one-way communication or information giving should be eliminated in favor of memos or e-mail. Face-to-face meetings should be held when there is a need for dialogue and problem solving. The team should review its goals, purposes, and expected outcomes and determine the most appropriate method to get the intended work completed. With this information, the team can determine if face-to-face or electronic communication or a combination is the most useful. Electronic communication should never replace situations in which healthy dialogue is needed. Electronic and face-to-face communication both have advantages and disadvantages.

Scenario 10: Nurse–Nurse–Organization. The manager is very concerned about overtime and has instructed nurses to clock out at the end of the shift. If there is more work (charting) to be done, the nurse is told to work on personal organization and priority setting skills and complete the charting off the clock.

Comment: The pressure to meet budget targets should never override acceptable practices. The practice described is not acceptable for two reasons. First, it is inconsistent with federal labor laws; second, failing to understand and manage the workload reflects a serious leadership need. This practice reflects the larger, unresolved and ever-present problem of too much work and too little time. The manager is challenged to evaluate the work that is being done to ensure that it is appropriate and positively impacts patient outcomes. New strategies to manage the variance between the required work and available staff need to be created by the healthcare team, not the individual nurse at the bedside.

Scenario 11. Nurse–Organization. The manager consistently decreases daily staffing in order to meet budget guidelines. Errors are increasing and patient care is negatively impacted. The nurses are planning to file a complaint to the nursing board against the manager for failure to delegate and supervise and protect patient safety.

Comment: The first step in a situation like this is to discuss the issue with the manager and also inform her that you believe she is violating the nurse practice act. If that does not yield results and patient care continues to be negatively impacted, the nurse must then follow the chain of command and communicate the concerns and the evidence of poor patient outcomes. If these efforts do not yield changes that impact patient care positively, the nurse may choose to report the situation to the board of nursing on the basis of mandatory reporting requirements for unsafe patient care.

Scenario 12: Nurse–Nurse. Most nurses on the unit refuse to precept new nurses because they don't have enough time and also believe that nurses should be better prepared by the schools before coming to work. Nurses understand their professional commitment for the development of novice nurses; however, they believe their patients are compromised when they are assigned a preceptor.

Scenario 13: Nurse–Nurse–Diversity. The nurse manager is Filipino and shows favoritism toward other Filipino nurses. She believes that if she doesn't honor their request for scheduled days and lunch breaks, they will quit and there will be less diversity in the team.

Scenario 14: Nurse–Nurse–Delegation. Critical care nurses have refused to work with nursing technicians or nursing assistants because it requires time to supervise and delegate, and the competence of the assistants is not always above average. It is believed that approximately 25 percent of the work in the critical care unit could be done by assistants without compromising quality. In addition, significant cost savings would be recognized with a decrease in registry nurses.

Comment: When there is reluctance to delegate, the root cause is more often lack of knowledge of the delegation-supervision principles and accountability principles. Basic delegation skills include knowing one's state nurse practice act, assessment of the situation, planning for the delegation, ensuring appropriate accountability, supervising performance of the task, and evaluation of the delegation process. When any of these steps are omitted, nurses assume the burden and take on overwhelming workloads that are nearly impossible to complete.

Scenario 15: Nurse–Patient–Organization. An experienced nurse administered an overdose of medication that resulted in serious patient instability and the need for additional therapeutic interventions. Although this was the nurse's first medication error, she was suspended and eventually terminated for unsafe practice on the basis of hospital policy. It was learned during the investigation that several safety checks were missed in the pharmacy department.

Comment: No nurse ever enters the profession of nursing to harm a patient. Given the inevitability of error in a human system, reacting to mistakes punitively is unlikely to minimize their occurrence, even though our culture leads us to expect the assignment of blame, correction of the error, and, in most cases, punishment of those who make the mistake. Attaching blame to individuals creates a climate of shame and guilt and further decreases candid reporting and discussion of mistakes.

The punishment of those who make errors fails to produce the desired results, namely, the elimination of error. The emphasis should be on recognizing and recovering from the error, to learn from mistakes, to identify actions that will decrease the chance of repeating the same mistakes, and to improve performance. The goal should always be to strive for excellence, not the unrealistic expectation of perfection given the uncontrollable variables present in the healthcare system.

Scenario 16: Given the situation in number 15, the nurse informed the patient and family of the error. The physician and other nurses are upset and believe this was not necessary because there was not lasting harm.

Comment: Disclosure of errors and apology is becoming more acceptable. Errors do not necessarily constitute improper, negligent, or unethical behavior, but failure to disclose them may.

Scenario 17: Nurse–Organization. Many states are advocating for safe staffing legislation. Some leaders believe this has resulted from leadership ineffectiveness. Others believe that it is the only way to address safe staffing issues.

Comment: External agencies should not be required to do the work an organization has committed to do—yet failed to do. The strategy to enact legislation to ensure safe staffing is representative of leadership failure to provide adequate staffing resources. Rather than work to legislate safe staffing, healthcare leaders should work to create effective systems and manage the reality of the imbalance between supply and demand.

Scenario 18: Nurse–Nurse. Peer review is a process used for evaluations. Three colleagues provide input, but policy does not allow the nurse to know specific feedback from each individual providing input. Nurses think it is unfair to withhold such information; the manager wishes to provide anonymity to participating staff to get honest information.

Open, honest dialogue about performance leads to better performance. Withholding or masking feedback behind an average rating within a 360-degree evaluation decreases an individual's opportunity to modify behaviors and reinforces the standard that open, direct communication is not an expectation. This policy should be modified to require open, honest sharing of feedback. Holding back information is an oppressive leadership behavior and prevents others from managing their own behavior.

Common Barriers to Effective Relationships

When one of these behaviors is identified, confront the issue and begin discussion to overcome and eliminate the barrier.

Bringing up unrelated issues	Holding a grudge—never forgive, never forget
Insisting that the problem is entirely the other person's fault	Being sarcastic
Being defensive	Being self-righteous and convinced you are right
Using the silent treatment	Disregarding the other person's feelings
Pretending nothing is wrong	Saying or doing things that are hurtful or cruel

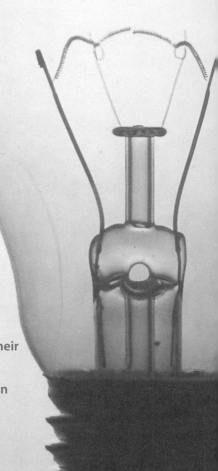

IF YOU WANT TO BUILD A SHIP, DON'T DRUM UP PEOPLE TO GATHER WOOD, SAW IT AND NAIL THE PLANKS TOGETHER. INSTEAD, BUILD IN THEM A PASSIONATE DESIRE FOR THE SEA.
—ANTOINE DE SAINT-EXUPERY

CHAPTER OBJECTIVES

Upon the completion of this chapter, the reader will be able to do the following:

» Understand the elements and processes associated with interdisciplinary team leadership and the particular role of the team leader.

» Define the role of the professional nurse as team leader and the unique skills necessary to make team leadership a basic expectation of the professional role.

» Enumerate the stages of the team process and the leadership skill capacity necessary to facilitate, coordinate, and integrate team action.

» Outline the characteristics of team dynamics related specifically to team roles, interaction, terms of engagement, and stages of team action.

» List at least 10 team fables that often impede understanding team process and obtaining effective team outcomes.

» State normative challenges teams confront in undertaking their work and identify mechanisms for managing them.

» Identify specific characteristics and skills of the team leader in relationship to collaboration, team dynamics, team decision making, managing conflict, and achieving team outcomes.

Team Leadership: The Foundation of Practice Effectiveness

All clinical activity essentially occurs in teams. In every work environment regardless of the unit of service, teams are key to work effectiveness (Losoncy, 1996). This is especially true in health care where the fundamental role of the nurse is to coordinate, integrate, and facilitate the activities of multiple players along the care continuum. As a professional nurse, it is critical to understand group dynamics, the essential characteristics of building the caring and clinical relationship, and the management and movement of effective teams.

While historic notions in health care set the physician as captain of the clinical team, both reality and practice demonstrate a more relevant notion of teams and leadership. Traditional configurations of teams having a single leader across the work spectrum and all team activities reflect an industrial model that is more historic than useful (Parker, 2003). This notion is also often reflective of paternalistic constructs for the leadership of teams. In more contemporary notions reflecting a deeper understanding of systems complexity, and using network metaphors as a frame, teams may take on a wide variety of forms. Teams are constantly in flux, shifting and changing members and processes depending on the character and emphasis of the activities to which teams are directed (Gratton & Erickson, 2007).

Because teams are social groups, they reflect the full spectrum of social life and human experience. Teams are sites for interaction, learning, communication, human expression, relationship building, and the expression of collective wisdom. Teams represent a central element in complex systems because they reflect a large number of interacting and intersecting components. These complex interactions lead to rich and important individual and group behaviors having specific and particular impact on the healthcare experience. From a variety of roles and perspectives reflecting the interaction between disciplines, the individual nurse, team associates, and patients, team dynamics are always at work.

REFLECTIVE QUESTION

How has the new digital world changed the way you interact and communicate with others? How will this digital reality affect the way you interact at work?

The Importance of Teams in Interdisciplinary Practice

Historically, in hospitals and health systems, teamwork has been often perceived as a departmental and unit function. Unit teams were generally made up of partners within the discipline including the registered nurse as team leader and associates and/or assistants as needed for the provision of clinical care (Barner, 2000). These discipline-specific teams rendered good care within the context of their own practice and functional work. These teams rarely included members from other disciplines. Broader notions of team involvement often meant utilizing the skill of other discipline resources when needed in a more incremental fashion representing more of a consulting relationship and interaction than inclusion in team membership and contribution (Ben Saoud & Mark, 2006). More recently, however, interdisciplinary team-based development has become a more critical notion of clinical care delivery. In the contemporary and more complex value-driven age of network systems, evidence-based practice, and clinical integration, the notion of broad-based team construction and clinical practice has emerged as a cornerstone in constructing the future of patient care (Curlee & Gordon, 2011). Digital technology, mobility-based communication systems, and the need to converge the work efforts of a wide variety of clinical members have coalesced to create the demand for a much more strongly defined foundation for interdisciplinary teamwork. Increasingly, the traditional historic biomedical model is giving way to a much more definitive complexity-based biopsychosocial model reflecting the intricacies and complexities of addressing and sustaining a health script along the continuum of care rather than simply undertaking late-stage incremental intervention in a tertiary care frame.

CRITICAL THOUGHT

In the 21st century, health care is quickly moving out of a biomedical model as its foundation toward a more complexity-based biopsycho-social model representing the intricacies of interaction and the interdependencies of the human network.

Because of the complexities of care, the need for interdisciplinary approaches draws upon the wide variety of expertise and specialties. They come from separate domains but link around patient problems and issues and intersect in a unique way that better addresses the substantive needs of patients. Driving much of this increased multilateral focus on patient care is the fact that much of the patient's own healing experience will occur in settings other than the hospital or healthcare system. The patient will need to engage significant others in managing his or her response to illness and the activities associated with either maintaining health or managing some level of their health status. Also, digitalization has created a social construct where the "user" becomes the owner of his or her own care and the intent and direction of technological application is to create more facility in this user for managing and directing his or her own care. This user-centric social reality shifts the accountability for impact, value, and sustainability from the provider to the individual and places full accountability for the ownership of health and the actions of the health journey on the individual rather than the health provider or the system. This shift in control from provider to user is perhaps the most significant driver of team-based interdisciplinary collaboration.

In this increasingly complex health environment, it becomes quickly apparent that no one discipline has all of the information, skills, and resources necessary to address the many intersecting needs of individual patients and patient populations. As the healthcare system continually recalibrates on substantive primary health and early intervention, an increasingly complex array of skill sets and team players will need to converge around the health script of patients and populations and work in highly collaborative teams through whose efforts clinical convergence and positive health outcomes will be achieved and sustained. Leadership of these teams will not be set by prescribed and fixed role delineations (e.g., physician directed); rather, leadership will be determined by the particular needs of the user and the combination of skills necessary to advance particular issues and concerns along the patient's continuum of care. This more emergent nature of leadership reflects a more self-organizing understanding of the dynamics of the team as it unfolds around specific needs or demands. Teams may therefore be led by a wide variety of different stakeholders, depending on at what point along the continuum of health service the intersection between health team and patient are located at any given time.

SCENARIO

Mrs. Wade, a 77-year-old long-term diabetic patient living alone in a high-rise apartment, is admitted to your unit because of complications related to uncontrolled glucose blood levels that appeared to have been poorly managed for some time. She is generally immobilized by neuropathic wounds on the ankles and metatarsals of both feet and appears also to have significant issues related to poor diet and malnutrition. She is alone yet alert and oriented and appears unable to continue to effectively self-manage her care.

Discussion Questions

1. As the attending nurse to Mrs. Wade, what interdisciplinary team members will need to be a part of your clinical team?

2. What role do you see for the physician on this team?

3. What team member will hold initial leadership on Mrs. Wade's clinical team?

4. What is the interdisciplinary team plan of care and how will you evaluate the synthesis of the efforts of all members in a way that shows how their care impacted the patient's experience?

The professional nurse therefore must recognize that a natural attribute of the nursing role in a complex system reflects historically held role competencies related to facilitation, coordination, and integration of clinical activities around a particular patient and his or her set of needs. This role delineation does not change in a complex environment; indeed, it becomes more critical. Essentially, the fundamental role of the professional nurse within the context of team-based collaborative approaches in primary patient care reemphasizes the centrality of coordination, integration, and facilitation of the activities of the team along the continuum of care. By both disposition and definition, the unique character of the role of professional nurse places the nurse at the intersection of the continuing care journey. The nurse operates at the interface between health system and everyone's response to the patient's needs. At this juncture between the disciplines, the nurse coordinates the need to address all the patient's needs and integrates the care of all the providers.

Team Construction

There are common elements in the construction of any team. Professional nurses must be aware that while teams may often form in a dynamic fashion, effective teams need design and structure in order to establish direction and evaluate progress with regard to team role and purpose. There are several elements essential for viable team construction. They are purpose, goals, roles, relationships, activities and functions, and coordination and leadership.

ELEMENTS OF AN EFFECTIVE TEAM

There are common elements in the construction of any team that must be the focus of development at the outset:

- Purpose
- Goals
- Roles
- Relationships
- Activities and functions
- Coordination and leadership

Purpose

Teams are formed in order to fulfill a specific purpose. There is a driving purpose for every team. The leader understands that the fundamental purpose for creating teams is to provide a general framework that advances the capacity of professionals to fully engage particular planning activities, decision making, and guide problem solving in a way that addresses patient care and improves team effectiveness. Engaging professional partners in team-based decision making helps them better understand decisions that are made, advances full participation in the process of making decisions, establishes a common frame of reference for problem solving, and ultimately advances ownership and investment in decisions and activities that relate to team activities. Team leadership and facilitation mean helping team members and stakeholders become clear about their reason for gathering and what end their collective deliberation will serve.

A statement of purpose is usually brief and focused. Although the statement of purpose will certainly evolve over time as work progresses, it does serve as an anchor to the work of the team and an indicator of the direction that is set for team activities. Examples of purpose statements are as follows:

- The purpose of this committee is to conduct a needs assessment of the clinical education priorities that better define the foundations of safe patient care on this unit.

- The purpose of this meeting is to finalize a clear decision regarding shared governance council meeting schedules for the next year.

The simpler and more direct a statement of purpose is, the clearer the work assignment becomes and the better understanding team members have of the direction of team activities.

Goals

After defining its purpose, every team has specific goals that are directed to fulfilling that purpose. The goal of clinical professional teams is generally to configure the provider members in a specific or unique arrangement around patient care processes or in specified efforts to meet the demands of advancing patient care. Specified goals enumerate the role and work of the team and, ultimately, the activities of each member in advancing that role. The establishment of goals is one of the more critical stages in team development. Goals give the team clear and specific direction and create a point of reference where teams can effectively evaluate their progress and determine movement toward completion. Goals involve both the team and individual members in defining the performance expectation of the team and when broken down can more clearly indicate the efforts and activities of individual team members. Congruence between team goals and individual member activities is essential to fulfilling the success of the team.

CRITICAL THOUGHT

Every team is simply the aggregation of the skills, talents, and behaviors of its participants. It is critical that the roles of all team members be clear and understood at the outset of team formation. It is ambiguity around role and contribution that can create the largest number of difficulties in making teams effective.

With clear goals the team leader can help the team avoid frustrations around ambiguity and lack of clarity as well as uncertainty in terms of specific activities and expectations of team members. Goals are tied to the purpose insofar as they become the tools for translating purpose into action in moving the team to some level of accomplishment. Here again, the simpler and more straightforward the goal, the clearer the expectation and the more likely it can be achieved.

Using the participatory process, the team leader generally engages the team in establishing goals. Because the goals provide the road map for the team's action, it is critical that everyone feel that they have participated fully in establishing direction and clarifying expectations of both members' actions and goals. The leader generally establishes goals and makes them visible through use of a white board or flip chart. The dynamics of the process contains basic elements the leader can use in helping the team focus on goals development:

- The team leader asks each team member the single most important activities that must be done in order to address the team's purpose.

- Team members should be given time to reflect on their responses and put them in writing in order to be clear about their own positions related to the goals.

- Identify congruence between goals and establish priorities with regard to goal activity and their relevance and relationship to the purpose.

- Prioritize goals as they relate to the goodness of fit with purpose and establish staging of goals in a trajectory that leads to fulfillment of the team's purpose.

- Clearly identify timelines and end dates related to specific accomplishment and fulfillment of the team's purpose.

- Be clear about the consequences of both performance and nonperformance. Usually the purpose defines the inherent deliverable or value of the team's action and therefore suggests the positive consequence. However, the negative consequence needs to be identified using terms such as "if we don't accomplish [a goal] what will happen or not happen; what will be the consequence; or what will be the impact?"

- When goals are clarified and established, and performance consequences and a timeline are determined, the team leader verifies understanding of goals, commits the team to achieving those goals, and finalizes the goals as the action steps enumerating the priorities and processes of the team's work (Curseu, 2003).

SETTING GOALS

1. Do the goals relate to the purpose?

2. Are the goals mutually supportive?

3. Are the goals clear and specific?

4. Do the goals relate to a specific action?

5. Can the goals be achieved by the work team?

6. Is there a way to measure points of progress and outcome?

7. Do the goals fit well together and aggregate in a way that fulfills the driving purpose?

It is always wise for the leader, after goals have been established and clarified, to obtain affirmation of understanding from each team member and specifically direct each team member to indicate how he or she understands the goals, what personal meaning the goals have in light of his or her own role, and a personal commitment to working with the team in achieving those goals.

Roles

The nurse team leader must sort through the participants on the team to determine what particular skills they could bring to problem solving. A lot of teamwork can be allocated and delegated to specific individuals or groups on the team with specialized skills (Chrispeels, 2004). Constructing team membership carefully is a major task of the nurse team leader. Aligning skills with specified work tasks on the team is a part of the role of the leader as he or she discerns the character of the work, the distribution of that work, and the best way to break down elements of the work into meaningful components. When the objectives are clearly ascertained, there are specific elements of work on the team that generally are not best done by all team members working together. Depending on the size of the team, much of the work that has been delineated through the setting of objectives can be accomplished through the use of smaller work groups.

TEAM TIP

Leaders always need to prepare for the team's work before the team ever meets. For team effectiveness the leader must establish the following:

- Rules of behavior
- Purposeful information
- Requisite financial data
- Good deliberation processes
- Clear sense of the role of members
- Information
- Terms of engagement

In performing against the objectives set by the team with regard to specific work, it is important that the work is closely aligned with the skills available on the team. While members of the team must have particular responsibilities in terms of meeting goals and objectives, it is not necessary that they simply meet those objectives through their own efforts. An effective team leader knows that there may need to be additional participation in team activities and that team members who are assigned specific additional work with regard to a goal or objective have the right to also access additional resources that will help inform or advance these specific tasks (Belbin, 2010). Making specific assignments that address core objectives and goal activity with regard to the purpose of the committee, the nurse leader needs to be sure the following elements are included in the assignment of work:

- Individuals who are charged with the responsibility for a particular goal need to be clear about what those specifics are and what the expectations are related to progress.

- A clear delineation of the action steps associated with fulfilling the purpose of the group's work must be determined and specifically enumerated by team leadership.

- Members working on particular goal-directed activity need to be clear about the time and resources they need to undertake the work and to effectively deliberate and act in a way that fits their assigned responsibility.

- The determination of the specific timetable and clear expectations with regard to the completion of the action related to a goal must be established early and related to the time parameters within which the goal must be achieved.

- Measures of success with regard to the specific goal must be incorporated into the team member work so that markers that indicate progress toward success can be used as definitive points of measure with regard to appropriate progress or real challenges to meeting the work group's performance expectations.

CRITICAL THOUGHT

Team leadership and working well with others is always a learned skill. No matter how well we know other team members, working in the context of a team requires a higher level of managing relationships and building team effectiveness. This work will consume much of the energy of the leader.

Relationships and the Terms of Engagement

The overall success and effectiveness of a team depends predominantly on the relationships and interactions through which the team does its work (Dunin-Keplicz & Verbrugge, 2010). Maintaining positive team dynamics and healthy interactions form the foundation for successful communication and progress with regard to team efforts and accomplishments. A major part of successfully moving the team is making sure that all members understand the rules of engagement and communication in order to make sure that the team remains positive and constructive in both its relationship and its work.

Terms of engagement are those general rules of relationship and interaction that the team adheres to as a way of maintaining a positive communication and interaction environment within the context of the team as it completes its work. Teams are driven by human dynamics and are therefore subject to the foibles and challenges of making these dynamics effective and productive. Therefore, the nurse team leader needs to be aware of his or her role in firmly enumerating the rules of communication and interaction that are critical to maintaining balance, equity, and fairness in team processes. Some of those might include the following elements:

- Members should be required to stay within the context of the issues and deliberations currently on the table. Reaching far afield in dialogue and in making points rather than sticking specifically to the points being discussed at the table wastes time. It causes anxiety with regard to maintaining focus on the specific work of the committee or team. The chair works to maintain focus on the issues at hand and limit the amount of peripheral or far-reaching dialogue that may not relate specifically to the efforts being undertaken at that time.

- The nurse team leader works diligently to make sure that judgment-laced language is not a part of the team's interaction or deliberation. Avoiding judgments about others' views or what they say is important in constructing an even table and advancing positive contributions.

- Team leaders always work to make sure that all participants are expected to contribute fully to the dialogue and processes associated with the team's work. It should be clear to team members that presence on the team does not simply mean a warm body sitting at the table. Team member presence means full engagement, investment, and pursuit of the team's objectives demonstrated by fully participating in the dialogue and interaction necessary to good teamwork.

- It is critical that team members avoid judgment words that reflect other people's thoughts or contribution to ensure that everyone's participation is honored. The nurse leader should help team members avoid moderating and judging language that negatively impacts individual contributions. Words such as "I agree," "I disagree," "you are right," "you are wrong" (almost any "you" statements or judgment statements) should be carefully identified as unacceptable and eliminated from the dialogue among team members.

- Establishing interaction parameters for communication should be done early in the team process and incorporated into a team communication charter as the foundation for established team communication behavior. Enumerating these elements and carefully affirming them as a part of the foundations of team processes is important to the effective work of the team and may need to be frequently referenced as they get forgotten at varying moments in the team process.

Issues related to challenges, problems, or emergent concerns are challenges that are generally a part of effective deliberation in teams. The nurse team leader should be aware that these are normative factors and to be expected as an ordinary operating part of a functioning team. The moderating role of the team leader is to not only be aware of these potential realities but to access the terms of engagement periodically as a reminder of the methods of communication that have been established by members as their way of doing business when individual members continue to either flaunt or ignore the terms of engagement (Salas, Goodwin, & Burke 2009). The team leader must have specific and focused conversations with that individual. These help challenge and remind the person of the obligations of membership or encourage them to alter aberrant behavior in order to better facilitate the work of the team. Consistent failure on the part of a team member to adhere to the terms of engagement, despite counseling, becomes

SCENARIO

You have been a member of the nursing unit for the past 12 months. The staff get along very well and there is a lot of team commitment to patient care. However, there has been a great deal of difficulty with appropriate shift staffing coverage, and staff members' commitment to their schedules appears to be passive, almost lackadaisical. The nurse manager works diligently to develop the schedules but appears to have a great deal of difficulty getting staff acceptance of schedules and making sure the staff follow their schedules. The problem with staff variable response to the schedule is evident in misunderstanding of work times scheduled.

You have agreed to lead the exploration of a self-scheduling process. It is agreed that a team of staff members will work together to develop a self-scheduling methodology, and you have been appointed the team leader. Explore the following questions as they relate to your role as team leader of this work group.

Discussion Questions

1. What will be the purpose statement for your team's action?

2. What reflection will you make with regard to who needs to be members of the team?

3. How large should the team be?

4. What information do you need to have available prior to the first team meeting?

5. What decisions will you make about personal characteristics of participants and how will that influence your effort to create sufficient diversity on the team?

6. Who would you select as your advisor/mentor to assist in your own team leadership development and assessment?

a disciplinary issue and needs management intervention and involvement as a final stage of resolution.

Don't Be Trapped by the 10 Team Fables

As a team leader you will need to confront much of the mythology and fable around the process of building effective teams. While there is much literature and documentation on creating effective teams, there is also a need to be aware of what impedes good team effectiveness. The following are 10 key moderators of effectiveness that should be addressed and kept in mind by the team leader:

Fable One: Team Members Always Feel Committed to Implementing a Good Team Process

This fable represents a myth that is really quite dangerous for the leader. Most people on health-related teams come from a clinical frame of reference. While they may have worked with each other, they have not necessarily related to each other in a formalized team process. Working with each other in the same place, within the same department, and even with the same patient population does not guarantee that the people work together well in a structured team format. Constructing a team-based frame for understanding the collective work of the service is very different from simply doing clinical work with other people. Also, the team leader should be careful not to be deluded into believing that people really want to work well in teams. Often, while well intentioned, they are really not clear about what teamwork entails. Most people have not learned how to work within the context of formalized teams. Just as leading a team is a learned skill, so is membership on the team a learned capacity. However, given appropriate time and use of the developmental and implementation tools available, carefully constructing a realistic approach to building team effectiveness helps facilitates staff coming quickly on board. Understanding that team construction includes development for team members will be an important beginning insight for developing an effective team.

Fable Two: All Team Members Are Created Equal

Perhaps one of the most dangerous considerations in building teams is the belief that all team members will have something of value to contribute to the team just by virtue of their presence. Keep in mind, the team members come to the role of team interaction with different beliefs about their own person, contribution, interactional skills, and the relationship to others on the team. The leader should have some early concerns around creating the foundation of equity, balance, and involvement of members on the team. As is outlined more specifically in other parts of this chapter, physicians come to the team with an entirely different sense of self and role perception than does the professional nurse, respiratory therapist, or physical therapist. On the other hand, the nurse comes to the team with a unique understanding of his or her role. The nurse needs to be able to participate from a strongly facilitative perspective. Each member will come to the team process within individualized insights, precepts, and levels of self-confidence regarding the expression of member roles that will need to be understood and clarified at the outset of the team formation. Many of the early developmental processes associated with growing an effective team will have the team leader working through issues of participant equity in an effort to build effective and truly collaborative team deliberation.

Fable Three: People Really Want to Reach Agreement and Move Past Their Issues of Concern

REFLECTIVE QUESTION

Is it possible to influence and change team behavior through preplanning and building good structures and processes within which the team will work? In other words, can good structure determine good team behavior?

One of the most difficult elements of team process the leader will confront relates to effective decision making and the ability to build consensus around meaningful decisions. The truth is, most people who come to a team do not know how to make good decisions. Members often do not understand the process of consensus building nor do they recognize that consensus can be obtained through a number of techniques and applications that, once learned, are very effective in moving the group to make good decisions. Clearly, for the team leader, knowing these techniques will be critical to team effectiveness and advancing decision making. The team leader must learn the techniques and approaches to moving the team to successful decision making and problem solving. For the team leader this is an early learning requirement and is a process that will require some concerted and intentional effort. The new team leader must be devoted to early learning activities around the techniques and modalities of good team decision making and build personal and collective skill, develop insight with regard to progress, and accelerate the capacity for leading effectively.

Fable Four: Team Members Generally Use Good Critical Thinking to Resolve Their Questions and Issues

Initially one of the more disheartening realities of team management is the leader's eventual recognition that team members do not necessarily exhibit the capacity for problem solving or the skill set for structured thinking the leader might have hoped for early in the team construction process. Often, analytical, objective, deductive, or reductive processes are not used by team members in the process of doing this new and more disciplined, collective work. Much of the skill that is reflected in team members' own patient care activities tends to be intuitive and responsive, a key reflection of their talents and skills honed over time that are second nature to their practice work. On the other hand, in team-based activities the discipline of critical thinking and problem-solving applications becomes more visible and is more essential in effective team deliberation and organized problem solving. While this may not be initially exciting work, refining deliberative and critical thinking skills within the team's activities will be important to effective skill development. The nurse leader must see at the outset of teamwork that time must be spent in verifying and advancing the team's problem-resolving skills. Where the effort of reflection, discernment, and discourse articulates well with the functions, activities, and priorities of good teamwork, good results can be achieved. Using good techniques that reflect evidentiary dynamics, the utility of accurate and timely information, good analysis and rationale development and decision-making synthesis will be important initial activities in ensuring the effectiveness and sustainability of the team's work.

Fable Five: Team Members Will Set Aside Their Emotional Issues in the Interest of Effective Team Decision Making

Of course, it is ideal to expect that team members are able to balance their emotional sensitivities with the requirements of the team and the elements of good team decision making. While this can ultimately happen with regard to team effectiveness, the team leader should not expect emotional maturity to be generally present at the outset. This kind of balance is as much a learned skill as any other and requires some specific focus and even some developmental activities on the part of the team. Early team facilitation should include from the leader a careful dialogue around the role emotion plays and the impact of feeling, expression, and the obligations of healthy communication in team dynamics. The team leader must remember that people work never ends in team dynamics and that individual circumstances and behaviors will always be a part of the team management process. However, making space for dialogue around the impact and implications of member feelings, emotions, interactions, and ownership is all a part of the dynamics of team interaction and therefore should be expected, even encouraged, as well as effectively managed by the team leader.

CRITICAL THOUGHT

Each of us develops our patterns of behavior over the years of our lives. It is a false expectation that we always know why we do what we do. Careful and caring attention to addressing the habits and rituals of others is important to building team effectiveness. Good leadership and facilitation techniques and methods can make the process work of teams operate effectively and create an open and responsive framework for accommodating the delicate personal issues that are always a part of good team function.

Fable Six: Each Team Member Fully Understands Why They Act as They Do

One of the mysteries of human relationships is the recognition that people bring different meaning, value, behavior, and insights to their activities and to their team interactions. While much of this behavior is unconscious activity, all individual behavior affects collective behavior. Surprisingly, many people do not fully understand the impact of their individual expressions on others. Human beings behave in ways that may make sense to themselves but do not necessarily positively impact their relationship with others. In team interaction, however, the unconscious must be made conscious. The team leader attempts to identify and advance normative interactions and minimize aberrant behavior, whether it be conscious or unconscious, that in any way fails to support good communication and effective deliberation as a member of the team. Certainly, terms of engagement help establish effective rules of communication and interaction. The team leader must depend on these interactive principles as a way of guiding appropriate dialogue and discussion and minimizing communication that is either negative or poorly expressed.

Fable Seven: People Always Want to Work with Others

While we often idealize the notion of team-based behavior, the truth is that people do not necessarily either want to, or know how to, work well with others. In clinical environments, much of the work that is done is driven by individuated action. Team-related interaction is often a secondary consideration of individual work. Teamwork is significantly different from unilateral action. Recognizing the unique character of a team and the characteristics of work in team relationships is very different from working in loose work groups. Team participants are not always precisely clear about the dynamics of teamwork and what is necessary to create and sustain an effective team. Becoming a functional, well integrated, fluid, effective, and synergistic team represents personal effort to tame unhealthy unilateral characteristics. The working synergy of a good team has a major influence on the achievement of positive outcome. However, this synergy is not achieved quickly nor is it easily effected by the team leader. Synergy develops over time and through the effort of good team interaction, deliberation, and decision making. Here again the team leader must develop the facility to build team congruence, effective interaction, good deliberation, strong decisions, and critical outcomes.

Fable Eight: Effective Teams Grow Naturally

The truth is, teams do not grow accidentally or naturally. Teams are constructed groups that undergo disciplined development before they can contribute to the fulfillment of the purposes for which they have gathered. Teams, much like other aspects of life, grow intermittently and incrementally; they do not grow in a straight line. Teams experience pushes and pulls, ups and downs, flurries of positive and meaningful activity, and periods of dormancy and nonproductivity. Incremental, intermittent processes and energy associated with teamwork represent highly variable elements of human relationship and interaction. Therefore, the team leader should not expect good team processes and effective deliberation to flow in a seamless continuum of good deliberation without anticipating the many challenges brought by a collection of a wide variety of competing human behaviors.

Fable Nine: Building Trust Is an Important Role of the Team Leader

The truth is, trust cannot be built. Trust actually represents or demonstrates something that's already in place. Trust is actually a visible representation of the work and methodology already underway whose effectiveness and success indicate the presence of trust. Trust is therefore a reflection of all the elements that give evidence of its presence. The only thing the leader can do to effect trust is to undertake the positive and productive activities that result in the sense of inclusion, engagement, openness, confidence, and good feeling among members of the team. For the team leader, it is important to recognize that building the elements of team effectiveness and constructing a frame for positive relationships and safe dialogue create the conditions that are ultimately demonstrated by the trust people have that the team is a safe and positive place where one can contribute, be valued, and make a difference. Just as trust can reflect what is good in team dynamics, it can be broken through major breaches in good process in broken relationship or through a series of minor breaks in the interactions among team members at any point along the continuum of team processes. The effort of the team is not so much in building trust but more in generating relationships processes and methodologies that address the circumstances and conditions that best demonstrate that trust is present. The role of the leader in this scenario is to advance the integrity and strength of the relationships of team members, advance their ability to problem solve and seek solutions, build the team's skill in dealing with performance issues and challenges and, finally, advance the team's ability to consistently obtain expectations and outcomes. Progress in each of these arenas will be critical to the sustenance and advancement of the conditions that ultimately demonstrate the presence of prevailing trust.

CRITICAL THOUGHT

Trust is not something that can be created. Trust is evidence of what is already present between people. If there is a safe, effective, rewarding, and well-functioning team with confidence of value and positive continuing relationships, that will be the evidence that trust is present.

Fable 10: Team Members Will Always Focus on the Outcomes to Which Their Effort Is Directed

Team members will not always focus on their work or their outcomes. Indeed, frequently group members will become unclear about what their purpose is and the related activities and even forget the outcomes to which their efforts are directed. A good part of the functional work of the team leader is to help the team continuously renew its understanding of its purpose, the value of its processes, the direction of its work, and the proximity of the team to its outcomes. Building in a continuous mechanism for evaluating place and progress is a good way for the team leader to check in with regard to where the team is in its work and progress against expectations and purpose. Achieving short-term or small outcomes may be a sign for the team leader to move on to the next phase, step, or goal of the team's effort to fulfill its purpose. Furthermore, team leaders remind their teams of specific conditions or circumstances impacting the purpose and goal in a way that helps the team continually evaluate process and outcome. Teams often find themselves so tied up in their process and activities that they often forget the ends to which their work leads. In this case, the work often becomes an end in itself, and purpose and meaning get lost inside activity and function. Reacquainting team members with the questions related to purpose and value helps the team reaffirm its work and firmly establishes a goodness of fit between what it is doing and the values it is seeking to advance.

Team Progress

Progress in teamwork is not always a straight line from initiation to success. Most human teams experience varying degrees of progress over increments of high achievement intertwined with times of minimal progress (Chau & elibrary, 2008). The leader must expect that these vagaries operate in the course of any level of effective teamwork and plan for them accordingly. Teams are also unusual insofar as they often reflect working relationships or a set of interactions that are not experienced in the same way as individual work. Teams are essentially an artificial construction that are neither permanent nor represent the usual or traditional relationships and interactions in the workplace. Often members of a team may not work with each other regularly and may only have interaction with each other during the course of the team process. While there are both strengths and deficits with regard to this particular dynamic, it is important for the leader to recognize these forces are at work during team activities. As the teamwork progresses constructively with some measure of success, these more negative dynamics sometimes operate just below the surface and should be anticipated so people are not surprised by them. Accordingly, as these forces make team progress challenging, or make progress difficult or slow, recognizing them as a normative part of team dynamics helps create a more positive frame for the issues (Parker, 2008). This allows team members to see the possibility of getting past them or even resolving the issues they may engender, creating a positive frame for team relationships compensating for the negative behaviors or interactions that can represent people's level of frustration, lack of progress, and difficulty in working through apparently intractable problems with each other.

It is the role of the nurse team leader to both monitor and moderate the effect of progress and challenges to an effective team dynamic. First, the team leader must not be overwhelmed by the seesaw between small successes as they intertwine with moments of challenge. This is normal and usual in the efforts of teamwork directed toward specific goals. In fact, the team leader should anticipate these swings and affirm to members that these elements will be a part of the team dynamics at a number of points in the team process. What is important is for the team leader to anticipate these events and to plan for them with appropriate responses anticipated in advance of their occurrence (Mash et al., 2008).

TEAM TIP

In an effort to be thorough, team leaders and members often construct more priorities for the team than they can ever address. Team leaders should create an agenda with no more than three to five items around which focused work activities are centered. This helps ensure that the goals for the meeting can be addressed in the time available.

The team's small successes should be celebrated by members as they progress. Success should not be saved only for the major accomplishments. Instead, the team leader should provide opportunities for the team to take time out at times of small successes to enumerate them, to identify and position them as critical steps along the trajectory of major progress, and to celebrate them as indicators of positive movement toward goal completion. Surprisingly, the same approaches taken with regard to momentary challenges are just as important. The leader needs to point out to the team members that these challenges are also signposts of significant moments and signs of progress that simply need further refinement, deliberation, clarification, and renewal of effort in order to better direct the team's work toward the goals or as a part of the effort to clarify different strategies necessary to keep the team moving (Rondeau, 2007). Through these actions, the leader recalibrates the team's action steps toward particular efforts and achievements. In these moments of challenge or team delay, the team leader needs to take on the relevant issues with transparence and specificity. Some immediate response strategies the team leader could initiate within the team process are as follows:

- Reaffirm specific goals and activities that were identified as essential to the team's progress toward fulfillment of the purpose of the team. Reaffirmation of the goals and stages of the team's work helps reestablish their relevance and affirm the direction of the team in relationship to its purpose.

- Place the problem, barrier, or challenge specifically within the context of particular stages or elements of change management in order to enumerate the particular context within which the problem falls to help prevent the generalization of the problem to the whole purpose and progress of the team.

CRITICAL THOUGHT

From time to time the team may need to access external consultation to help provide information or impetus regarding a particular deliberation. The team leader should always seek whatever resources and support are necessary to help inform or advance the team's thinking and work.

- When the context of the issue has been delineated, help break the problem down into smaller issues so it can be better understood and more specifically dealt with within the context of the stage, gap, or elements of the goal affected by the problem. Here again, the team leader attempts to see the problem in context and to suggest that no one particular problem can by itself be a threat to the purpose or goals of the team. Instead a problem may merely be an issue that helps the team refine and hone its focus. These smaller issues may actually move the team forward more effectively, addressing concerns that affect progress and/or affirm direction.

- When team goals and efforts have been reaffirmed by the team and articulated by the team leader, identifying particular responses and solutions helps keep the team's effort focused and enables clear delineation of team-derived responses and opportunities and removes the issue as a barrier.

- It is often helpful for the team leader to bring in experts and skilled problem solvers that can help reinform, broaden the insight, present new information, or help the team recalibrate efforts and strategies that overcome problems or barriers in a more creative and unique manner. New insights and understanding of the problem help reenergize the team and bring to bear a new focus on solutions that will further the process and move the team forward.

The nurse team leader must be aware of the various strategies that can help the team advance critically toward fulfilling its purpose and achieving its goals. It is important that the team leader recognize that he or she must be flexible and fluid in terms of anticipating challenges and changes within the team process. This leader must be consistent with and faithful to the team's purpose and goals and be willing to make necessary adjustments in approach to advance the interests and competence of the team, maintain a high level of commitment and energy to the work of the team, and help the team undertake new and different strategies that can ensure successful movement toward goals and the fulfillment of the team purpose.

When the Problem Is a Team Member

The nurse team leader will often find challenges emerging from members on the team either by virtue of individual patterns of behavior, problems in relationships among team members, or varying levels of commitment or contribution of team members to the purposes and efforts of the team. Here again, this is not an uncommon set of circumstances and should be seen as a normative expectation in the course of any interactive, relationship-based process. However, even though such dynamics are normative, the team leader should develop strategies for addressing these challenges early. The leader's effort must support team interaction over the course of the team's work. When the problem is individual team member behavior, early engagement and intervention are critical to the progress of the team and for ensuring that the negative impact of the anomalous team member's behavior does not have lingering effects on the integrity and effectiveness of the team's work.

There will always be challenging elements of human behavior the team leader must be prepared to address. Professionals need to be aware of the reality that even the best-intended members will represent challenges to team leader activity and team member progress. These challenges reflect the dynamics inherent in human interaction and simply demonstrate the need for continuing good facilitation, problem solving, and competence building. When aberrant behavior arises, none of these circumstances should be seen as a terminal event for the leader and team effectiveness; they are simply human characteristics that are part of the collective work of deliberation and teamwork. Their occurrence also reflects the need of a good team leader to have facilitation skills that help address the noise of human dynamics and team interaction (Rouse, 2007). Skill development is the most critical component of successfully addressing team relationship and interaction problems. These skills develop over time with maturation, experience, and personal experimentation. The good team seeks leader mentorship and guidance in the process of learning and exercising the leadership role. The openness of the team leader to accessing expertise and guidance from mentors and leaders in the organization provides valuable resources as the team leader builds skill competence in team facilitation. The positive development of talent in dealing with personal conflict challenge and anomalous team member behaviors can be addressed with good technique, opportunity, patience, and continuous and faithful application of honed skills, which can make all the difference in facilitating team interaction and performance effectiveness.

TEAM TIP

In order to minimize misunderstandings and problems with individual team member behavior, the team leader should clearly review and affirm the operating expectations of team members, including each of the following:

- Functions
- Activities
- Relationships
- Interaction
- Processes
- Expectations
- Outcomes

Collaboration

The development and use of teams for decision making and work processes could fill many textbooks, and have. While this is simply an introduction for the professional, team-based dynamics is the preferred method through which he or she will work for the full course of professional life. Historic leader learning has not emphasized the critical understanding that team-based work frames are the primary way in which professionals advance decision making and work processes. Collaboration is the essential central methodology through which the diverse team stakeholders work in order to advance the interactions that both define team response to patient needs and advance the team's competence in serving their population well.

Collaboration implies the capacity to have team members work well together, deliberate purposefully, and decide and act in ways that are in the best interest of both the patient and the team (Peterson & King, 2007). The team leader has the responsibility for ensuring that the structure and framework of the team's action represent what is necessary to advance the collaborative care process.

COMMON MYTHS ABOUT TEAMS

- Good teams don't need strong leaders
- Teams can always be self-directed
- Failure is a sign of an ineffective team
- Good teams don't experience conflict
- Teams should never experiment
- Individuals, not teams, are important
- You cannot really evaluate teams
- Left alone, teams get into trouble
- Teams are always well supervised
- Individuals perform better than teams
- Team players are compliant and quiet
- Teams who err are failures

Teamwork operates very much like a well-designed and structured symphony. The discipline of effective teams very much represents a dance. It is the obligation of the team leader within a collaborative work model to carefully and judiciously plan the character and content of the team's work and anticipate how the team will accomplish that work. The discipline of good planning for collaboration requires that the team leader utilize the necessary skills to facilitate the initiation of good team collaboration.

Decisions

The most important aspects of the team leadership is the team leader's clarity with regard to the decisions around which the team will gather. One of the great errors of teamwork is the often idealized belief that teams really do gather to undertake processes that will result in the achievement of some goal or outcome. Actually, the true foundation of team effectiveness is bound up in whether that team is dealing with the right questions and that the questions are clear enough to the team such that they will bring the right answer to those questions. Therefore, the team leader must make sure everyone is consistently certain of the purpose around which the team is gathered and the questions that initiate that work. Team questions can range anywhere from organizational objectives to clinical behaviors and personal fulfillment of standards, practices, or activities. Whenever the team is forming and questions arise about what decision making will be used, the selection of approach should be clear and precise. The sooner the leader learns that his or her focus is on a question specific to each stage of the deliberative process, it helps the group focus on doing its work (Porter-O'Grady, 2009).

TEAM LEADER'S CHECKLIST

- Make sure all the elements of the team and team performance are acting congruently.
- Maintain a consistent leadership style that best fits the character and content of teamwork.
- Make sure the team adheres to all the rules of engagement that they have developed and corrective action is undertaken early when there are breeches.
- Manage team error and conflict early and well, establishing processes that address these issues calmly as a normal part of team processes.
- Watch for individual behavior that acts in opposition to the synthesis and effectiveness of team performance.
- Meet frequently with individuals and the full team to assess progress, confront issues, undertake learning, and measure goal achievement.

Setting the Table: Overcoming the Uneven Table

When the questions around which the team will gather are clear to the facilitator, it becomes important to make decisions about how those questions are best constructed to address the diversity at the table. The team leader's interest is in ensuring that the questions driving the team's work are broadly enough informed and served by the breadth of membership at the team table. **Setting the table** means knowing how all the decisions need to be served, what talent or expertise needs to be gathered, the size of the team in relationship to the issues it will be addressing, and what particular gifts and skills will be available to the team as they deliberate the questions before them.

Breadth of representation on the team is important and must be reflected in the kind of people selected to deal with those issues. One of the greatest difficulties in team management is focusing the team on its work with an adequate array of resources at the table. Often teams will be formed because of the relationship of members to particular disciplines or to a geographical location or even some affinity to the issue itself. These are not the best reasons for gathering people together in a team process. If the table is to perform its work effectively, that work must be well served by the right skills, talents, and team capacity in order to address the issues before the members. This process of careful selection based on the members' personal alignment and commitment to the team goals helps establish the strength of the team before it even begins to do its work and provides a healthy backdrop for ensuring that the collaborative process can work well. Aligning membership with team goals and work is one of the most critical elements in ensuring team effectiveness.

Just as diversity is essential to the decision-making process and team collaboration, it is also vital in terms of the kinds of team members around the table regarding or related to particular behaviors they will bring. Nothing is worse than having a team's patterns of behavior limiting progress and challenging good relationships, thus making it difficult for the facilitator to coordinate and integrate the decision-making process with the collaborative team. Behavior patterns are critical to the success of deliberation and of team processing. Bringing behavioral balance between representing the breadth of skills and personal dynamics will be important to good team dynamics even before the team has formed (Larson, 2011).

CRITICAL THOUGHT

All teams experience conflict. All conflict has value. The good team leader looks at conflict as a normal part of team effectiveness and simply engages it early and often.

People bring as much diversity to their patterns of behavior as they bring diversity with regard to their personality characteristics. Setting the table for the kinds of personality characteristics that need to be present in the deliberation of an issue requires that the nurse leader carefully reflect on the dynamic that needs to be expressed in order to make the deliberation process effective and move the team in a valid direction. Loading a team with highly articulate dramatic and aggressive operators will create a lot of action on the team but will not yield much consensus. On the other hand, loading the team with highly reflective, thoughtful, and nonexpressive people means the team will be deliberating a great deal but will not necessarily move to decision and action in a timely fashion. The goal is to be able to mix actors and reflectors in a broad diversity of representation so that significant balance is brought between those who can well articulate the drive to decision making and action with those who can thoughtfully and carefully reflect on the meaning of the discussion and the implication the discussion might raise for people and for organizations.

In addition to care and caution with regard to table setting for personality and behavioral characteristics of team members, the attitude of team members with regard to the team and the issues it will address is an element of team facilitation that is frequently underaddressed. The team leader needs to be aware that in every deliberation process there are negative elements that operate. At a minimum this negative undercurrent can slow the team's progress or cripple its deliberative dynamics. Negative behaviors and responses can create a milieu for the team that discourages team membership participation, diminish the energy necessary to address critical issues, and often delay the effectiveness of the team's deliberation and decision-making process. Here again, the team leader must be prepared for the negative dynamics that are inevitably present in the course of almost any kind of teamwork. Preparation in advance means the leader develops the techniques and skills necessary for dealing with negative behaviors and for establishing terms of engagement about team processes to which all team members will adhere. These terms of engagement are critical to the collaborative dynamic because they provide the frame for dialogue and establish a rule set within which team members can operate and with which team members can build a sense of personal safety and trust in the process of heavy, diverse deliberation. These terms of engagement serve as a discipline for the team and a framework for the team leader to access when team behaviors do not act consistent with the standards established by team members at the outset.

SCENARIO

Sam is the leader of a relatively new team. The team is finishing the first stage of development and is developing rules of engagement, performance expectations, and common goals. The team has been making good progress with regard to its formation activities; however, it is having some difficulty dealing with conflict emerging between two strong team members. Sam sees this conflict coming fairly early in the process, but he is a little concerned about how to properly address it. Two other team members are becoming aware of the conflict between the two strong personalities, and both have come to Sam mentioning their concerns that this problem may be growing and is beginning to have an effect on team cohesiveness as well as their team processes.

Sam wants to take care of this problem as quickly as possible. In the past, Sam has always taken care of these issues in a one-to-one exchange, exerting his personal leadership. He realizes, however, that this is a team issue and should be addressed within the context of the team. He knows that the team must own its relationships between team members and work to resolve this conflict as soon as possible. Furthermore, Sam knows that, as team leader, he must facilitate the processes that will lead to confronting this issue, ultimately creating a framework for the team's ability to work together and achieve outcomes. Sam feels struck and needs some insight and assistance. He has come to you for guidance.

Discussion Questions

1. What are the elements of the conflict resolution process that Sam must be aware of as he walks through the stages of addressing the conflict between these two individuals?

2. How does Sam engage the team in owning and investing in this conflict resolution process?

3. How does Sam keep the environment safe yet push for resolution among team members as well as ensure a successful conflict resolution process?

4. How does Sam evaluate the effectiveness of the process used and whether it made any difference?

Some terms of engagement contain some of the following elements:

- Each member of the team will have an opportunity to speak. A procedural caveat: when that opportunity is presented, the individual who has spoken is challenged by the discussion facilitator not to raise his or her issue again or respond to it until at least one or two other team members have responded to the issue.

- Avoid the use of judgment terms, such as "I agree" or "I disagree." These judgment statements at no time are relevant to the deliberation nor do they contribute content to the discussion. They are instead simply fragments of personal judgment that are not essential to the value of the common good at the table. Members should be encouraged to simply share their views rather than reflect those views as a reaction to others' views.

- Team members should be encouraged to use "I" statements as a way of expressing their thoughts or notions so that their ownership of them can be quickly established. Participants should always be expected and encouraged to operate from the perspective that reflects their personal ownership for their views and contributions made to the group deliberation.

- The use of appreciative strategies in conversation (those techniques that add value to the conversation rather than react to the prevailing negatives in a conversation) should be encouraged and stimulated. Participants must be continually seeing themselves contributing to further deliberation and refinements of decision making in a way that moves them forward rather than reacting or acting on negative statements regarding the process or the deliberation before them. Keeping this appreciative frame recalibrates the discussion within the context of the possible and the relevant in a way that positively grows the team's efforts to advance meaningful change.

- The chair makes regular time available to the team to take momentary time out to evaluate the team's sense of its own progress and its operating dynamic. This process of checking in helps the team reanchor its deliberations and make some judgments with regard to progress and challenges in the team's work.

Interdisciplinary Alignment

Clinical teams in health care have some unique issues that need to be the specifically addressed prior to the team undertaking work. Historically in health care, hierarchy has been a significant impediment to the collateral horizontal nature of collaborative relationships. Historically, specific healthcare individuals have had a different level of status and relationship in the system, creating issues of equity, value, and integration of decision making in the system. For example, physicians have historically been outside the employee category in hospitals and healthcare systems. For the most part, the majority of physicians have been self-employed and have a different relationship to the hospital or healthcare community than any of the other players that comprise the deliberative team. This is an important consideration when one includes physicians in the deliberative work group because the implicit character of the physician's role is one that has traditionally been perceived as leader or director of healthcare decision making. Whether or not there is any evidence of the truth of that notion, it is a commonly perceived characterization within the healthcare system. This role identity places in the center of the team's deliberation a mental model contributed to by both the physician and other team members that may create some difficulty in establishing common ground, equity, and respect for all contributions on the team. Furthermore, what often occurs in team dynamics is evidenced when the physician member of the team is not happy with the team's work. Because of historic preset notions of the physician's role and position in health care, the team often assumes that the physician's nonapproval serves as a veto of the team's direction, decisions, or progress. Subordinating characterizations and behaviors make it difficult to get equivalent value from all team contributions at such an uneven table. The team leader must recognize some of these historic role presets with regard to expectations, performance, and behaviors and be able to address them at the outset of the team's deliberative process. Simple rules need to be established. Matters such as how people on the team will be addressed (everyone's use of first names, for example) in order to ensure that there is a common understanding of how people are recognized on the team, the role team members will play with regard to each other within the team dynamic, and the expectation of equal contribution and value of all members and contributions of the team needs to be clarified as the team begins to do its work (Finkelman, 2011). Teams often fail because this step has not been carefully deliberated and decisions related to the team's processes haven't been well articulated in a way that sets the team up for sound collaborative processes and for good decision making. This effort at creating an even table is one of the most critical formative steps of the team leader in ensuring an effective framework for team dynamics (Kritek, 2002).

Focus on the Team Leader

The team leader has huge implications with regard to the power of influence that can drive the team toward effective and responsive processes and ensure the good alignment among reflection, group energy, engagement, coordination, and communication (Yukl, 2009). Early commitment on the part of the team leader is vital to ensuring the team is structured appropriately and has the information it needs to do its work and get access to resources, processes, and creativity necessary to advance the best outcome. All of these relate to the talent of the leader in his or her successful effort at structuring teamwork in a way that can ensure effective processing and meaningful outcomes.

The team leader essentially creates the facilitating context, conditions, and circumstances that lead to effective team performance (Plsek, 2010). Construction, structure, purpose, and team dynamics all converge to create the conditions that positively predict effectiveness. In addition, the team leader is aware of the need to maintain as much membership stability on the team as is necessary for the team to work effectively. High team member turnover usually reflects underaddressing many of these forces and the resulting negative impact on the value and relevance team members feel about their membership and contribution to the team's work.

Team leaders should consider mentoring advisement as a part of their own developmental program as they develop their team leadership skills. Personal team leadership coaching helps serve to construct a frame for both evaluating the behavior of the team leader and assessing the effectiveness of the team leader within a particular team format. The mentor should be encouraged to assess the utility and effectiveness of the team leader's work by targeting the team leader's capacity, approach, and affect, assessing it within the context of the team's progress toward fulfilling its purpose and goals. In addition, mentors can help team leaders in skill development and in creating more effective interaction between team leader capacity and the overall effectiveness of team dynamics and goal achievement.

Long-term team effectiveness reflects the team leader's ability to further encourage and develop team members in their own effectiveness as participants in processes of interaction, relationship, and collective deliberation (Wolfe & Sparkman, 2010). The team leader must see his or her role as an opportunity to help team members develop higher levels of contribution and, therefore, more strongly influence long-term potentials for team effectiveness and individual member contribution. In addition, mentors can help the team leader assess and translate personal effectiveness into measures of team effectiveness in the achievement of the team's purpose and the desired product of its work. The three major factors that are critical to the effectiveness of the team leader's role relate specifically to the adequate structuring of the team, the use of good process, and the progress of the team toward its goals or in fulfillment of its purpose. Here a mentor can be helpful in assessing strengths and challenges with the team leader and address specific arenas of talent development that can guide the team leader to higher levels of competence.

RESOLVING TEAM PROBLEMS

- Identifying the problem: All teams have the potential for difficulty and for challenge. In the context of all human relationships, the potential for conflict always exists. The leader knows this, anticipates it, and is constantly prepared to deal with it. The leader, therefore, always has a focus on the potential for problems, helping the team with the awareness of that potential and in identifying those problems as soon as possible. Problems left too long or dealt with too late have the potential for greater impediment to accomplishing the work than those addressed early.

- Creating individual awareness and ownership of problems: After the problem or concern is identified by the leader, it is vital that it be shared with individuals or a collective body of team members. The leader must always remember that team members own their own problems. The team leader never makes the problem his or her problem. When this occurs, a transfer in the locus of control for its resolution also occurs. The solution is always operating within the context of the team members and in the process of their work. The leader facilitates dialogue, discernment, and problem solving with the appropriate owners of the problem.

- Moving the group to resolution: Resolution is more a journey than a destination. The leader is helping the team assess the most appropriate responses to problems or concerns and the identification of the best strategy for addressing the problem in a particular time frame or within the context of a particular circumstance or process. Here the team leader is always concerned about techniques and methodologies that might be applied to problem solving as a set of tools for the team members in creating an objective format for problem solving. The team leader draws from these objective processes, helping the team focus these techniques in a way that can address the issue, find the solution for the problem, and help the team move toward its goal.

REFLECTIVE QUESTION

When you anticipate yourself filling the role of team leader, what are your own personal developmental and role skills you need most help with developing?

It cannot be understated that the motivation, energy, and commitment of the team leader establishes an emotional frame for the team and helps create a milieu that reflects the kind of personal energy that demonstrates commitment, enthusiasm, and a strong desire for the team to be effective in its work (Northouse, 2007). These personal attributes of team leaders help establish a positive, energetic, and safe context for team members that can translate into a culture of collective value in the broad-based sense of the real potential for contribution that comes from each team member. The confidence and trust of team members can be assured if there is a broad sense in the team that each member is valued, that the work of the team is purposeful, that the team is a safe space for collective interaction and engagement, and the team actually achieves its intended ends.

Virtuality and Team Performance

Digital technology has created significant shifts in the way in which teams are constructed and the processes through which they do their work. Although many of the dynamics of good team construction and management are similar between geographical and virtual teams, there are some obvious differences. The medium of technology creates an environment that is structurally and emotionally neutral and often ameliorates the human intensive patterns of visceral responses that simply can't be as well noted in the digital team environment (Gibson & Cohen, 2003). Although the relational challenges are more obvious, what is also clear is that digital team processes and dynamics have the potential for moving more quickly, deliberating more succinctly, and moving faster with regard to specific task performance. The counter to this prevailing potential is that levels of depth of understanding, uncertainties, or challenges that are normally visible through critical assessment of body language and emotional interactive cues are less available to the team leader. Compensating for the more two-dimensional team interaction, team leaders must check in more frequently to determine the insight of team members with regard to their sense of the team process and their evaluation of its progress (Singh & Waddell, 2004).

CRITICAL THOUGHT

The team leader is always sensitive to including team members in decisions that affect what they do. The wise leader never acts unilaterally or in any way that does not demonstrate team ownership and team value.

Spatial and temporal differences in team interaction will cause the team leader to be more purposeful in articulating the progress of the team. The leader must check in to validate general consensus of the team's sense of effectiveness or progress. Thinking through the structural elements of team dynamics and creating a rubric for monitoring and evaluating team interaction and task progress creates an objective tool for team leaders to more accurately determine team members' sense of engagement and progress with the team effort.

In the 21st century digital environment for teamwork, team leaders must recognize that unilateral team direction that was once successful in more vertical and geographical team processes may not be as effective in the digital infrastructure. Teamwork must often be broken down into smaller components, and leaders and small groups of team members must become more focused on particular goals and tasks associated with the team's progress. Breaking down task function and leadership engagement spreads the expectations for performance and progress among team members and develops the notion of leadership that is itself more collective and engaging. These smaller work groups with more narrowly designated team leaders are now more able to focus specifically on particular dialogue, tasks, and goals. Smaller work groups can take ownership for components of the process where there can be quicker success and team member contributions can be more easily enumerated in the context of this small work group dynamic. The team leader must develop more effectiveness in coordinating and integrating the work of smaller digital work teams. Team leaders must help to ensure that each smaller work group produces outcomes that can represent a goodness of fit with the broader objectives for the team when well integrated into the full team's effort. Effective smaller teams demonstrate a subsequent positive contribution, more quickly moving the whole team more strategically to the accomplishment of its collective goals.

Chapter Summary

Teams are more generally the basic unit of contemporary work, especially in knowledge-driven work settings. There are broad and intensive elements and characteristics of teamwork and effectiveness that are elemental to the role of the nurse leader. The professional nurse will respond to a lifetime of opportunity and challenge to lead many team efforts in advancing the interests of healthcare organizations and the obligations of the profession for addressing all areas of patient care. Every professional nurse must expect that he or she will play a major role in team processes as both leaders and participants. The critical factors related to the nurse's role on teams and as a team leader are reflected in the leader's capacity and skill to construct the team effort around a clear purpose, goals, and processes. Building on functional clarity for the team, the team leader demonstrates the value of constructing a well-functioning team by aligning team members with the specific breadth, capacity, and range of skills necessary to address the team's work focus in an effective way (Porter-O'Grady & Malloch, 2010).

The team leader focuses on setting the table for effective team functioning through clarity around equity and membership, terms of engagement, team process dynamics, and effective relationship building and management of the interaction of team members. The development of personal leadership skills creates a demand for the nurse team leader to be aware of personal attributes, and identify and work with a mentor to help grow the facilitation, integration, and coordination skills necessary for effective personal team leadership. The wide variety of team approaches includes a growing emphasis on digital team activities, which means that the team leader must develop a range of approaches that best reflect the kind of team and its characteristics through which the team leader will work. As teams become a more common medium for deliberative work processes, the professional nurse must come to expect that he or she will need to develop a wide array of team leader skills as the nurse's role in coordinating interdisciplinary team dynamics becomes a more central aspect of the clinical work environment.

CHAPTER TEST QUESTIONS

1. Teams are the central component of the delivery of healthcare services. True or false?

2. Healthcare reform and transformation have made teams less important, instead advancing the value of individual clinical functions over team activities. True or false?

3. The professional nurse is a critical and key leader on clinical and health delivery teams. True or false?

4. Purpose, goals, roles, and relationships are the four central elements upon which team effectiveness depends. True or false?

5. It is the obligation of the team leader to establish the goals for team members and make it clear to team members their relationship to meeting the obligations of these goals. True or false?

6. Conflict is always a barrier to team effectiveness and success and, therefore, it is the role of the team leader to eliminate conflict from the team so it can proceed to successfully complete its purpose. True or false?

7. Team members need a clear understanding of their individual roles so they know what they are committing to and the expectations of their participation in team activities. True or false?

8. Measures of team success are identified only after the team has made progress with regard to its goals and therefore have a foundation in measuring the team's degree of success. True or false?

9. The team leader must reaffirm the team's purpose and its progress frequently in order to help team members understand where they are in the team process, the progress they have made with regard to their goals, and the need for adjustments and accommodations to changes affecting the team's action. True or false?

10. All team leaders should have external mentoring, guidance, or advisement directed to helping advance personal insights and skills for team leadership. True or false?

> **WWW** For a full suite of assignments and additional learning activities, use the access code located in the front of your book to visit the exclusive website: http://go.jblearning.com/leadership. If you do not have an access code, you can obtain one at the site.

References

Barner, R. (2000). *Team troubleshooter: How to find and fix team problems.* Palo Alto, CA: Davies-Black.

Belbin, R. M. (2010). *Team roles at work* (Online resource). Oxford, UK; Burlington, MA: Butterworth-Heinemann.

Ben Saoud, N., & Mark, G. (2006). Complexity theory and collaboration: An agent-based simulator for a space mission design team. *Computational and Mathematical Organization Theory, 13*(2), 113–147.

Chau, V. S., & elibrary. (2008). Relationship of strategic performance management to team strategy, company performance and organizational effectiveness. *Team Performance Management, 14*(3–4), 111–191. Bradford, Emerald.

Chrispeels, J. H. (2004). *Learning to lead together: The promise and challenge of sharing leadership.* Thousand Oaks, CA: Sage.

Curlee, W., & Gordon, R. L. (2011). *Complexity theory and project management.* Hoboken, NJ: Wiley.

Curseu, P. (2003). *Formal group decision-making: A social cognitive approach.* Cluj-Napoca: ASCR Press.

Dunin-Keplicz, B., & Verbrugge, R. (2010). *Teamwork in multi-agent systems: A formal approach.* Hoboken, NJ: Wiley.

Finkelman, A. W. (2011). *Case management for nurses.* Boston, MA: Pearson.

Gibson, C. B., & Cohen, S. G. (2003). *Virtual teams that work creating conditions for virtual team effectiveness.* San Francisco, CA: Jossey-Bass.

Gratton, L., & Erickson, T. (2007). Eight ways to build collaborative teams. *Harvard Business Review, 85*(11), 100–111.

Kritek, P. B. (2002). *Negotiating at an uneven table: Developing moral courage in resolving our conflicts.* San Francisco, CA: Jossey-Bass.

Larson, W. J. (2011). Team member characteristics contributing to high reliability in emergency response teams managing critical incidents. Tucson, AZ: University of Arizona: 215.

Losoncy, L. (1996). *Best team skills.* Boca Raton, FL: St. Lucie Press.

Mash, B. J., Mayers, P., Conradie, H., Orayn, A., Kuiper, M., & Marais, J. (2008). How to manage organisational change and create practice teams: Experiences of a South African primary care health centre. *Health Education (Abingdon), 21*(2), 132.

Northouse, P. G. (2007). *Leadership: Theory and practice.* Thousand Oaks, CA: Sage.

Parker, G. M. (2003). *Cross-functional teams: Working with allies, enemies, and other strangers.* San Francisco, CA: Jossey-Bass.

Parker, G. M. (2008). *Team players and team work new strategies for developing successful collaboration.* San Francisco, CA: Jossey-Bass.

Peterson, L., & King, S. (2007). How effective leaders achieve success in critical change initiatives part 4: Emergent leadership—an example with doctors. *Healthcare Quarterly, 10*(4), 52, 59–63.

Plsek, P. (2010). Directed creativity: How to generate new ideas for transforming healthcare. In T. Porter-O'Grady & K. Malloch (Eds.). *Innovation leadership: Creating the landscape of healthcare* (pp. 87–106). Sudbury, MA: Jones and Bartlett.

Porter-O'Grady, T. (2009). *Interdisciplinary shared governance: Integrating practice, transforming healthcare.* Sudbury, MA: Jones and Bartlett.

Porter-O'Grady, T., & Malloch, K. (2010). *Quantum leadership: Advancing innovation, transforming healthcare.* Sudbury, MA: Jones and Bartlett.

Rondeau, K. (2007). The adoption of high involvement work practices and Canadian nursing homes. *Leadership in Health Services, 20*(1), 16.

Rouse, W. (2007). *People and organizations: Explorations of human-centered design.* New York, NY: Wiley.

Salas, E., Goodwin, G. F., & Burke, C. S. (2009). Team effectiveness in complex organizations cross-disciplinary perspectives and approaches. *The Organizational Frontiers Series* (pp. xxxiv, 589). Hove, UK.

Singh, M., & Waddell, D. (2004). *E-business innovation and change management.* Hershey, PA: Idea Group.

Wolfe, B. D., & Sparkman, C. P. (2010). *Team-building activities for the digital age: Using technology to develop effective groups.* Champaign, IL: Human Kinetics.

Yukl, G. (2009). *Leadership in organizations.* New York, NY: Prentice Hall.

Appendix A

Sample Techniques for Team Decision Making

There is a whole range of approaches to disciplining decision making and incorporating the team within the decision-making process. Processes such as flowcharts, workflow diagrams, Pareto charts, cause-and-effect diagrams, matrices and stratification instruments, checklists, scatter diagrams, brainstorming, and multivoting are just a few of the tools that teams can use in making good decisions. The team leader carefully makes choices with regard to what decisions need to be made in the processes that support decision efforts.

Some decision-making techniques are as follows:

Nominal group technique:

- Useful when time is a concern
- Controls for issues of power
- Helps establish priorities
- Can aggregate ideas
- Builds group acceptance
- Is transparent

Affinity groups:

- Builds consensus and acceptance
- Uses a smaller group for process
- Lets participants know how broadly the idea is supported
- Offsets power
- Effective use of time
- Values and supports individual and group ideas
- Takes more time than nominal group technique
- One idea helps spark others

Delphi technique:

- Can use to gather information from outside team
- Good for brainstorming
- Key ideas are identified and related ideas are drawn
- Good for gathering much information from a broad group
- Participants feel safe to share controversial ideas

Appendix B

Team-Based Decision-Making Process

Team decision making is always a structured process and is therefore a learned skill exercised by all members of the team.

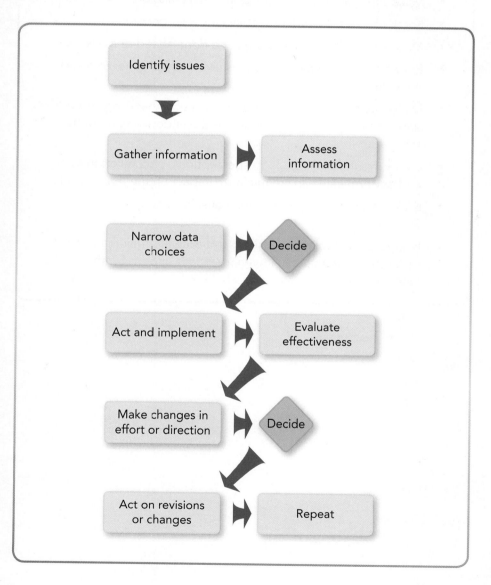

Appendix C

Keeping the Team Focused

- Make sure the team is always aware of its mission.

- Know who has what accountability for what decisions.

- Make sure planning is thorough and done ahead of the work.

- Ensure that each team member is aware of his or her role and individual contribution to the team's work.

- Do frequent consensus testing to make sure that every individual's understanding of the work matches the understanding of the team as a whole.

- Clarify misunderstandings, misperceptions, or conflicts in roles and performance early to minimize impact on the team's work.

- Evaluate the team's process, relationships, and progress frequently.

- Integrate the efforts of the team and evaluate their interface in order to ensure that each team member's effort is synthesized with the work of the team as a whole.

Appendix D

Some Dos and Don'ts of Team Leadership

Dos	Don'ts
Give the team the information it needs to work well.	Oversupervise the team and control the team processes.
Help the team with skill building in relationship to its work.	Criticize or punish team members in the presence of others.
Build effective communication mechanisms among team members.	Personally own the work of team members as though it belongs to you.
Undertake corrective action potentially impeding teamwork as early as possible.	Ignore internal or external dynamics with the potential to impact team effectiveness.
Evaluate the effectiveness of the team as you go—do not wait.	Let the team get tangled up in peripheral and nonessential issues that impede their work progress.
Confront conflict early and assess often.	
Review goals and progress toward them with team members regularly.	Let the team forget that their work serves a purpose and has value.
Reward and encourage team members' successes frequently and well.	Take all the credit for the team's work and identify them as "my" people.
Assess external and internal impediments to team effectiveness and remove them as soon as possible.	Overwork the team without providing ample time for relationship building, social interaction, and celebrating successes.
Celebrate team successes frequently.	Limit information or access to resources that might affect team goal achievement.

Appendix E

Creating Team Infrastructure

- For teams to be successful, they must be the way of doing business and a part of the continuous dynamic of the organization from the inside out.

- Teams are a strategic imperative.

- Senior management supports the team approach.

- All leaders operate within the context of team processes and are skilled in team management.

- Staff operating in teams is the expectation of the organization and is supported through continual team learning.

- Team processes are used for all decision making and problem solving and are evaluated for effectiveness.

Appendix F

Considerations for Team Effectiveness

As teams move through their specific stages of development, the team leader, working at the periphery, is constantly monitoring and measuring the effectiveness of interactions, relationships, problem solving, and work processing. The team leader recognizes that resolving issues in any of these arenas early creates a frame for team effectiveness and success that can operate over the long term. Creating a culture of openness to issues of concern with regard to problem solving, work processes, and relationship building establishes a frame of reference for the team that is positive, disclosing, and safe. Through this early engagement of issues, the leader sets up a foundation upon which subsequent problem solving can build and team success can be ensured.

- Forming: The initial stage of team development in which rules are uncertain and team expectations, rules, and roles are unclear.

- Storming: The formative stage of the group process, filled with conflict as the group begins to establish roles, relationships, and rules around purposes and the work of the team.

- Norming: Work processes are established, rules are agreed to, systems are set up, and creative work patterns emerge in ways that more clearly define the team.

- Performing: The team now begins to work well together, undertake processes, work through difficulties, achieve objectives, and measure results.

- Evaluation and retooling: The team assesses internal and external dynamics, makes decisions about more effective processes, and refines the team work rules, roles, and relationships.

IT'S NOT ENOUGH TO BE BUSY, SO ARE THE ANTS. THE QUESTION IS, WHAT ARE WE BUSY ABOUT?
—HENRY DAVID THOREAU

CHAPTER OBJECTIVES

Upon completion of this chapter, the reader will be able to do the following:

» Understand the six basic categories of resources associated with the provision of healthcare services.

» Describe the interactions among the economic concepts of demand, supply, and price from a healthcare perspective.

» Compare and contrast the purposes, utility, and importance of value and volume measurements in health care.

» Understand basic data measurement concepts, analysis, and interrelationships in determining healthcare value.

» Explain the importance of variance management and the role of the clinical nurse leader in responding to variances in financial, productivity, and performance data.

Resources for Healthcare Excellence

In order for the healthcare system or any healthcare organization to function effectively, resources for personal, fiscal support, physical settings, supplies, technology, and time to do the expected work are needed. These six major resource categories are incredibly complex and intertwined. While it is important to understand current practices, it is far more important to be thinking about how to dramatically change how we will manage our resources in the future. Current practices and policies on how we finance, organize, deliver, and evaluate health care serve only as an informational baseline. Working to sustain most current practices will result in reinforcing our less than effective healthcare system; thus there is an urgent need for us to be rethinking how we select, manage, and evaluate our resources. Current practices must change dramatically if system quality, cost, and value are going to improve.

In this chapter, the foundations of our current practices in managing resources are presented along with new ideas to consider for the future. An overview of basic economic principles specific to price, supply, and demand; discussion of major resource categories in health care; differences in value and volume measurements; as well as the basics of budgeting, data analysis to inform decisions, and managing variances will be discussed.

Basic Economics Are Not So Basic: Price, Demand, and Supply Complexities

A basic understanding of **healthcare economics** is helpful for clinical nurse leaders to advance their understanding of the complex nature of the workings of health care. There are multiple resources available to study healthcare macro and micro economics in greater depth if the reader is so interested. The accompanying box includes a selected list of current resources available. To be sure, healthcare economics is a fascinating field that provides vital insights in managing resources and advancing change in the marketplace.

SELECTED HEALTHCARE ECONOMICS RESOURCES

- Feldstein (2012)
- Folland (2010)
- Getzen (2010)
- Shi & Singh (2011)

Healthcare economics is described as a branch of economics focused on efficiency, effectiveness, and behavior in the production and consumption of healthcare goods and services (Shi & Singh, 2011). It is the study and science of how human needs are perceived in relationship to what supply is available. Price is always a factor and changes based on the dynamics of supply and demand. In the early 1960s, Arrow distinguished healthcare economics from other types of economics (Arrow, 1963). The involvement of the government, the intractable uncertainty in many healthcare areas, barriers to access to services, and third-party agents in brokering and managing funds distinguished healthcare economics from general economics and continue in current times. These distinctions further reinforce the complexities of healthcare economics. Price, demand, and supply are three basic concepts in the economic model.

In general, *prices* for healthcare resources, such as supplies, people, and physical settings, are based on what one has to give up to buy a good or service. The price is also based on available dollars and the need for a good or service. Prices are considered from multiple perspectives: the actual costs of services, the actual charge determined by the seller of the goods, and the overall expenditures of dollars. Several factors impact the price of healthcare services and are intertwined in complex ways. Most notably, changes in the need for people (human) resources, materials, equipment, and technology will result in a price change.

The *supply* of goods or services is the amount that is available at a specific price. The supply of healthcare goods and services includes people, supplies, technology, and time, as well as the funds to pay for these services. Overall, supply includes all healthcare workers, the physical facilities for patient care, materials, equipment, technology, financial, and time resources required to provide health services.

Each of these different types of supplies reacts differently in the environment. For example, the supply of healthcare workers has ranged from undersupply to oversupply and tends to follow cyclical trends based on changing conditions in price and demand. The supply of nurses is a continual area of analysis and requires ongoing discussion and strategizing to ensure the right nurse is with the right patient at the right time. Both short-term and long-term nursing supply processes are important in allocating the appropriate numbers of nurses. Most recently, the demand and supply of nurses have been influenced by emerging evidence for safe staffing and staffing effectiveness. It is important to note that these staffing effectiveness studies still need to be customized to the individual facility, geographic location, and available technology in the determination of appropriate supply and demand projections.

Of interest is the traditional estimation of the demand for nurses. Currently, the average number of nurses per population is used to estimate the demand for and supply of registered nurses. This approach is limited in that it is only specific to the quantity of available nurses and does not include the types, education, skill levels, and clinical areas of need. For example, the average number of nurses per 100,000 population in the United States in 2010 was 860, but the average number of nurses in Arizona is 653 per 100,000 population (StateHealthFacts.org, n.d.). Figure 8-1 is a US map that depicts the current nurse supply for each state.

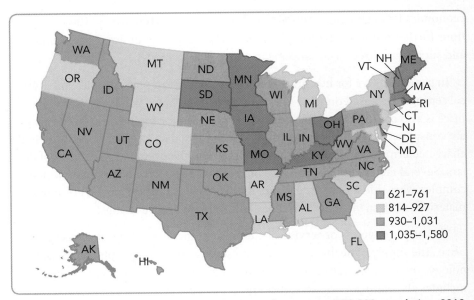

Figure 8-1 Registered nurses per 100,000 population, 2010.
Source: The Kaiser Family Foundation, statehealthfacts.org

To determine both the adequacy of the Arizona nurse population and a plan to change the number of Arizona nurses, more information is needed. Information about the patient population being served, skills and competencies of the Arizona nurse population, and geographic location of the nurses are needed to adequately inform the forecasting of nursing demand. It would be futile to increase the supply of surgical nurses if the supply was already in excess and surgical nurses were looking for jobs. An additional analysis of the supply numbers is needed to best determine the characteristics and geographic locations for nursing demand (Malloch, Davenport, Hatler, & Milton, 2003).

The supply category also includes physical facilities for patient services—the number, location, type, and quality of locations for healthcare services across the country. The numbers and locations of healthcare facilities are impacted by demand for services, geographic location, and available funding for services provided. The physical facilities are also impacted by changing technology, such as telemedicine and the model of care delivery. Most notable is the shift from medical centers to community centers and services.

SCENARIO

Your state supply of nurses is 10 percent below the national average. Your team has been asked to create a plan that will result in an optimal number of nurses that results in patient quality outcomes at the 99 percentile.

Discussion Questions

Create a plan that includes the following:

1. Rationale, metrics, and quality indicators, including target registered nurses per 100,000 population

2. Assessment of clinical specialties (adult, critical care, pediatric, behavioral health, rehabilitation, surgical, ambulatory, and community health) available to the state, specific to geographic regions

3. Areas of clinical need

4. Areas of geographic need

5. Timeline to achieve goals

6. Facilitators to this work

7. Barriers to this work

8. Plans to support facilitators and address barriers

Material supplies include those items most often used only once and then discarded. Examples include dressings, medications, and food needed for patient care services. Material supply levels are impacted by the types of services provided, the access to supplies, and the cost of supplies.

The supply of equipment includes several factors, such as items that can be used more than one time. Patient beds, wheelchairs, lift equipment, computers, and monitoring equipment are examples. The availability of equipment, the effectiveness of the equipment in advancing patient care, and the cost all impact the type and quantities of equipment supplies that are available in the healthcare system.

SCENARIO

The current conditions in many emergency centers reflect disparities in supply, demand, and price for the care of patients presenting to the emergency center for treatment.

Discussion Questions

1. Identify all of the issues or factors related to each of the three major categories of supply, demand, and price.

2. Based on your analysis, develop a plan to equalize supply and demand.

3. Identify the changes that would need to be made in each resource category to accomplish this goal.

The availability of financial resources is similarly complicated, and it is highly interrelated with the supply and demand factors. Financial resources are available from government and private resources. Federal healthcare spending is impacted by the types of programs approved by Congress and each of the 50 states as well as funding provided by employers to insure their employees. As pressures increase for reductions in allocations for healthcare insurance, the supply of financial contributions decreases, creating a higher and higher number of uninsured citizens.

Time is also a significant supply resource. To be sure, the time required to analyze, plan, and facilitate effective healthcare programs is significant and often overwhelming. The available supply of time is often not analyzed or categorized as an essential economic resource; however, an understanding of the available time to address supply and demand needs is critical for effective dialogue and evaluation of ongoing activities. Although it is difficult to accurately estimate the time required or needed, discussions and reflections specific to estimation of the capacity of individuals need to occur, and the supply of time for each one is finite.

SCENARIO

Change Healthcare is an organization dedicated to transparency in healthcare charges and costs. In a recent news release, the organization reported a wide range of prices within one town, from $230 to $1800, for a pelvic computed tomography (CT) scan.

Discussion Questions

1. Considering the supply and demand factors in providing healthcare services that could be involved in this situation, list at least five supply and five demand factors that created this situation.

2. Is it possible to standardize these prices?

3. What would be the facilitators and obstacles to standardization?

Sources: Adapted from Change Healthcare (n.d.); Kennedy (2011, June 30).

Demand for goods or services is generated by the number of consumers (patients in the healthcare model) who desire the available goods at a certain price. Demand is about the desire to own a good or service, the ability to pay for it, and the willingness to pay the asking price at a given point in time. Demand is influenced by available resources, prices of related goods, numbers of interested buyers, and preferences. There are multiple dynamic influences on the demand for healthcare goods and services.

In general, as the price increases, the demand for a good or service decreases; as the price decreases, the demand increases; and as the quantity of goods or supply increases, the price decreases. These relationships are studied extensively to better understand future prices, supplies, and demands from the healthcare economics perspective. Figure 8-2 illustrates these basic relationships in the economic model. In the next section, five resource categories within the healthcare marketplace that are continually influenced by price, supply, and demand are briefly described.

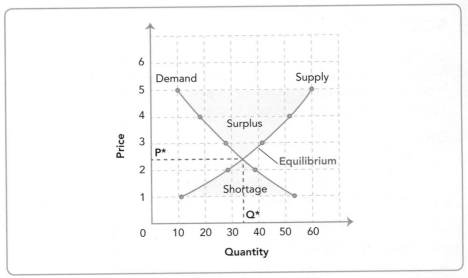

Figure 8-2 Supply and demand

Resource Categories: Human, Fiscal, Material, Technology, and Time

The first category is human resources or people resources and includes those individuals required to provide direct patient care and those who support patient care processes, or indirect care. The comprehensive management of human resources includes the recruitment, management, and retention of these people resources. Recruitment of individuals is based upon defined or anticipated needs for services. Advertising, interviewing, selecting, and hiring are included in the recruitment processes. The demand, supply, or availability of individuals for healthcare work varies by geographic region, type of worker, and wage and benefit levels.

To be sure, the more effective the recruitment process is in identifying and selecting individuals who closely match the needs of the unit and organization, the stronger the team will be and the higher the quality of patient outcomes will be. An ineffective recruitment process impacts the supply and demand cycle, resulting in increased work effort and unnecessary expenses.

Managing demand can be positively impacted by a strong, evidence-based retention program. Nurse retention is a basic consideration for all organizations and groups of nursing. Ensuring that competent nurses are satisfied and continue to thrive in their environment requires proactive planning and programming.

SCENARIO

Nurse retention is more than providing pizza and movie tickets to nurses. Recent research identified focused and structured processes with clearly defined evaluation criteria for effective nurse retention.

The following five practices have been identified as important in decreasing turnover:

- Onboarding: The early processes of socializing nurses into the workplace to achieve optimal employee engagement.

- Employee rounding: Regular rounding in work areas to identify employees' most critical needs, safety issues, and clinical concerns.

- Social networking: Specific social activities to support team building, seasonal challenges, and common needs.

- Employee recognition: Acknowledgment of outstanding behaviors, communication, accountability, valuing diversity, delivering excellence, and teamwork.

- Developmental stretch assignments: Assignments to improve employee satisfaction and engagement through autonomy and leadership practices.

Discussion Questions

1. In a team setting, make a list of activities specific to each of the five practices that are occurring in your organization.

2. Also make a list of activities that should occur in the next year for each of the five categories.

3. What are the facilitators and barriers to improving retention?

Source: Adapted from Hinson & Spatz (2011).

The costs associated with experienced nurse turnover are better spent in retaining competent nurse experts who are acclimated and socialized to the setting. Focusing on retention is especially important when resources are limited. According to Hinson and Spatz (2011), focused initiatives on retention can be quite successful in retaining nurses. The implementation of five retention concepts—**onboarding, employee rounding, social networking, employee recognition,** and **developmental stretch assignments**—reduced voluntary nurse turnover by 91 percent; 100 percent retention of 43 newly hired nurses and a savings of $655,949 (Hinson & Spatz, 2011).

The second resource category is financial resources. Fiscal or financial resources include the dollars required to purchase and pay for human, material, and technology resources. The current US financial system for health care includes financing, insurance, payment, and delivery (Shi & Singh, 2012).

COMPONENTS OF THE CURRENT US HEALTHCARE SYSTEM

- Financing: The payment of premiums to provide coverage for insured individuals
- Insurance: The vehicle to manage risk across populations
- Delivery: Provision of healthcare services by providers, hospitals, diagnostic clinics, and suppliers
- Payment: The process of reimbursement to providers for services rendered

Source: Shi, L., & Singh, D. A. (2012). *Delivering health care in America: A systems approach* (5th ed.). Sudbury, MA: Jones & Bartlett Learning.

The system has evolved over many years and is quite complex as well as costly. Some of the characteristics of the system are as follows:

- Public and private funding resources: Federal and state government and private insurance companies are the major financiers of health care.
- Insured and uninsured individuals: Insured individuals include those with employer-sponsored health plans and selected populations for government programs (older citizens, military, veterans, disabled citizens, and impoverished groups); uninsured individuals include those that do not fit into insured groups.
- Varying costs to individuals: Costs to individuals vary across plans (copays, deductibles, etc.).
- Financing models: A variety of models of financing, insurance, and/or payment that are not integrated across the healthcare continuum (managed care organizations, integrated networks, self-insurance by large employers, private insurance plans, etc.).
- State versus federal systems: Some states assume accountability for federal programs, such as Medicaid programs.
- Varying coverage: Coverage or payment varies across government and private insurance plans for selected conditions and procedures.

- Inconsistency: Charges are inconsistent for services and quality control mechanisms.

It is these widely variable characteristics in the financing of health care that spurred the passage of national healthcare reform. This national legislation, the Healthcare Reform Act of 2010, is intended to provide healthcare coverage to every citizen and eliminate many of the challenges of the existing system, such as disqualifications for preexisting conditions, portability of benefits, and lack of quality and cost control. Specifically, reform is intended to create an integrated network of interrelated components working together coherently and effectively.

GOALS OF 2010 AFFORDABLE CARE ACT

- Rein in the worst excesses and abuses of the insurance industry with some of the toughest consumer protections this country has ever known.
- Hold insurance companies accountable to keep premiums down and prevent denials of care and coverage, including for preexisting conditions.
- Make health insurance affordable for middle class families and small businesses with one of the largest tax cuts for health care in history, reducing premiums and out-of-pocket costs.
- Provide the security of knowing that if you lose your job, change your job, or start a new business, you'll always be able to purchase quality, affordable care in a new competitive health insurance market that keeps costs down.
- Strengthen Medicare benefits with lower prescription drug costs for those in the "donut hole," chronic care, free preventive care, and nearly a decade more of solvency for Medicare.
- Improve our nation's fiscal health by reducing our deficit by more than $100 billion over the next decade, and more than $1 trillion in the decade after that.

Source: HealthReform.gov (n.d.)

Interestingly, the management of fiscal resources continues to challenge the best healthcare leaders for several reasons. In addition to perceived limited resources, the wide variation in charges for similar healthcare services is especially problematic. It is important to note that the charges for healthcare services are different from the actual costs of specific healthcare products and services. The actual costs of products and services are difficult to determine given the need to include administrative and delivery costs for each product and service. The specific charge for a product or service thus includes cost plus administrative fees. Further, costs and charges vary by provider, geographic region, and type of organization providing the service. For example, patients may pay as much as 683 percent more for the same medical procedure, such as magnetic resonance imaging or a CT scan, in the same town depending on which provider they select (Kennedy, 2011).

The third category is material resources. Material resources for physical settings, supplies, and equipment include those resources needed for the environment and supplies and equipment to provide the required patient care. Similar to human and financial resources, there is significant variation in material resources and continuing demand for new and improved material resources. For example, as evidence emerges specific to the relationship between attributes of the physical setting and patient outcomes, redesigns in facilities are in demand. The accompanying box identifies many of the recent demands in healthcare facilities based on new research evidence.

PHYSICAL SETTING: CHANGES IN DEMAND

- Private rooms
- Patient rooms with views of nature
- Enclosed medication administration rooms
- Decentralized and centralized workstations
- Multiple hand washing dispensers located based on human factors research
- Multipurpose interventional suites for surgery, catheterization labs, endoscopy, and interventional radiology
- Admission units for all patients except critical care
- Family space in all patient rooms
- Healing modalities of music, water features, and gardens
- Attractive space for staff lounges
- Separated greeter and unit clerk space

The fourth resource category is technology. Technology resources include those resources required for the electronic or virtual management of information such as hardware and software applications for clinical documentation, data analysis, clinical monitoring systems, communication devices, and robotics. While most of the emerging technology provides improvements in selected patient care processes and supporting information processes, not every new technology is appropriate for the organization because of limited resources. The addition of technology must necessarily be evaluated for the fit with current technologies and manual practices, the anticipated value to patient quality and safety outcomes, employee safety and performance, physical setting safety and effectiveness, and affordability. The potential for saving time, reducing errors, and increasing the reliability of information management is an important consideration when the demand for new technology is being considered.

 ## SCENARIO

Adding technology resources to an organization requires careful consideration. There must be a clear understanding of the potential value of the technology specific to time savings for employees, quality improvements for patients, patient safety, cost savings, and overall satisfaction.

Several nurses just returned from attending a large national conference in which robots were featured for delivering pharmacy supplies, delivering and picking up medical records, and delivering and picking up food trays. The nurses believe that all three types of robots would benefit the unit in a variety of ways. The nurse executive is very interested and requested the nurses to identify the potential value for the organization.

Discussion Questions

On the basis of this information, develop a value-based proposal for each of the three robots and prioritize which robot should be purchased and why. Categorize your rationale into the following categories:

1. Improvements in patient care outcomes

2. Time savings for specific caregivers

3. Costs/cost savings including technology, maintenance of technology, patient reimbursements

4. Satisfaction of patients, caregivers, and providers

The fifth resource is time. Time resources include the available time to provide the care and support services for healthcare work. Very few individuals ever believe they have enough time to do the things they believe need to be done. Thus, time emerges as an important resource to manage. Learning to identify what needs to be done, the level of priority of work, who needs to do the work, and how to create boundaries between work and personal time is an underdeveloped competence for most healthcare workers.

CRITICAL THOUGHT

- Recognize that everyone has capacity for improvement in the use of time.
- Focus on the importance of balancing one's energy rather than efficiency.
- Share the spirit of the reality that there will always be a shortage of time and excess of desires—a never-ending struggle to close the gap!
- Stay focused and aware of personal performance.
- Support others who are less successful in time balancing, knowing there are opportunities to improve for all.

The following strategies are helpful in assessing and managing one's time. First, self-assessment is essential. Determine what your personal abilities are in managing your work across a span of time. Take into consideration both your own personal assessment and the feedback from others on your team. Personal reflection specific to meeting deadlines, feeling stressed or overwhelmed, managing interruptions, prioritizing, avoiding time wasters, idle chatter and complaining, focus on perfection, and procrastination are areas that should be considered. Second, develop a personal plan to optimize your time management. Select one or two strategies to address areas of concern. Do not overwhelm yourself with unreasonable goals and timelines because they will soon be forgotten and set aside. Consider planning at the beginning of a work period with a short time for reflection on the work to be done, prioritizing of work, and estimates of the time required for small blocks of work. Estimating time often provides invaluable insight into time requirements and helps to identify sources of overuse and underuse of time. The third activity is to review the results at the end of the work period and recognize what went well and what could be improved. It is important to remember that there are numerous techniques to improve time management; some will work for you and some will not. Being open to new ideas will provide insights into other successful approaches.

SCENARIO

Your team has a reputation for poor time management on some days and excellent time management on other days. Patient call lights are not always answered in a timely manner, pain medications are late, documentation is usually done after the shift, and overtime is above 5 percent.

For a clinical ladder project, you and two other nurses have decided to figure out how to learn from those that have excellent time management skills and those that are struggling. You believe you can learn something about work habits and systems issues if you work with both groups.

Discussion Question

Using the following categories, brainstorm with team members to create a plan to share ideas and improve management of time. Include both positive and negative behaviors. Ask each individual to create a personal plan for time management. Feel free to add other categories that you believe are involved.

- Prioritizing
- Planning
- Procrastination
- Interruptions
- Perfectionism
- Complaining
- Communication
- Feeling overwhelmed

Productivity: Value and Volume Measurements

Productivity measurement is a long-standing quantitative measure of the efficiency of the use of specific resources. Productivity is a ratio comparing what is produced to what is required to produce it. Usually this ratio is in the form of an average, expressing the output divided by the total. Productivity is also a measure of output from a production process, per unit of input (Shi & Singh, 2012). Aggregate productivity ratios are helpful in determining the overall efficiency of processes and individuals at a macro level. Productivity values generally increase as volumes of work increase. This infers that few obstacles or deviations from that standard process occur and that less time for a process will result in the desired quality outcome with higher volumes. Historically, higher productivity levels have been associated with higher profits. Examples of productivity metrics include the following:

- Registered nurse hours/patient day
- Registered nurse hours/treatment or procedure
- Admissions, discharges, and transfers/shift
- Direct care hours/total care hours
- Overtime hours/total worked hours
- New staff orientation hours/total worked hours
- Total salary cost/diagnosis-related group (DRG)

It is important to note that while emphasis is often placed on productivity targets, it is only one part of the picture and more information about processes and outcomes is needed before a determination is made that the productivity level is either positive or negative. The out-of-range productivity result may in fact be more than acceptable if the patient care conditions (demand) exceeded the standards in the productivity target calculations.

Historically, many healthcare workers have confused high work volumes or high productivity with high quality and value. Also, some have considered completion of process requirements, such as completion of a checklist, with high levels of quality and value. Completing checklists 100 percent of the time or distributing healthcare information to all patients with a certain disease is not enough to determine valued outcomes. What is needed is to know what value was produced from completing the checklist or from distributing healthcare information. The value outcome is specific use of the data from the checklist to better plan patient care or improvement in patient knowledge and healthy behaviors. Specifically, it is essential to know if patient care was positively impacted in a way that the patient care provided an outcome that was significant and valued by the patient.

Another challenge in measurement is the use of single or multiple related measures. Single metrics are limiting and provide only one aspect of the overall performance of the organization. Not only are single metrics limiting in the information that can be produced, but the type of analysis is also limiting. Traditionally, a return on investment or cost–benefit analysis is done to determine if there is worth or value in expending resources; spending resources will result in increased financial value. However, there is more to analyze in expending resources. Consider expending resources for a women's wellness service. The financial outcome is positive; however, it is not known if changes in women's level of wellness are achieved. Knowing the value and achievement of the goals of a program in addition to the financial benefit is an essential analysis that is needed to support effective allocation of resources. Figure 8-3 summarizes five types of value analyses that should be considered when expending resources.

1. Cost-minimization analysis (CMA)

Assumptions in CMA:

- The emphasis is on keeping costs as low as possible.
- Only costs are evaluated.
- Assumes that clinical outcomes are the same.
- Example: Practice guidelines for thrombolytic therapy; streptokinase via tissue plasminogen activator (TPA).

2. Cost-consequences analysis (CCA)

Assumptions in CCA:

- Consequences of two or more alternatives are measured as well as the costs, but costs/consequences are listed separately.
- Example: Comparison of early discharge of low-birth-weight infants whose care was managed by advanced practice nurses compared to traditional physician care.

3. Cost-effectiveness analysis (CEA)

Assumptions in CEA:

- Outcomes are measured in the same units between alternatives, such as dollars per life-year gained or cases avoided.
- Example: Evaluation of pain management interventions for patients with chronic arthritis.

4. Cost-utility analysis (CUA)

Assumptions in CUA:

- A special type of cost-effectiveness analysis that includes measures for both quantity and quality of life.
- Individual preferences for different health outcomes are sought and included.
- A difficult comparison; the goal is to compare $/Quality Adjusted Life Years.

5. Cost-benefit analysis (CBA)

Assumptions in CBA:

- Outcomes are measured according to some monetary unit.
- A single dollar figure, representing cost minus benefits, is calculated.
- Example: Is the cost of a pain management clinic covered by revenue generated?
  Cost: $500.00
  Revenue: $750.00 = 50% ROI

Source: Adapted from Buerhaus (1998).

Figure 8-3 Five types of evaluations

The addition of measures that identify the quality of the processes and the outcomes of providing patient care are gaining attention, particularly in light of the goals of healthcare reform. Value or the specific positive impact on functionality, reduction of pain, and time expended for care must be included in determination of value along with costs, reimbursement, processes, and completion of procedures. For example, while the charges and reimbursement are available for a surgical procedure, there may be no value to an elderly individual who is in the hospice stage of life. The surgical procedure meets all of the quality parameters for a safe procedure; however, no value or change in functionality or pain level is experienced by the patient. Table 8-1 is an example of a multilevel measurement evaluation for macro patient, employee, organization, and payer categories. Using the same framework, Table 8-2 compares quality, productivity, and cost indicators specific to a pain management program.

According to Porter (2010), healthcare value should always be defined around the patient and in a well-functioning system; creating value for the patient should be the determiner of rewards for all others in the healthcare system. Value in

Table 8-1 Value evaluation: Multiple measures for consideration

	Quality	Productivity	Cost
Patient	Clinical outcome	Length of stay	Cost of service
	Functionality	Length of procedure	Charge per case
	Comfort status	Time to treatment	Out-of-pocket
	Satisfaction		expenses
Employee	Competence, credentials, certifications, experience	Hours per unit of service	Wages and benefits
		Skill mix percentages	
		Turnover	
	Level of education	Registry staff %	
	Satisfaction with work	Overtime %	
Organization	Reputation in the community	Full-time equivalent (FTE)/Adjusted occupied bed (AOB)	Net income margin
	Licensure status		Departmental margins
	Accreditations		Available capital
Payer	Reputation with providers and organizations	Claims processed per 24 hour period	Cost of claims

Table 8-2 Value evaluation: Pain management program

	Quality	Productivity	Cost
Patient	Satisfaction increased 10% specific to level of pain relief Clinical documentation indicates pain relief from level 3 to level 2 on a 10-point scale	Length of stay decreased 0.5 day for 2 DRGs	Charge per case decreased 10% in past 12 months
Employee	Pain specialist provider and direct caregiver satisfaction increased 4% in past 12 months	No change in turnover, skill mix or registry nurse hours Overtime decreased 10% in the past 6 months	Increased cost of $50.00 per day per patient on pain protocol to cover pain specialist
Organization	Reputation in the community improved as a result of the availability of a pain management clinic No deficiencies in licensure review specific to pain management	No change	Margin for 2 DRGs increased 10%
Payer	Positive reputation with providers and organizations for reimbursement practices	No change	Cost of claims decreased because of decreased length of stay

health care should be determined by the achievement of the desired outcomes, not by the volume of services delivered or the number of checklists completed. Thus the goals of the patient become the unifier for all providers and caregivers across the system. Porter further states that the overarching goal of healthcare delivery is high quality value for every dollar spent. What is important in this discussion is to recognize the need for multiple measures in determining the effectiveness and efficiency of the complex healthcare system as well as the specific value to the patient.

The shift to a value-driven system from a quantitative-driven, financial model in which meaningful measures guide the work is a complex process that requires time, patience, and willingness to challenge many current assumptions. Focusing on patient-centered value outcomes requires all members of the healthcare team to identify what outcomes are important to the patient and which interventions should not be considered because of the lack of expected value.

The Consumer-Purchaser Disclosure Project (CPDP) provides a model for consideration and includes 10 criteria for assessing and monitoring meaningful measures (2011). The criteria include the following:

- Prioritize consumer and purchaser needs
- Use direct feedback from patients and their families in measuring performance
- Use dashboards of measures to monitor a complete picture of patient care
- Focus measurement on areas where there is a potential for improvement in outcome quality
- Ensure that measures generate the most valuable information
- Require that all patients fitting clinical criteria be included in analysis
- Assess whether treatment recommendations are followed
- Deemphasize check-box documentation measures
- Measure provider performance at all levels
- Collect data efficiently

Value can also be conceptualized on the basis of what the specific caregiver role contributes to the overall organizational outcomes. With the multiple levels of preparation for registered nurses, the licensed practical nurse role, and other technical support positions, the question is often asked as to what difference the registered nurse makes to the overall provision of patient care. To be sure, this is a complex question that deserves careful consideration. Recent studies of the significance of nursing by Shaha (2010) documented the quantification of the relationship among nursing, financial success, and nurse and patient satisfaction. The study examined measures of quality and clinical excellence, specifically acute myocardial infarction (AMI), heart failure (HF), and community acquired pneumonia (CAP). Financial performance measures were extracted to compute costs per adjusted discharge and case mix adjustments as well as nurse and patient satisfaction from a third-party survey. The impact of nursing on outcomes from a value perspective was significant. Both financial performance and satisfaction were positively affected; costs decreased, profitability increased, and satisfaction increased (Shaha, 2010).

In another study by Kohlbrenner, Whitelaw, and Cannady (2011), the contributions of nurses specific to quality performance standards for venous thromboembolism, patient safety, quality of care, and financial performance were identified. When nurses spent increased time with patients to avoid the preventable complication of venous thromboembolism, a positive and direct financial impact resulted.

There are numerous methods to identify value from the use of resources; each method provides information to clarify what should be done and what work is no longer needed. These different value considerations provide an overview of the need for and challenges in shifting the focus from solely volume measurements to multimeasurement systems that are driven by patient value. To be sure, as healthcare reform efforts move forward, clear valuation of healthcare work will be multifaceted directly related to reimbursement.

Basics of Budgeting

Every organization develops a plan that includes anticipated volume of work, the cost of the work to be accomplished, and the expenses required to make that work a reality. At best, this plan or budget serves as a guide to the allocation of resources. While the basics of budgeting remain quite stable, the regulatory requirements for specific fiscal transactions change frequently and require higher-level financial expertise. The following is a list of additional resources for budgeting:

- Dietrich & Anderson (2012)
- Dunham-Taylor & Pinczuk (2010)
- Finkler, Kovner, & Jones (2007)
- McCue & Glick (2009)

There are also numerous, more in-depth resources on specific and detailed aspects of budgeting in healthcare organizations. Interested nurses are encouraged to access current references. A basic understanding of the budget is an expectation for all healthcare workers while the complexities and intricacies of forecasting and accounting should be understood only at a general level, referring questions to the financial experts. Appendix A includes descriptions of common financial reports.

SCENARIO

Your team has identified a need for an additional nurse and a new piece of equipment that has been documented and published in other facilities to save costs and improve quality. In an informal setting, you requested consideration of this idea and expenditure and were told that it was not in the budget. You really believe this should happen for several important reasons.

Discussion Question

Work with 2–3 team members. Using financial principles, value-driven outcomes, and multilevel measurements, build a convincing case to present formally to the supervisor.

At the unit or department level, several items of information are required for the basic budget. These include *projected work volume*; the *operating budget*, which includes required supplies, equipment, and support for the physical setting to provide patient care; and a *personnel budget* that includes required personnel to provide and support the identified patient care. Within each of these three major categories, it is important and helpful to forecast needs across a 12-month period to support balancing of revenues and expenses. Regular adjustments of expenses based on actual patient volumes are expected and necessary for effective resource management.

In addition to the operating and personnel budgets, there is a capital budget. The *capital budget* is distinct from the operating and personnel budget in that the source of funding for these items is from previous year organizational profits. A capital budget includes larger items that generally exceed a certain cost and are expected to last beyond 1 year. Typical items include diagnostic equipment, furniture, and technology hardware and software.

Dashboards and Measures

In this section, the use of dashboards and analysis of variances from targeted data are discussed. Dashboards and scorecards have become useful to leaders in managing the plethora of data in a strategic manner. Typically, **dashboards** are a combination of graphics and numbers to quickly display important data elements. Basic information, technology considerations for accessibility to data, and meaningful measures that users have some control over are important considerations when constructing a dashboard ("Effective Dashboards," 2011). According to Mick (2011), administrators and stakeholders want to know if financial investments in programs are achieving the desired outcomes as well as compliance with regulatory requirements. Thus dashboards with a combination of financial, performance, and productivity measures reported in real time become critical resources for clinicians. Continually monitoring progress and data allows for course corrections or changes in strategy in a timely manner.

Effective dashboards include data that individuals can react to and have control over. For example, a unit clinical dashboard would include the number and type of caregivers present; a summary of the levels of education, experience, and expertise; and comparisons to target hours of care and cost projections. Another dashboard would be specific to patient feedback and satisfaction with specific areas of care, such as caregiver responsiveness, information provided, and level of pain relief achieved. Using a focused method that attempts to select those most critical variables is an important first step. Appendix B includes an example of multiple metrics to analyze staffing effectiveness. Figure 8-4 provides an example of a dashboard focusing on critical measures for the nursing staff on an oncology unit.

The greatest difficulty with dashboards is to identify and measure what really matters—which metrics are the critical variables that indicate value, service, and cost outcomes accurately and comprehensively. As previously noted, multiple related metrics are required to explain the causality of relationships; seldom does one variable explain one outcome. By its very essence, the complex and dynamic nature of health care renders it resistant to simple linear, cause-and-effect metrics. For example, no one intervention is accountable for the resolution of a patient's pneumonia; diet, fluids, medications, and activity all contribute to the resolution of the chest congestion. Similarly, the hours per patient day (HPPD) metric cannot be linked simply and traced to the activities of a single unit leader; the competence of staff, level of illness of patients, number of interventions required, and availability of equipment and supplies all impact the level of HPPD.

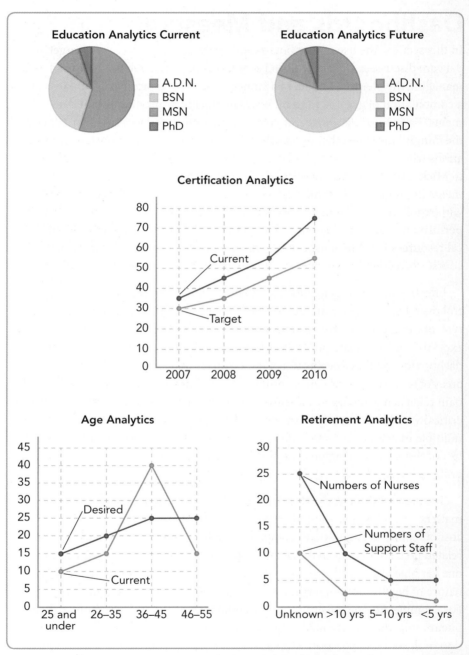

Figure 8-4 Dashboard: Oncology unit retention

It is seldom readily apparent which combinations of metrics provide the desired information. Further, as the work of health care continues to evolve, the evidence changes and the metrics will also need to change. Appendix C provides an overview of evolving metrics resulting from innovation specific to documentation.

Comparing multiple metrics often provides new insight to performance. For example, safe medication administration is a major challenge for all healthcare workers in the United States. Multiple structure and process variables interact to produce safe medication administration. Working to decrease preventable adverse drug events (PADE) without additional changes to structures and/or process variables could be futile. For example, increasing nursing hours of care without adding electronic processes to support patient identification and ensure legibility of orders could result in no change in the number of PADEs. To effect change, combinations of variables known to impact the structure and processes are needed. In Table 8-3, scenario 1 reflects the optimal conditions scenario for medication administration patient excellence based on the structure and processes available.

Another important issue is the fact that focusing on the combinations of metrics or aggregate metrics has advantages and disadvantages, supporters and nonsupporters. Supporters see the value of assessing multiple perspectives, and nonsupporters prefer one metric, usually a financial metric, to provide the essential information in a simple and straightforward manner. It is always important to identify the critical variables, build the case for the selected combination of variables and their associated metrics, and document the results.

Table 8-3 Preventable adverse drug events (PADE): Multiple inputs, processes, and metrics

Structure	Processes	Metrics	Expected level of performance
Scenario 1			
• Electronic health record	• Computerized physician order entry with standard order sets	• Number of PADEs	• Fewer than 4 PADEs/month or 0.001 error/100,000 doses
• Enclosed medication preparation rooms		• Nursing hrs of care per patient day	• Nursing hrs less than 6.0 hrs/patient day
• Bright task lighting at least 1400 lux	• Computerized medication administration documentation	• Pharmacist hrs/patient day	• Pharmacist hrs less than 0.2 hr/patient day
• Single bed rooms		• Total cost of care/patient day	• Cost of patient day < $240.00/day
• Decentralized pharmacists	• Bedside documentation	• Number of verbal orders	• < 2% verbal orders
• Positive patient identification	• Patient/medication bar coding	• Turnaround time from order to dispensing for first dose, non-stat medications	• Turnaround time (TAT) < 60 min for first dose, non-stat medications
Scenario 2			
• Manual documentation system	• Manual documentation at central station	• Number of PADEs	• Fewer than 20 PADEs/month or 0.005 error/100,000 doses
• 75% single bed rooms	• Handwritten physician orders	• Nursing hrs of care per patient	• Nursing hrs less than 6.2 hrs/patient day
• Centralized pharmacy services	• Manual order transcription	• Pharmacist hrs/patient day	• Pharmacist hrs less than 0.25 hr/patient day
• Overhead lighting less than 1400 lux	• Visual patient name identification	• Total cost of care/patient day	• Cost of patient day < $300.00/day
		• Number of verbal orders	• < 10% verbal orders
			• TAT < 3 hrs for first dose, non-stat medications

Structure	Processes	Metrics	Expected level of performance
Scenario 3			
• Electronic medication administration record	• Manual documentation at central station	• Number of PADEs	• Fewer than 15 PADEs/month or 0.004 error/100,000 doses
• 75% single bed rooms	• Handwritten physician orders	• Nursing hrs of care per patient day	• Nursing hrs less than 6.1 hrs/patient day
• Centralized pharmacy services	• Manual order transcription	• Pharmacist hrs/ patient day	• Pharmacist hrs less than 0.22 hr/patient day
• Overhead lighting less than 1400 lux	• Electronic documentation/ reconciliation of medications	• Total cost of care/ patient day	• Cost of patient day < $275.00/day
	• Visual patient name identification	• Number of verbal orders	• < 10% verbal orders
			• TAT < 2 hrs for first dose, non-stat medications

Variance Management

It is rare for there to be a perfect match between desired and actual outcomes. Once the data are gathered, available, and displayed, they can be interpreted for potential course correction action. Variance between needs and resources is a reflection of the realities of forecasting human behaviors. Important information can be gained from analyzing, monitoring, and adjusting system elements in a timely manner.

CRITICAL THOUGHT

One must ask if variance is indeed a forecasting problem or merely a reflection of a living system.

Variances occur routinely in all of the major resource categories: personnel, finances, technology, equipment, and time. The information specific to the variances or differences between desired outcomes and actual outcomes is an essential data point for system effective evaluations. Variances occur at the individual, unit, and system level, depending on the type of analysis. Once a significant variance is identified, it is important to determine if the variance is natural or artificial. According to Long (2002), natural variances occur in levels of competence, responses to treatments, timing of interventions, and communication styles. In contrast, artificial variances are those that one wants to eliminate, such as errors, lack of knowledge, or ineffective scheduling. The goal is to work to minimize the natural variances and eliminate the artificial variances to improve forecasting accuracy (Long, 2002).

Examination of the required staff needed for care and the actual staff is a routine activity of nurse leaders. What is not routine is the systematic documentation of the difference between required and actual hours and the interventions to address and mediate the variance or gap. Note that both positive and negative variances need to be addressed and documented.

Staffing variances are of great concern to caregivers. In spite of the efforts to plan and project adequate numbers of staff, variances continue. The identification and management of the variance between needed staff and actual staff hours can be helpful to improving and decreasing future variances. At some point in time, there should be a team discussion to ensure inclusion of issues from the direct caregiver perspective as well as the manager perspective. Managing the difference between actual hours of staff and required hours of care requires analysis of individual caregiver variances well as total variance hours. Figure 8-5 presents a variance analysis template that displays the actual, required, and variances in the hours of an evening shift. When a significant variance is determined, variance actions are implemented and documented. Most organizations select a reaction point when action will be taken, such as plus or minus 5 percent or 10 percent variance. These data provide valuable trend information for nurses as they continually work to create effective workload management systems.

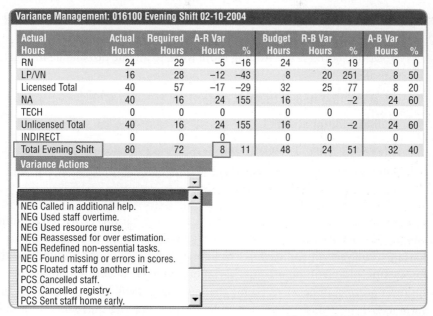

Variance Management: 016100 Evening Shift 02-10-2004

Actual Hours	Actual Hours	Required Hours	A-R Var Hours	%	Budget Hours	R-B Var Hours	%	A-B Var Hours	%
RN	24	29	−5	−16	24	5	19	0	0
LP/VN	16	28	−12	−43	8	20	251	8	50
Licensed Total	40	57	−17	−29	32	25	77	8	20
NA	40	16	24	155	16		−2	24	60
TECH	0	0	0		0	0		0	
Unlicensed Total	40	16	24	155	16		−2	24	60
INDIRECT	0	0	0		0	0		0	
Total Evening Shift	80	72	8	11	48	24	51	32	40

Variance Actions

NEG Called in additional help.
NEG Used staff overtime.
NEG Used resource nurse.
NEG Reassessed for over estimation.
NEG Redefined non-essential tasks.
NEG Found missing or errors in scores.
PCS Floated staff to another unit.
PCS Cancelled staff.
PCS Cancelled registry.
PCS Sent staff home early.

Figure 8-5 Variance analysis

Eliminating non-value-added work is an intervention that is often overlooked. Typically, new interventions and processes are added to work lists without removing outdated processes. Also, system inefficiencies are often not recognized and continue to require time that is not adding value to the outcomes. Efforts to identify and minimize time spent in searching for supplies and equipment, inefficient handoffs at shift change, waiting because of lack of response, waiting for transportation, and work-arounds are important in increasing efficiency and effectiveness as well as in reducing the gap between required and actual staff (Korner, Hartman, Agee, & McNally, 2011; Storfjell, Ohlson, Omoike, Fitzpatrick, & Wetasin, 2009).

There are several strategies to address staffing variances. Examples of interventions to address the variance or gap between needs and actual staffing include the following:

- Work as a team, not as individuals, when there is a gap. Be proactive together. Working as an individual can be isolating, impulsive, and highly stressful.

- Prioritize together as a team. Identify patient care issues that require immediate attention and those that can be safely postponed until later in the shift or until the next shift. Postpone nonemergent patient care.

- Delegate and supervise to the best of your ability.

- Communicate regularly during the shift. Arrange for short, frequent updates with the team to assess how well things are going and reassign and reprioritize as needed.

- Postpone admissions. Adding more work to an out-of-balance unit is unsafe.

- Float existing staff to the unit in need.

- Call in additional staff.

- Reevaluate patient acuity ratings.

- Document variance management that includes actions taken, patient care concerns, safety issues, and other events.

In summary, managing the difference between what was projected or anticipated and what actually occurred is an essential step in managing resources. Variance analysis with all resource categories is important and strengthens the forecasting and planning process. Variations typically occur in finances, personnel, and/or supplies. Everything that has a target will have a variance. Zero variances, as previously noted, are most unlikely. Practice and geographic variations are also significant. Variations in finance can result from greater or lesser revenues and greater or lesser expenses. Analysis of variances is best focused at the micro level, the point at which a meaningful interpretation can be made as well as a focused intervention. The goal of variance analysis is to strengthen the accuracy of predictions and minimize crisis management and intervention when there is a gap between what was available and what was needed.

In most cases, variation that exceeds resources is problematic. The delicate and dynamic challenge to balance variation and standardization is forever present. Expert clinicians must determine the basic principles that should be standardized and also when to vary in the application of those principles.

Variations in practice patterns also have an impact on price, supply, and demand. Wennberg, the principal investigator and series editor of the *Dartmouth Atlas*, has documented significant geographic variations in medical practice since the early 1970s. According to Wennberg and colleagues (2004), Medicare patients with similar chronic conditions receive strikingly different care, even among hospitals identified as "best" for geriatric care. The studies show that the frequency of physician visits, the number of diagnostic tests, and the rate of hospital and intensive care unit (ICU) stays vary markedly (Table 8-4). The studies show that a higher intensity of care and higher level of spending are not associated with better quality or longer survival times even in the most renowned teaching hospitals.

Table 8-4 Comparison of provider services for cancer, CHF, and COPD (risk adjusted)

	Lowest	Highest	% Variation
Days in the hospital	8.5	32.3	25%
Days in ICU	0.6	13.4	45%
Physician visits	13	99	37%

Source: Wennberg et al. (2004).

The variation documented by Wennberg and colleagues (2004) is difficult to explain or justify. The same analysis of caregiver variation is also needed to identify which standards of care represent best practices and best outcomes. In light of the variations in provider practices, the work of caregivers must necessarily vary in response to the variations of length of time in the facility, in the ICU, and in assisting the physician during rounds.

Concluding Thoughts: The Role of the Clinical Nurse Leader in Resource Management

Managing healthcare resources is a complex and at times unwieldy process. The goal of having the right resources for the right patient can be overwhelming at best. The clinical nurse leader is ideally positioned to regularly identify and share needs with those managing resource processes; it is the content of the resource needs that the nurse is able to provide. In many organizations, staff create a documented process to communicate the effectiveness of the categories of financial, staffing, equipment, technology, and time for managers and leaders. This is a vital process because clinical leaders are the only ones who can identify the specific impact on patient care processes; managers and leaders can only infer and speculate based on observations of clinical leaders. Finally, be sure to provide both positive and negative feedback on resources—the team needs to know when things are going well and when they are out of range.

CHAPTER TEST QUESTIONS

1. The interactions among price, supply, and demand in health care are (a) usually linear and driven by prices, (b) highly interactive and unpredictable, (c) currently driven by the demand for technology, or (d) are unrelated to healthcare quality.

2. Healthcare economics provides (a) guidance for healthcare reform, (b) information about the current status of national spending, (c) an overview of the study of supply, price, and demand interactions, or (d) information about the motivations for spending in the United States.

3. Calculation of the demand for nurses is (a) a state function, (b) a national function, (c) still to be done accurately, or (d) essential for funding of national legislation.

4. Uninsured populations are the result of (a) excessive costs for coverage, (b) excess demand for insurance coverage, (c) lack of employment, or (d) illegal immigrants.

5. Time resources (a) can be controlled with time management training, (b) are not as important to understand and manage as human and financial resources, (c) will never be adequate given the complex world of health care, or (d) are needed to adequately plan, analyze, and provide services.

6. The current healthcare system (a) provides health care that is costly and inconsistent in quality levels, (b) while costly, provides the most accessible care in the world, (c) would benefit from a national healthcare system, or (d) reflects a system in which price, supply, and demand are out of balance.

www

7. Productivity monitoring is intended to provide (a) a snapshot of the quality of care being delivered, (b) one metric specific to efficiency of output to total work, (c) the cost of current supply and demand for healthcare services, or (d) a metric used by the financial services department.

8. Dashboards are (a) management tools created to display multiple metrics specific to an area of interest, (b) limited to executives because of patient privacy regulations, (c) another management fad that will soon be replaced by another fad, or (d) difficult to create because of the extensive amount of data available.

9. Variance analysis (a) is additional work after the shift has ended and is often forgotten, (b) results in useful information about performance specific to a target, (c) requires high-level financial experts to complete adequately, or (d) should be completed at least monthly.

10. Value measurements are intended to identify (a) the cost–benefit ratio of dollars expended, (b) a record of process measurements and outcome measurements, (c) the positive change in a patient's health status or functionality based on expenditures of resources, or (d) the savings resulting from excess demand over supply.

> **WWW**
>
> For a full suite of assignments and additional learning activities, use the access code located in the front of your book to visit the exclusive website: http://go.jblearning.com/leadership. If you do not have an access code, you can obtain one at the site.

References

Arrow, K. (1963). Uncertainty and the welfare economics of medical care. *American Economic Review, 53*(5), 941–973.

Buerhaus, P. I. (1998). Milton Weinstein's insights on the development, use and methodologic problems in cost-effectiveness analysis. *Journal of Nursing Scholarship, 30*(3), 223–228.

Change Healthcare. (n.d.). The actionable cost transparency solution. Retrieved from www.changehealthcare.com

Consumer-Purchaser Disclosure Project. (2011). About the disclosure project. Retrieved from http://healthcaredisclosure.org/

Dietrich, M. O., & Anderson, G. D. (2012). *The financial professional's guide to healthcare reform.* Hoboken, NJ: Wiley.

Dunham-Taylor, J., & Pinczuk, J. (2010). *Financial management for nurse managers: Merging the heart with the dollar* (2nd ed.). Sudbury, MA: Jones and Bartlett.

Effective dashboards: What to measure and how to show it. (2011, June). *Hospitals & Health Networks.*

Feldstein, P. J. (2012). *Health care economics* (7th ed.). New York, NY: Delmar Cengage Learning.

Finkler, S. A., Kovner, C. A., & Jones, C. (2007). *Financial management for nurse managers and executives.* St. Louis, MO: Saunders Elsevier.

Folland, S. (2010). *Economics of health and healthcare* (6th ed.). Upper Saddle River, NJ: Prentice Hall.

Getzen, T. E. (2010). *Health economics and financing* (4th ed.). Hoboken, NJ: Wiley.

HealthReform.gov. (n.d.). About HealthReform.gov. Retrieved from http://www.healthreform.gov/about/index.html

Hinson, T. D., & Spatz, D. L. (2011). Improving nurse retention in a large tertiary acute-care hospital. *Journal of Nursing Administration, 41*(3), 103–108.

Kennedy, K. (2011, June 30). Health care costs vary widely, study shows. *USA Today.* Retrieved from http://www.usatoday.com/money/industries/health/2011-06-30-health-costs-wide-differences-locally_n.htm

Kohlbrenner, J., Whitelaw, G., & Cannaday, D. (2011). Nurses critical to quality, safety, and now financial performance. *Journal of Nursing Administration, 41*(3), 122–128.

Korner, K. T., Hartman, N. M., Agee, A., & McNally, M. (2011). Lean tools and concepts reduce waste, improve efficiency. *American Nurse Today, 6*(3), 41–42.

Long, M. C. (2002). *Translating the principles of variability management into reality: One physician's perspective.* Boston, MA: Boston University School of Management, Executive Learning.

Malloch, K., Davenport, S., Hatler, C., & Milton, D. (2003). Nursing workforce management: Using benchmarking for planning and outcomes monitoring. *Journal of Nursing Administration, 33*(10), 538–543.

McCue, M. J., & Glick, N. D. (2009). *Financial management of health care organizations: An introduction to fundamental tools, concepts and applications.* San Francisco, CA: Jossey-Bass.

Mick, J. (2011). Data-driven decision making: A nursing research and evidence-based practice dashboard. *Journal of Nursing Administration, 41*(10), 391–393.

Porter, M. E. (2010). What is value in health care? *New England Journal of Medicine, 363*(26), 2477–2481.

Shaha, S. H. (2010). Nursing makes a significant difference: A multihospital correlational study. *Nurse Leader, 8*(3), 36–39.

Shi, L., & Singh, D. A. (2012). *Delivering health care in America: A systems approach* (5th ed.). Sudbury, MA: Jones & Bartlett Learning.

StateHealthFacts.org. (n.d.). Registered nurses per 100,000 population, 2010. Retrieved from http://www.statehealthfacts.org/comparemaptable.jsp?cat=8&ind=439

Storfjell, J. L., Ohlson, S., Omoike, O., Fitzpatrick, T., & Wetasin, K. (2009). Non-value added time: The million dollar nursing opportunity. *Journal of Nursing Administration, 39*(1), 38–45.

Wennberg, J. E., Fisher, E. S., Stukel, T. A., Skinner, J. S., Sharp, S. M., & Bronner, K. K. (2004). Use of hospitals, physician visits, and hospice care during last six months of life among cohorts loyal to highly respected hospitals in the United States. *British Medical Journal, 328*, 607–612.

Appendix A

Common Financial Reports

Balance Sheet (Statement of Financial Position)

A **balance sheet** is a financial statement that includes assets, liabilities, and equity. It is a snapshot of the organization's financial position at a specific point in time. Current assets include cash, accounts receivable, inventories, income taxes receivable, investments, intangible assets, and other. Property and equipment assets include property, land, buildings, equipment, construction in progress, and accumulated depreciation. Liabilities include accounts payable, accrued salaries, long-term debt, professional liability risks, and other. Equity is the difference between assets and liabilities.

Income Statement

An **income statement** is a financial statement that includes information about revenue sources and expenses at a specific point in time.

Cash Flow Operating Activities

Cash flow operating activities is a financial report that shows the cash inflow and outflow activities or financial stability of the organization.

Source: Dunham-Taylor, J., & Pinczuk, J. (2010). *Financial management for nurse managers: Merging the heart with the dollar* (2nd ed.). Sudbury, MA: Jones and Bartlett.

Appendix B

Staffing Effectiveness: Scorecard

Evaluation of resources and their impact on outcomes is an essential attribute of cultures supportive of professional accountability. In this analysis, the human resource indicators reflect the inputs that produced the clinical outcomes on the right side of the table.

Human resource indicators		Clinical indicators	
Hours of care: % Registered nurses	850 hours/62% RN	Number of patient codes	8
Hours of care: Respiratory therapy	125 hours/2% RT	Patient falls with injury	2
Hours of care: Social worker	50 hours/0.5% of patient hours	Medication omissions	30
Hours of support: Advanced practice nurses	150 hours/10% APN	Medications late (greater than 60 minutes)	55
% Core staff	80%	Surgical site infections	0
% Registry staff	20%	Patient satisfaction with skill of nurses	88th percentile
Admission support	55% admissions completed prior to unit	Employee satisfaction	75th percentile

Appendix C

Evolving Metrics

In this table, the evolution of documentation from the paper and pen to the mass storage device or memory stick, associated expectations of the innovation, and the metrics to evaluate the innovation are identified. Each evolving change or innovation requires reconsideration of the expected metrics to accurately identify the real value of the innovation. It is important to note that continuing to use the same expectations and metrics for paper and pen handwriting for voice recognition would be an incomplete recognition of the benefits of voice recognition. The metrics must reflect the expectations.

Innovations to improve the process, quality, and storage of information have evolved over time. Each new documentation innovation is associated with new expectations and new metrics. The continuing challenge is to review and revise the expectations and then modify the metric to reflect the outcomes.

Innovation	Expectation	Metric
Paper and pen to record information/handwriting	Documentation of the information that can be retrieved	Amount of paper/ink used Amount of time to document
Electronic writing/typing	Documentation of the information Retrievable from paper file Legible Correct spelling	Amount of paper Cost of device/keyboard technology Decreased time for documentation
Computer programs for data/word processing to include storage devices 3-inch floppy disk Zip drive/CD/DVD Mass storage device/ memory stick	Large file data storage Portable High-speed access Retrievable from multiple access points File backup device Device compatibility	Data storage capacity Cost of hardware, devices, and software Size of devices Productivity; number of pages produced
Voice recognition documentation	Elimination of typing Device compatibility Increased speed for documentation	Productivity Number of pages produced Cost of recording/ interface devices

LEADERSHIP IS A NOBLE CALLING. IN ADDITION TO MEETING WELL-DEFINED STRATEGIC OBJECTIVES, LEADERS MUST ALSO HELP THEIR ORGANIZATIONS MAKE MEANINGFUL CONTRIBUTIONS TO SOCIAL ISSUES, ECONOMIC GROWTH, AND POLITICAL STABILITY. THAT'S WHY EFFECTIVE ORGANIZATIONAL LEADERSHIP PLAYS A VITAL ROLE IN SHAPING OUR WORLD. —ROBERT L. JOSS

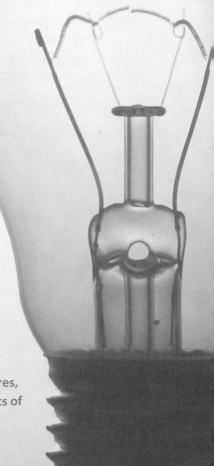

CHAPTER OBJECTIVES

Upon completion of this chapter, the reader will be able to do the following:

» Understand the fundamental networks and organizations that support professional practice.

» Define the relationship among structure, profession, practice, and the individual in ways that reflect contemporary structures for health care.

» Enumerate the elements of complex adaptive systems and the frames they create for professional practice.

» Outline the characteristics driving a stronger fit between the demands of the external environment and the internal organization facilitating health transformation.

» List at least five major elements of shared governance as a reflection of how they advance professional practice.

» State the considerations related to structures that support professional practice and the interface among those structures, individual behavior of the professional, and the requirements of the profession.

Organizations as Networks: Creating a Context for Professional Practice

Leadership isn't just about changing things; it's about changing the world. Every person who has any level of awareness recognizes that the world is in the midst of major social transformation, the transformation that extends to every component of our sociocultural experience, including today's major transformations in health care (Kaufman, 2011). American health care has come to the major work of transformation much later than other segments of the social and global community. It is now deeply in the throes of a dramatic shift from a vertically oriented, tertiary-care, pay-for-procedure, illness-focused system toward a system that represents the social value of health, engages every citizen, and provides access to the most basic of health services (McClellan, McKethan, Lewis, Roski, & Fisher, 2010).

CRITICAL THOUGHT

Leadership isn't just about changing things; it's about changing the world.

Although the political process within which transformation unfolds is noisy, messy, competitive, and challenging to work through, people of every political stripe recognize that the old system is no longer viable or relevant for the future. The design, structuring, funding, and operation of the transformed system will go through many iterations as what works and is sustainably effective gets clarified and validated through the process of experimentation, application, and evaluation.

Much of the effort to move toward a transformed generative healthcare model includes creating a system that represents a foundation grounded in general access, service synthesis, critical health impact, resource and service value, impact on sustainable social health, and evidentiary foundation, which advances practice based on the evidence of impact. Each of these are small components of the broad dynamic shift in health care and will transform the way in which it is organized and structured and, ultimately, the way it is delivered. Although broad disagreement exists as to which strategies might work to get us to this outcome, the effort to move toward that goal is clearly underway.

As the healthcare system works to recalibrate itself for a more viable and relevant future, every clinical professional plays a role and has a stake in both the process and the outcome of this change. Changing service means adjusting structure to support it. Building access and equity into the service framework requires that equity, ownership, and engagement are required of every professional role as an interdisciplinary design emerges as one of the nonnegotiable elements that underpins all efforts at building truly effective value-based health care (Pauly, 2010) (Figure 9-1).

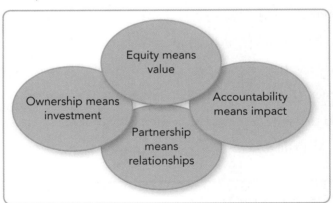

Figure 9-1 Four professional requisites

The structures that will best support this effort and role characteristics of healthcare leadership that will guide its implementation require role clarity, autonomy with integration, professional team-based performance, the structure for shared decision making, and the means to ensure that the clinical work done is resource-effective, timely, value-based, and works to advance the mission and vision of the healthcare system. Good clinical structure requires that leaders lay the foundation for embedding the expectation that evaluation will be ongoing, work will be continuously modified based on the evidence, and the work and the structure necessary to support work will be flexible and adaptable enough to meet the demand for change that evidence requires (Rapp et al., 2010).

As the vision and value of a health-based future unfold, become more clearly articulated, and achieve a level of agreement, new structure will evolve to support it. Historically leadership was based on the idea that form or structure follows function; however, the reality is that both the structure and function are dynamically intertwined and constantly work to affect each other. In **complex adaptive systems** this relationship between an environment and a system is like a continuous dance; each brings something to the partnership and both are dependent on the action of the other. Ultimately, synthesis is the product of the action on both. Rather than directing deliberation, decisions, or work processes, structure should provide a framework for dialogue, deliberation, gathering, deciding, and acting on the part of the stakeholders. They can then represent through both their collective wisdom and individual contribution a synthesis among them that demonstrates a sound reflective process, effective dialogue, evidence-driven decision making, integrated action, and coordinated effort in evaluating impact in changing practice. This network of intersections, interactions, and interrelationships is the place where the vast majority of the work related to deliberation, design, and doing occurs (Miller & Page, 2007).

REFLECTIVE QUESTION

Is collective deliberation and decision making always better than individual decision making? The answer is no, but why? In what circumstances is collective deliberation wise, and in what other circumstances is collective decision making not appropriate?

Structure is the format within which the dynamics of human interaction unfold. Structure either supports that confluence of activities or intends to impede it. Like the work itself, effective structure involves and is constantly re-created to adjust to changes in the relationship between the environment and the organization. This relationship is not fixed. It reflects all of the vagaries and dynamics of the continuous development and advancement in the human community, and the mechanisms of that advancement work on changing who people are and what they do. Organization calls for constant alignment among power, authority, decision making, innovation, control, roles, work processes, and the mechanisms for evaluating effectiveness (Tolbert & Hall, 2009). These more fluid structures, often called networks, for contemporary healthcare organizations now necessarily consider the work of healing and health as a transdisciplinary, integrated, partnership activity. These networks represent the confluence of the efforts of each member around the commitment of all to have an impact on health. The people of these networks ensure that those who are served in the healthcare system demonstrate the best values of health in their own life and experiences. It is the network structure that supports this level of integration, collaboration, and the therapeutic interactions that advance the achievement of health, both personal and societal.

Complex Adaptive Systems

Complex adaptive systems theory is grounded in work generating out of biology, mathematics, physics, and complexity science (Miller & Page, 2007). Complexity science as applied to human behavior is represented in the study of a number of different approaches to understanding the relationship among behavior, organizations, and the larger systems that form the context. Predominantly many of the foundations within complexity science that apply to human behavior and health care fall into the areas of behavioral economics, networks, evolution and adaptation, pattern formation, systems theory, nonlinear dynamics, and game theory. Although they share many foundational principles, each of these arenas of study focus on a different element of complex patterns, networks, interactions, intersections, and processes that represent how systems behave.

Of special interest to the study of organizations is the understanding of sociotechnical systems and their impact on human dynamics. Because health care is one of the strongest representations of the interaction of social and technical forces, it is clear that there is a direct link between those forces and organizational design and performance (Resinicow & Page, 2008). Although there are certainly linear cause-and-effect relationships, the predominant relationships are nonlinear, complex, unpredictable, and highly interactive. The failure to build organizational structures to recognize these complex sets of interrelationships and to design work models that reflect them has had a dramatic impact on work processes, patient care, quality, and health outcomes (Paley, 2007). It is suggested in complex thinking that focus on either social (organizational) or on technical (functional/applied) processes actually increases the unpredictable, uncertain, uninformed, unstable forces impacting systems, organizations, and work groups. Optimization in the system is a reflection of the strong goodness of fit between the human organizational dynamics and the technological functional processes that comprise the overall structure of the work environment.

CRITICAL THOUGHT

The strong interdependence of all knowledge workers implies a powerful need for organizational designs and structures that support collaborative relationships.

One of the interesting factors affecting organizations demonstrates that the traditional compartmentalization that is historically evident in organizational structures has actually paradoxically contributed to their own decline in productivity and effectiveness (Rouse, 2008). These paradoxical observations have indicated that regardless of improvements in technology, systems, productivity, benefits, value, and outcome have diminished measurably over the long term. Unless there was a goodness of fit between the structure of the organization, the dynamics of human behavior, and the processes and tools used to undertake work, any one of them taken alone would negatively diminish value and outcome. This is especially true in systems where the predominant activity is knowledge work (Bennet & Bennet, 2010). Health care is clearly one of those arenas.

Structuring and organizing for knowledge work is one of the fundamental functional capacities of complex adaptive systems. Healthcare organizations are fundamentally driven by the application of complexity science as evidenced by the breadth and depth as well as variability of complex clinical activity and the intersecting impact of systems and structures that either support or impede it. The heavy interdependence that knowledge work suggests also indicates the need for organizational structure that supports and advances interdependence, interactivity, and integrating activities around a common user (the patient) in an environment where the outcome is the evidence of the convergence of the effort of many stakeholders, rather than the results of the efforts of any one stakeholder (Leon, 2011).

Complex adaptive systems are living organisms whose structures very much represent the same characteristics as biological systems (Ang & Yin, 2008). Although they are not directly linked and are certainly not an exact replica, these complex living systems represent a model of organization that more closely represents the dynamic and interacting forces influencing systematic and individual human behavior (Figure 9-2). The traditional organizational structures of hospitals and healthcare systems presented organizations as great machines in a way that reflected the central themes of Newtonian physics (Kelly, 2005). Complex adaptive systems reflect a deeper understanding of complexity science and quantum mechanics as applied to human behaviors and human organizations.

This more living, fluid, relational approach to dynamic systems serves as a better metaphor within which organizational structures unfold and represent the closer characterization of how complex systems actually operate (Bjorn & Persson, 2009). We see complex adaptive systems in a wide-ranging set of exemplars in the broader society. From stock markets, to societal networks, to information systems, all the way to every level of biology of living things, the "adaptive" in "complex adaptive system" implies the ability to continuously and dynamically change when the relationship between the system and its environment shifts or is altered either by action in the relationship or circumstances beyond it (Marshall, 2011). In the system, there are a number of interdependent things, and these are identified as agents. A complex adaptive system is a densely linked, intersecting, and interacting connection of agents, each making their own contribution and acting both independently in making that contribution and interdependently in linking that contribution to the independent but related contributions of other agents (Shanine, Buchko, & Wheeler, 2011).

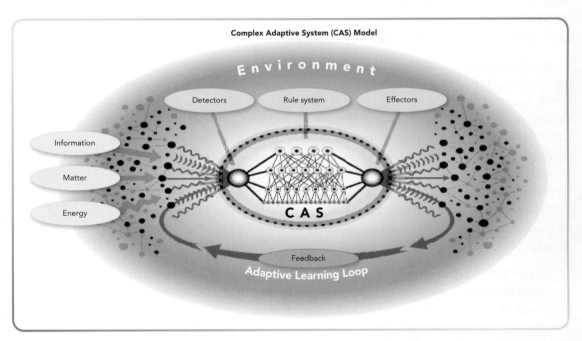

Figure 9-2 Complex adaptive systems network

Placing Power Where the Action Is

In complex adaptive systems, power is relocated out of the formal structure and is more closely aligned with the point-of-service decision making (Styer, 2007) (Figure 9-3). Although this occurs in many organizations, it is especially important in hospitals and healthcare systems. As these organizations begin to move away from a strong, clearly defined hierarchical infrastructure and management-only-driven frame for decision making, moving into more clearly knowledge-driven and point-of-service models, they will have to reformat their strategic, operations, and services processes to become more effective (Malloch, 2010). Increasingly short-term and responsive action must occur at the point of service in a way that can quickly adjust changes in strategy, tactics, programs, policies, and practice in a way that responds more effectively to the needs of the user.

> The framework for clinical excellence begins with structure that supports work processes that are fluid, flexible, and supportive of practice excellence in the organization. Building excellence into the fabric of an organization requires a supportive structure for caregivers as well as the commitment and engagement of individuals to the work of healing. Today's nurses are seeking work environments in which excellent patient care is supported, effective communication occurs, and caregivers are acknowledged for their positive behaviors and negative behaviors are addressed quickly.
>
> A structure that allows for change and supports efficient work processes and satisfaction is essential to achieve the desired excellence. A flat, decentralized structure is the hallmark of organizations who have achieved Magnet accreditation and high levels of excellence (ANCC, 2010).

Figure 9-3 Power and authority

Recalibrating decisions to be more effective means shifting the design and operation of the infrastructure by moving structure and supporting decisions to more facilitate their operation at the point of service. In complex adaptive approaches, integration of services and provider relationships along the user's continuum of care requires that organizations recalibrate their infrastructure; revise service delivery, interdisciplinary relationships, and work processes that demonstrate the effective convergence of their efforts; direct the relationship of effort to outcome; and evaluate practices and their impact in order to create sustainability.

These changes in the organizational structure and relationships now call for full engagement of all stakeholders in the elements of design, partnership, accountability, and ownership for effort and outcome (Porter-O'Grady, 2009). New frames of references and terms of engagement must reflect the measured affect on delivery, impact, and outcome, creating a clear relationship between the structure process and outcome of work in a manner that represents their synthesis. As organizations, for example, move into completely digitally driven documentation and clinical systems, new ways of practicing, interacting, communicating, working, and evaluating impact require modified vertical constructs, altered lines of authority, more localized locus of control, stronger unit-based collaborative models of deciding and acting, and better intersections and handoffs among providers and with users (Gunter, 2005).

Understanding How Clinical Work Changes

SCENARIO

Mary Cumming, RN, is trying to implement the use of texting for communicating changes in patients' conditions between registered nurses and physicians. The medical and nursing staffs are both thrilled with the idea because it makes communicating so much easier and response times to changing conditions quicker and more efficient.

However, Mary is receiving a lot of push back from the administration, legal, and quality departments because of the potential for Health Insurance Portability and Accountability Act violations related to confidentiality, consistency, and appropriateness. An additional problem is that younger staff are already texting in the workplace regarding patient care, and the more mature staff have not engaged it and are not thrilled with the idea.

The shared governance leadership has asked you and your colleagues to form a texting task force to deliberate this issue and to discuss all the variables and complexities that influence making a wise decision about what to do. They have asked that you establish a texting standard for the organization and present it to the Practice Council.

Discuss the issue with your colleagues, sort through the complexities, and construct a protocol/standard that could be presented to the Practice Council and have your team present and defend it with all your supporting rationale and evidence.

The emerging clinical leader must be increasingly clear about shifts in the environment that suggest a different calibration of work, workplace, and relationships (Porter-O'Grady & Malloch, 2010). These emerging leaders must be willing to explore self-directed, seamless, and integrated mechanisms for practice, interdisciplinary relationships, delivering care, and evaluating their relationships with the user (patient). Each of these practitioners must recognize that practice now represents a just-in-time dynamic that reflects the reality that current real-time practice serves as a baseline for changing next-time practice. For the practitioner there is a strong relationship between the work I did today and how it informs how I will do that work differently tomorrow. Much more horizontal and collaborative interaction around this work and how it performs will be a fundamental expectation of the professional worker. Furthermore, individuals at the point of service will need to be more self-directed and require more integrated and supported unit structures. Staff will need a stronger, more seamless, and horizontal set of relationships, interactions, and structures to support the collaborative point-of-service models of decision making, care delivery, and impact evaluation. These much more self-directed, relational structures will require a different management capacity and framework for advancing effective and integrated patient care.

The Changing Nature of Clinical Work

In the contemporary transformation of health care, traditional approaches to clinical delivery of service are no longer supported. In the contemporary age clinical work is reinventing ways that will provide new support for a different understanding of clinical work, of healthcare service, information management, definitions of quality, delineations of outcomes, kinds of clinical relationships, and the necessary intersections that will be required in order to advance effective, evidence-based delivery of care (Chalkidou et al., 2009). These changes will no doubt result in a changing organizational structure, altering the numbers and roles of managers in significant ways. Furthermore, clinical leadership will become increasingly important as more point-of-service decisions, actions, and relationships will form the centerpiece of the activities of patient care (Solow & Szmerekovsky, 2006). In health care there a number of significant shifts already under way that the clinical leader must incorporate into his or her understanding of leadership in practice. Some of these are as follows:

- Tertiary care is slowly being deconstructed as the ship of health care turns around to better provide a full range of service to every citizen in a much stronger primary-care-driven model.

- Accountability and value are now requiring a much stronger goodness of fit among services around patient populations in a way that demonstrates a net improvement in the health of these populations.

- Digital technology is making it possible to create an increasingly portable diagnostic, therapeutic, and interventional environment making it increasingly mobile, fluid, flexible, and portable.

- Organizational and management models now must reflect a higher degree of engagement and ownership of professional teams at the point of service because much of the ownership and the locus of control for effective decision making, practice, and measurement will be driven from that point of service.

- Increasingly, systems compete for value and quality; these systems will be measured based on their health impact, healthy status of the populations they serve, and the effective use of resources as it relates to their use and the difference they make.

- The fundamental value of practice is no longer embedded in volume measures related to how much an individual has done in the interests of patients. Instead measures will be based on what difference and impact action had and the efficient and effective relationship between clinical action and patient impact.

There are many critical influences that are driving these specific shifts in function activity and health care with which the clinical leader must be grounded. These changes in the environment are driving changes in the healthcare system. Creating a stronger fit between the emerging environmental conditions and the required organizational changes in health care will be important in healthcare services to thrive and to demonstrate its real value in the lives of those it serves:

- Change forces are now global; changes in the greater environment create the need for changes in the local setting. Clinical leaders must be aware of these environmental demands.

- The infrastructure and organization for health care must reflect a lean relationship between management, support, and providers in a network that represents their intense interaction and the need for sustaining their relationship.

- The financial model now reflects a strong emphasis on value rather than the volume. Doing more does not mean doing better. The most effective mechanism for doing better depends on the judicious use of time and resources. Using more resources does not demonstrate better outcomes.

- Focus of healthcare system structures, processes, and evidence is reflected in dynamics that clearly demonstrate impact, effectiveness, and significant measures of levels of health. Enabling and sustaining health is a social, structural, and functional aim of all healthcare services.

- Evidentiary dynamics and improvement science now guide mechanisms of advancing practice within the context of a strongly interfaced digital information infrastructure. The relationship between human action and digital infrastructure is now so critically aligned that one cannot proceed without connection to the other.

- Clinical leadership is mostly emergence, derived from the point of service, and clearly directed to specifically advancing decisions, relevant work action, changes in practice, and evidencing positive impact on health (Porter-O'Grady & Malloch, 2010).

 REFLECTIVE QUESTION

Can behavior be changed in any sustainable way simply by inviting people to change? Reflect on your answer carefully. What role does structure play in influencing behavioral change, and how does the impact of structure on behavior alter your approach to undertaking change?

From a Medical Model to a Health Model

The medical model requires an organization; the health model requires a network (Liebler & McConnell, 2012). The very foundations of the structure that supports the drive toward creating true and sustainable health are so different from the existing infrastructure that radical organizational surgery will be required to create an effective health model. In this future healthcare delivery system, unfolding now, there is a requisite for growing dependence on a primary infrastructure and, ultimately, a preventive health service structure. Primary service models require that health providers access the user earlier in the cycle of health long before the traditional high-intensity, high-intervention, and high-cost illness-based system normally addresses the needs of patients. Just imagine the complexity and detail of leadership work that must be undertaken in order to create a truly effective health-based delivery system for the whole nation (Figure 9-4).

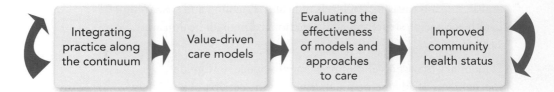

Figure 9-4 Contextual/environmental shifts

All of this transformation of health care occurs within the context of our broader social shift—one that is predominantly user driven (McStay, 2010). In user-driven systems, individual users hold the primary obligation for access, use, account-ability, and full participation in the actions that affect their lives and, in this case, their health at every level of society. User-driven models reflecting many of the principles of behavioral economics are emerging in support of this user-driven societal construct. Digitalization, information, and social networks all created the underpinning for translation of these approaches into a broader sociopolitical model that reflects a growing foundation for individual choice and social action. The natural and normative response to this sociocultural shift is greater intensity of interaction, integration, sharing, and social interdependence.

Ending Medical Separatism

Historically in the United States medical practice was the predominant paradigm for the health system. Physicians historically remained unilaterally directive and controlling as managers of medical and health decision making (Joint Com-mission, 1991; Mazur, 2003; Rivington, 1879; Taylor, 1974; Waddington, 1984). Because much of the unilateral control remained in the hands of physicians, broad-based, specific, and personal performance and outcome accountability have been relatively subjective. In this model, the public have viewed medicine as cloaked in the mystery of the incomprehensible, scientifically inarticulate, pro-fessionally protective, and compartmentally shrouded practices that could only be communicated effectively to each other (Mazur, 2003). Further enabling this protective pattern are broadly permissive state medical practice acts that serve to codify these mysteries and practices, protecting them from encroachment, question, or compromise. Over the years, a wide range of laws and regulations of every stripe emerged from the states that insulated physicians further from external influence or compromise and frequently shielded them from ques-tions and challenges to patterns of practice and professional behavior (Nelson, 2006a). Although much of this has changed considerably as a product of the emergence of the digital age, the effort to break through the shield is still chal-lenging and fraught with difficulty as the legal system slowly works to chip away at the bricks and mortar of professional entitlement, protectionism, and social nonaccountability (Nelson, 2006b). Adding to the effort to broader accountability is the increasing transparency created by the availability of digital information and increasing access and knowledge available to people who seek it and use it to make healthcare decisions.

Value-Driven Health Care

Within the context of the digital age, the transparency and availability of information are daily reminders of the increasing user locus of control (Kamae, 2010). In the healthcare world where the digital infrastructure now makes it possible for evidence-based, value-driven decisions to be made, conditions are now created for reorienting the delivery system to a much stronger point-of-service construct making it more functional, cost effective, and increasingly service sufficient (Aziz, 2006). The demand for quality now invariably includes the requisite for value, focusing on the relationship between performance and achievement. The achievement of value from the perspective of the user requires a stronger integration and linkage between providers. This interface between providers now more clearly defines expectations from the perspective of the user. Individual provider-driven expectations for outcomes mean nothing to the user if they do not coordinate well and synthesize in a way that has a net aggregated positive impact on the patient's experience.

CRITICAL THOUGHT

In the near future the entire health system will be reconfigured on achieving health values for the community. The nurse leader must put value at the center of practice and ask the question "why?" before responding to the question "what?"

This user-driven service model now requires a stronger linkage and integration among the disciplines, reflecting a deeper value and understanding of each others' contribution to the complex interaction positively affecting the patient experience. The organizational structure now requires that interdisciplinary team-based relationships be constructed and that the work of the disciplines be integrated in a way that is mutually supportive. Equity and value of the unique contribution of each discipline at the point of service now must be clearly articulated, and every element must converge around particular patient or population groupings in a way that demonstrates impact, difference, and resulting in better health (Wright et al., 2008).

Traditional organizational structural models cannot support this much more fluid, flexible, user-driven, provider-related model of health service delivery. These structures now must be carefully deconstructed as newer frames are created to help organize human action into a contributing, systematic, linked, and integrated pattern of practices and behaviors that when coalesced come together to make a significant difference in the health of those served.

This means that highly vertical, structured, department-oriented, silo-based models to clinical work must disappear into the shelves of history as new constructs are created. The challenge here will be the confrontation of old rituals and routines, patterns and practices that reflect the long history of people's accommodation of such structures and organizational frames. The ability to be flexible, accountable, and evidence driven will create much noise in the system as the professions attempt to adjust the dance of building truly equity-based balanced relationships among the disciplines. It will be fraught with its own contentions and challenges as new kinds of relationships are configured (Malloch & Porter-O'Grady, 2009a). This resulting structural and political noise will result in some organizational schizophrenia as clinical work groups attempt to move forward and confront those things that tend to move them backward. However, new roles will unfold, and new intersections and interactions will also emerge and interdisciplinary team-based dynamics will ultimately become the normative pattern of behavior at the point of service (Figure 9-5).

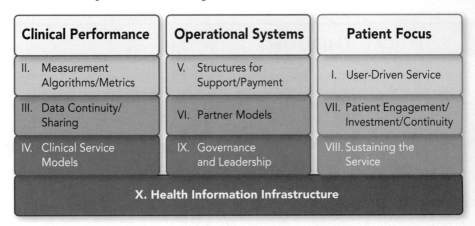

Figure 9-5 Accountable care systems

The nurse leader will be at the center of this journey to new relationships. Indeed, this leader will likely coordinate, integrate, and facilitate the journey just by virtue of position and role in the new organizational construct. The nurse leader will be central to the shift because of the unique nature of the nursing role in the central positioning it holds at the point of service (Shifflet & Moyer, 2010). This leader will require a different focus with regard to his or her self-perception, role characteristics, and willingness to engage the development of new models of relationships, interaction, communication, and clinical practice. More emphasis will be on the clinical leader, requiring the nurse with the bachelor of science degree to be better prepared in understanding these organizational shifts; interacting with other disciplines; more clearly delineating functions, roles, and expectations among the members of the clinical team; and more fully utilizing the digital tools necessary to facilitate and to advance the relationships and practices of these many professionals. This new structure creates a demand for the clinical leader to act as a catalyst and an agent of a much more collateral, collaborative, and horizontal set of relationships that creates an environment for shared decision making, mutual accountability, interdisciplinary practices, and integrated evaluation of the collective impact on the patient experience and the quality of health. This professional shared governance, shared decision making, and shared interaction become the framework for structuring the delivery of healthcare services in a much different way.

Elements of a New Kind of Structure

In a professional organization where integration partnerships are critical, vertical structures and command and control management methodologies are no longer relevant frames for organizational design (Zerwekh & Garneau, 2012). In professional organizations, the unique contribution of each member of every discipline is critical to the value of the work and to creating the context for service. In a patient care environment this criterion is especially important. The wide ranging number of disciplines having something to do with patient care must, at some point, intersect, interact, and create a convergence of effort that positively impacts the patient's continuum of care.

In this integrated professional organization structure, there must be a framework that supports activities at the point of service and sustains the clinical work processes of the professions in a meaningful way. Much of the interaction, relationships, and communication follow a horizontal trajectory requiring from the organization a strong commitment to equity, partnership, accountability, and ownership (Porter-O'Grady & Malloch, 2010). These driving principles are essential to creating a sustainable interaction among the professionals in a way that respects the contribution of each, the value of each to the other, the interdependence represented in the collective work, and the commitment of each discipline to working with all disciplines to converge their effort in a meaningful way to successfully address the issues of patient care. These are the foundations of the organizational structure commonly referred to as shared governance, a framework that provides the support of the professions, their interaction, and their collective obligation to advance the interest of health care.

There are specific reasons why a shared governance organizational structure operates effectively in complex adaptive systems such as a healthcare environment. First, the sustainability of healthcare services fully depends on how the point-of-service professionals function individually and collectively. Complex adaptive systems are user driven and require the inclusion and ownership of users as a system addresses their needs along their healthcare continuum. The traditional historic model of compartmentalized, nonintegrated, unilateral role characteristics and performance factors representing a more vertically designed organizational framework does not work to support the necessary relationships between disciplines in a way that advances the health needs of the user. Shared governance serves to build a stronger, more effective frame for the interactions necessary to operate in this more integrated environment (Bednarski, 2009).

Clinical knowledge is forever changing, growing, adapting, and improving. The structures of complex adaptive systems and the components necessary to operate effectively within them call for interdisciplinary equity and collective engagement with all stakeholders in the decisions and actions that represent the life of the system. In a complex organization the expression of ownership from the participants best demonstrates the organization's ability to adapt and thrive and respond to the call for change and transformation. Compartmentalized, vertically oriented, and unilateral operating systems often found in traditional organizational models are clearly inadequate to support the kinds of relationships and infrastructures that are required to provide and improve health care. Membership in professions implies a personal and collective level of ownership in the work of the profession. Membership requires a structure that recognizes this ownership, engages it, and invests in decisions and actions of the system and provides the demand for and integration and coalescing of efforts at the point of service around the needs of those the system serves (Batson, 2004). This linkage from all members who contribute to this work operates at a level beyond simple and arbitrary hierarchical and position-oriented structures and decision models and favors instead a collateral, integrated, invested model of ownership and engagement where providers and users converge in the dynamic interaction that meets the purposes of the system.

Secondly, the emergence of knowledge organizations demonstrates that knowledge is not fixed or finite and does not operate simply as a capacity. Knowledge, instead, is a utility; therefore, distance between the needs of knowledge workers and the supporting knowledge system and the design and structure of the organization can create significant impediments to the creation, generation, utility,

SCENARIO

Frank Taylor, RN, is the discharge planning coordinator on the geriatric diabetic services team. He is also chair of the service's Practice Council. Because of the changes stimulated by healthcare reform, the unit leadership has begun working on developing a continuum of care geriatric diabetic services model to ensure adequate services are available to geriatric diabetics across their continuum of need. Focusing on this population's continuing healthcare needs requires Frank and his colleagues to reflect on the model of service that would integrate the disciplines and link a variety of geriatric services in a model that would support geriatric diabetic patient care needs along their health continuum. The task appears complex and challenging, but Frank and his colleagues sense that it is the right priority to address.

Discussion Questions

1. Because this will require interdisciplinary team deliberation and decision making, who should be at the table? How do they reflect the continuum of care for this patient population?

2. Because Frank and his team are building a continuum of care service structure for this patient population, what are the services that will be provided and how does that reflect the continuum of care for this population?

3. What is the specific role of the nurse both in developing this continuum of care model and in its coordination, facilitation, and integration once the team has designed and formulated their desired approach for this population?

After responding to the above questions, create a map of the continuum of care services for this population, then identify who the key players are along the various stages of the continuum and what services they might provide for this population.

and evaluation of that knowledge (Bennet & Bennet, 2010). In a value-driven health system, narrowly vertically controlled structures now must move into multimodal, multidirectional integrated systems that accommodate the growing need for interdependence, integration, and building the capacity for judgment on the part of knowledge workers. This growing in importance of the character of the collective work of the professions and the increasing complexity of healthcare delivery now require that there be congruence and confluence among the organizational structures of the systems, the contributions and interface of the professions, and the impact of their collective effort in creating the conditions for sustainable health.

For these complex adaptive systems to thrive and for the professions within them to cooperate within an effective shared decision-making framework, the following principles must operate:

- The whole is always greater than the parts but also serves to define the parts.

- Every element and component of the system is a part of the whole system and must collectively support that system.

- A problem in any one part of the system ultimately affects the whole system.

- An effective user-driven system always operates from its point of service where the system lives and where the forces converge to have an impact and fulfill the purposes of the system.

- All disciplines serve the user and/or serve someone who serves the user.

- In complex adaptive systems, form and function interact with each other; otherwise they are not a dependent relationship.

- In a complex adaptive system, all members have ownership of their work and contribution to the system. The structure of the system must provide opportunity for full engagement of the owners and representation of the stake they hold in the work of the system.

- In a complex adaptive system, the managers are facilitators, integrators, and coordinators of the system, providing resource support and enabling the stakeholders to be successful in fulfilling the purposes of the system.

- Impact and outcome are always the locus of value. Decisions and actions are directed toward fulfilling and supporting a systems value.

In evidentiary dynamics and improvement science, evidence-based health practices require a more intensive and relational set of interactions that form a fundamental part of the processes and work of determining, undertaking, and validating the value of health care and of services provided (Malloch & Porter-O'Grady, 2009b). This evidence of value and impact required is the aggregation and integration of data that support the contribution of each professional and the collective integration of that contribution in a manner that clearly demonstrates the difference that makes on the services that it provides. This evidence-driven effort is simply not successful if it is not unfolded in a context that supports the collective, integrating, collaborative trends and the professional processes necessary to coalesce efforts that define the difference made and the impact obtained. In a digital infrastructure, information structures and data generation require that the collation, integration, and generation of relevant information reflect the evidentiary dynamic of the organization and the processes and functions that demonstrated action and advance its impact in the system. The accuracy of the relational work of the disciplines, its effective integration, and its value impact on the health of the population become the source point that demonstrates data utility, value, and impact on health (Parmelee, Bowen, Ross, Brown, & Huff, 2009).

CRITICAL THOUGHT

This emerging postdigital age moves everything toward more control by the user. User-driven service structures include health services. The nurse—indeed, all providers—now must focus on constructing patient-driven, user-friendly clinical models and service processes in a way that empowers users to manage their own health.

The third critical point reflects the reality that in a continuum of care approach, no one healthcare organization can own, control, or unilaterally mandate all of the service linkages and connections necessary to fully serve a specific population at any level of adequacy. Partnership, relationship, interaction, and collective correlation of effort along the horizontal continuum will be key to comprehensive and integrated population service. Increasingly the health of the population will demand relevant partnerships across the continuum of care, coordination and integration of the service continuum across partnerships, and the shift or change in the comprehensive provision of services as the health demands of the population change. Therefore, systems and the professionals that comprise them must always be fluid, flexible, focused, portable, mobile. These organizational and behavioral characteristics provide the contextual framework for the effective delivery of population health care and complex adaptive systems within which that service will be provided. These three frames of reference constitute the foundations upon which shared decision making emerges in a shared governance structure that supports it. Regardless of what terms are used for shared governance in an interdisciplinary environment, the designated type of structures must reflect the principles of partnership, equity, accountability, and ownership if the behaviors, practices, and clinical activities necessary to fully achieve an integrated, evidence-driven, valued-based health system is ever to be achieved.

In complex adaptive systems, the reformatting of clinical services from an interdisciplinary intersection calls for clinical reformatting of the organizational design in a way that is more oriented to supporting decisions and actions made at the point of service. The place where the patient and the provider meet is the critical intersection in the healthcare organization; it is the centerpiece in the construct around which all structures in the system are built (Patlak, Balogh, & Nass, 2011). However, for this transformation to operate effectively, organizational structures must be reconfigured substantially around point-of-service design modeling in a way that allows the system to actively operate from the point of service. For this system to be effective, the following considerations must be addressed:

- The primary driving point of decision making in a complex clinical delivery system is the place where the provider and the user meet.

- Complex adaptive system providers are integrated in a collaborative and linked relationship that synthesizes well around the needs of the user.

- In complex service-based approaches, the provider and user need as much freedom as their relationship requires to make the necessary clinical decisions that will positively advance the potential for health.

- A full and appropriate range of data points must converge around the point of service to support the collaborating decision makers, inform their clinical activities, and provide the requisite information to evaluate impact and value.

- The purpose of organizational structure in a complex adaptive health system is to ensure that there are no impediments to the seamless interface of people, data, and systems supporting the value of health delivery at the point of service.

- Point-of-care linkage and interface in a complex adaptive system are structured in a way that ensures the engagement of all members, stakeholders, and users in a way that encourages them to undertake relevant processes that result in meaningful and sustainable value.

- The complex adaptive clinical system is constructed from the core point of service outward into the system, such that all structures, formats, processes, supports, operations, and clinical systems converge to serve the primary purpose of the organization as exemplified by the activities that occur at the point of service.

Clearly, the transformation of existing control-structured organizational systems alone is not adequate to configure or support an integrated continuum-based value-driven healthcare system (Figure 9-6). Although some might question the importance of structure in a complex system, it is central to creating a framework for patterns of sustainable interactions, intersections, and collaborative behavior as represented by the action of its members. The primary purpose of structure in a complex adaptive system is to provide a broader framework for the relationships and interactions among human systems behavior, digital systems behavior, patterns of supporting resource distribution, and the consonants of all elements of the system around the work it does at the point of service. Indeed, the capacity to create sustainable patterns of interaction and behavior depends on the veracity and consistency between the system structure and the interfacing human reflecting the synergy essential to advance the continuum of health care (Molter, 2007). A well-defined and fluid system infrastructure provides the frame, the vehicle within which best practices and behaviors are exemplified. This dynamic relationship between structure and action allows for the essential range of necessary connections and behaviors that converge to contribute to the purposes of the system and the work that reflects them.

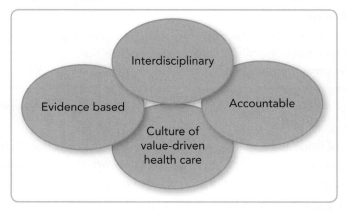

Figure 9-6 Value-based system drivers

The Premises of Professional Shared Governance in Health Care

Shared governance represents a professional structure of relationships in a complex adaptive healthcare system that enables knowledge work and advances the interaction, collaboration, and action of the disciplines in advancing health care. Professional shared governance in a complex adaptive health system reflects the following premises:

- All structures must serve the purposes of the organization and directly support the work that fulfills those purposes. Any part of the organizational structure that does not specifically support the organization's purposes and work automatically impedes it.

- What actually goes on at the point of service in a complex organization defines the reality of the organization's life and reflects its real purpose.

- The power of every profession is embedded in its practice, and its practitioners represent the expression of that power. Organizations must be configured in a way that does not empower the profession to fully express the obligations of its practice (Figure 9-7).

- Professional knowledge and skill
- Defined area of practice
- Desire for autonomy
- Responsibility and authority to make decisions based on professional knowledge and skill and the ability to execute these in practice
- An environment that supports professional practice and respects the professional's individual and collective right to challenge circumstances and decisions

Figure 9-7 Critical attributes of autonomy

- Clinical value and impact are the product of the convergence of effort requiring the confluence of transdisciplinary work and the synthesis of the collective contribution of each discipline.

- In any knowledge-based system (such as a professional organization), all knowledge workers contributing to the value of the system have both the right and the obligation to fully participate in the life of the system—to own their own decisions and to control that which advances their work. Nothing in an effective complex system should ever arbitrarily or capriciously moderate, remove, or impede the rights and obligations of the knowledge worker to fully express the contribution that they make in partnership with other stakeholders in fulfilling the purposes of the system.

- In a multimodal system (multidirectional flow), emphasis is placed on interface, intersection, integration, and relationship. Consequently, a multimodal complex adaptive system must adapt to a structure that facilitates real autonomy through interaction, communication, partnership, collaboration, and the confluence of effort around a mutually derived value (Figure 9-8).

Structural and work autonomy: The worker's freedom to make decisions based on role requirements.

Attitudinal autonomy: The belief in one's freedom to exercise judgment in decision making.

Aggregate autonomy: Encompasses attitudinal and structural dimensions, the socially and legally granted freedom of self-governance and control of the profession without influence from external sources. Autonomy is viewed as self-determination in practice according to professional nursing standards.

Professional nurse autonomy: The belief in the centrality of the patient, when making responsible decisions both independently and interdependently, that reflect advocacy for the patient.

Figure 9-8 Characteristics of real autonomy

- There are three major components of convergence in a structure necessary to ensure structural integrity in the system: governance, operations, and service. In a complex adaptive healthcare system each of these components is seamlessly linked to the other in a way that supports the purposes of the organization, the needs of the service, and the values to which it is directed to advance (Klein, 2008). A complex adaptive health system's predominant purpose is to address the health of the populations it serves. This health system demonstrates its purpose at the point of service where the living community of the system needs to fulfill the values of the system. The provider–user relationship has the same constituents at the point of service as does the community–system relationship at the level of the systems environment. Therefore, the mandates, principles, processes, and values that govern the relationship of the point of service are precisely the same as those that govern the relationship at the level of environment–system.

- An effective complex adaptive health system is an open system. This means that there is a seamless connection among decisions, decision makers, purpose, and value, representing essential membership in the system, ownership of its values, and full and active participation in its decisions related to strategy, tactics, goals, and practices directed to fulfilling the purposes of the system and obtaining its defined values.

- Management roles in the system reflect both stewardship and servant leadership. The primary role of management in a complex adaptive system is to ensure the seamless interface between the system's purpose and its resources, both directed to advancing that purpose and obtaining its full value.

- Accountability drives the work of professionals in complex adaptive systems. Accountability is the foundation for all knowledge work performance. Every member of a complex adaptive system has both rights and obligations that generate from the full participation in the life and activities of the system. Every member of the system must fully contribute to the extent of his or her capacity in a way that ensures that the system thrives and fulfills its essential value.

- Effective complex adaptive health systems provide a sustainable format for the essential work of the system. Every system creates its own structural scaffolding that serves as the framework for the intersecting structures, processes, relationships, and behaviors in a seamless and intersecting dynamic flow whose effectiveness is continuously demonstrated by its fulfillment of purpose and advancement of value.

These premises underlie the foundational understanding of knowledge work in a complex adaptive health system. They also reflect the transforming notion of the relationship between components of the system and elements of its impact within the context of a shared purpose (Figure 9-9). Furthermore, "system-ness" redefines the relationship of the stakeholders to the system and to each other. The direction to which each of these premises points leads to the construction of a complex adaptive organization that operates synergistically to fulfill its purpose and to advance its value in the larger social environment.

- Evolves from accountabilities sustaining it
- Enhanced by full accessibility to organization
- Grows along with commitment and ownership
- Becomes more central with staff involvement

Figure 9-9 Achieving shared purpose

The Individual and the Organization

In knowledge-work-driven organizations, the complex relationship among individuals, knowledge work, and team integration becomes obvious. Within this framework the contemporary professional worker must demonstrate the fluidity, mobility, flexibility, and portability that characterize the emergent role of the clinical provider (Figure 9-10). Individual human behavior is a complex and dynamic process emphasizing the difference each individual represents in the community of relationships. The challenge of an effective knowledge-driven organization is in successfully matching the knowledge worker with the work, with colleagues, and with the organization (Alvesson, 2004). In a complex adaptive system, the ideal situation includes careful on-boarding and analysis of the relationship between individual and the defined knowledge work expectations. Foundational expectations reflect the need for the individual to demonstrate full accountability for the products of work and specific competence necessary for the process of work.

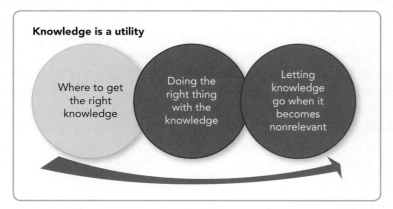

Figure 9-10 Components of effective knowledge work

Inherent in individual contributions is the strength of the enriching and supporting environment that facilitates individual contribution, inclusion, and demonstration of impact. This synergy of forces is essential to demonstrate the facility among each of the elements that advance the individual's role in relationship to the team and the organization. In complex adaptive systems, a fluid and dynamic interface among the network, the individual as agent, and the obligations of the impact on the outcome are critical to effectiveness. Clearly, the abilities of the individual and the capacity of the organization to use them are important interfaces that facilitate the goodness of fit and value of the individual in the work system. Knowledge workers have a unique role to play and specific contributions to make to the organization within the context of the knowledge they bring to the organization and the expectations that the individual and the organization have with regard to its applications and impact (Bennet & Bennet, 2004). Clinical leaders must always be aware that the notion of "fit" is really critical in assessing the work and role of an individual within the complex array of factors influencing and moderating their success.

Individuals must know that they are accountable for advancing the work of the organization and through their membership in the work community agree to participate in individual and collective deliberation and action in applying the work of the profession, advancing the patient care aims of both the profession and organization. This partnership between individual and profession and profession and system is the critical context for ensuring fit, effectiveness, and sustainability. If individuals are not committed to the work of the discipline and the goals of the organization with regard to advancing the health of the community both serve, evidence of the noncommitment becomes apparent as witnessed by their nonenergy, lack of convergence with the standards and expectations for performance, objections to full participation in the work of the profession, and limited expression of the gifts and talents the individual brings to his or her work. The dramatic opposite of these behaviors are the drivers of true professional behavior: collaboration within and between the disciplines, effective use of data systems for both decisions and actions, grounding practice in evidence, reflecting contemporary and relevant standards of care, ensuring that professional nursing efforts result in a positive impact on the patient's health experience, and demonstration of a shared collaborative relationship across the continuum of care (Figure 9-11).

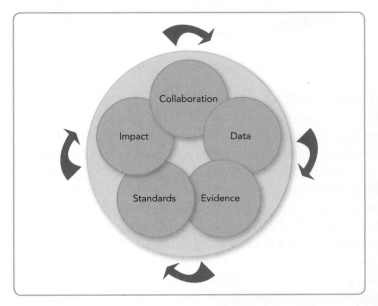

Figure 9-11 Integration of effort to advance value

Knowledge workers are members of the professional community; they do not merely do a job. Professionals must recognize that the expectations for their individual behavior are defined by the professional community to which they have the right to fully participate. Having that right and not fully exercising it is not the fault of either the profession nor the organization. The individual professional has an obligation to demonstrate contribution to his or her membership and evidence in his or her unique contribution to the work of the profession and the goals for advancing the health of the community. The profession always maintains the role of defining the parameters of practice; the individual does not. When the individual holds his or her practice standards in a way that unilaterally operates out of the context of those defined by the professional community, that person holds the community hostage and fails to demonstrate personal interest in advancing the work of the profession. If an individual gains insights and competencies that can advance the work of the profession, it is that person's obligation to join his or her effort with the professional community in incorporating those insights into the deliberations that define the parameters of practice for all community members. Failing to do so creates fragmented, discordant, and fractured clinical practices that fail to demonstrate an evidence-grounded effort to advance and improve clinical care.

Shared governance provides the opportunity for individuals to be fully empowered in the deliberations, decisions, and actions undertaken by the profession. The structure of shared governance clarifies and distinguishes between the accountability that belongs to the system and that which belongs to the

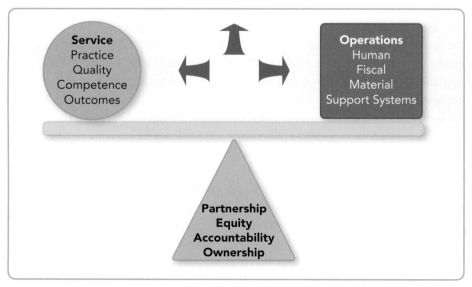

Figure 9-12 Clarity and convergence of system's accountability

Responsibility (20th Century)	Accountability (21st Century)
• Process	• Product
• Action	• Result
• Work	• Outcome
• Do	• Accomplish
• Task	• Difference
• Function	• Fit
• Job	• Role
• Incremental	• Sustainable
• Externally generated	• Internally generated

Figure 9-13 Differentiating between responsibility and accountability

practitioner. The structure of shared governance, reflecting the principles of partnership, equity, accountability, and ownership, clearly enumerates the locus of control for practice accountabilities and for organizational (management) accountabilities (Figure 9-12). The expectation of shared governance is that every individual will demonstrate personal accountability by fully engaging and participating in decisions affecting the practice of the profession in advanced clinical care for the patients (Figure 9-13). If individuals do not render as much care for the profession as they do for their patients, both suffer and the standards necessary to truly advance the delivery of care become deficient. The mechanisms available to each professional staff member aggregate to the whole and begin to empower the profession in ways that demonstrate equity, value, and contribution. Behaving in a way that demonstrates professional characteristics, interactions, and demonstrations of impact creates the conditions for equity and establishes a framework for value-driven interdisciplinary models of effective patient care. The resulting congruence and partnership between professional caregivers and the shared decision-making structure through which they operate create a means for sustainable collaboration, cross-disciplinary evidence-driven practice, and, ultimately, a positive impact on advancing the quality of health of the community.

CHAPTER TEST QUESTIONS

1. American health care has come to the major work of transformation much later than other segments of the social and global community. True or false?

2. Building access and equity into the service framework requires that equity, ownership, and engagement are directed by the management role. True or false?

3. Unless there is a goodness of fit between the structure of the organization, the dynamics of human behavior, and the processes and tools used to undertake work, any one of them taken alone would negatively diminish value and outcome. True or false?

4. The foundations within complexity science that apply to human behavior and health care fall into the areas of behavioral economics, networks, evolution and adaptation, pattern formation, systems theory, nonlinear dynamics, and game theory. True or false?

5. Evidentiary dynamics and improvement science are the traditional mechanisms for changing practice within the context of a strongly vertical medical records structure. True or false?

6. In the healthcare world where the digital infrastructure now makes it possible for evidence-based, value-driven decisions to be made, conditions are now created for reorienting the delivery system to a much stronger point-of-service construct. True or false?

7. The emergence of knowledge organizations demonstrates that knowledge is fixed and finite and does not operate simply as the utility; knowledge, instead, is a capacity. True or false?

8. In complex adaptive systems, form and function interact with each other; they do not reflect a dependent relationship. True or false?

9. Clinical value and impact are the product of the divergence of effort requiring the deconstruction of transdisciplinary work and emphasizing the unilateral contribution of each discipline. True or false?

10. The centrality of shared governance to creating a framework for the pattern of sustainable interactions, intersections, and collaborative behavior as represented by the action of its members is beyond question the primary purpose of a professional clinical structure in a complex adaptive system. True or false?

References

Alvesson, M. (2004). *Knowledge work and knowledge-intensive firms*. Oxford, England; New York, NY: Oxford University Press.

ANCC. (2010). Magnet Recognition Program Manual. American Nurses Credentialing Center: Washington, DC.

Ang, Y., & Yin, S. (2008). *Intelligent complex adaptive systems*. Chicago, IL: IGI.

Aziz, S. M. (2006). *Citizen e-readiness for digital society*. New Delhi, India: Corniche Books.

Batson, V. (2004). Shared governance in an integrated health care network. *Association of Operating Room Nurses, 80*(3), 493–512.

Bednarski, D. (2009). Shared governance: Enhancing nursing practice. *Nephrology Nursing Journal, 36*(6), 585.

Bennet, A., & Bennet, D. (2004). *Organizational survival in the new world: The intelligent complex adaptive system*. Boston, MA: Butterworth-Heinemann.

Bennet, A., & Bennet, D. (2010). Multidimensionality: Building the mind/brain infrastructure for the next generation knowledge worker. *On the Horizon, 18*(3), 240–254.

Bjorn, J., & Persson, P. (2009). Reduced uncertainty through human communication in complex environments. *Cognition, Technology and Work, 11*(3), 205–215.

Chalkidou, K., Tunis, S., Lopert, R., Rochaix, L., Sawicki, P., Nasser, M., & Xerri, B. (2009). Comparative effectiveness research and evidence-based health policy: Experience from four countries. *Milbank Quarterly, 87*(2), 339–367.

Gunter, B. (2005). *Digital health: Meeting patient and professional needs online*. Mahwah, NJ: Lawrence Erlbaum.

Joint Commission. (1991). Medical Staff. 99–119. Retrieved from http://www.jointcommission.org/assets/1/18/MS_01_01_01.pdf

Kamae, I. (2010). Value-based approaches to healthcare systems and pharmacoeconomics. *Pharmacoeconomics, 28*(10), 831–838.

Kaufman, N. (2011). Changing economics in an era of healthcare reform. *Journal of Healthcare Management, 56*(1), 9–13.

Kelly, K. (2005). *Out of control: The new biology of machines, social systems, and the economic world*. New York, NY: Perseus Books Group.

Klein, J. T. (2008). Evaluation of interdisciplinary and transdisciplinary research: A literature review. *American Journal of Preventive Medicine, 35*(Suppl. 2), S116–S123.

Leon, R. (2011). Creating the future knowledge worker. *Management and Marketing, 6*(2), 205–222.

Liebler, J. G., & McConnell, C. R. (2012). *Management principles for health professionals*. Sudbury, MA: Jones & Bartlett Learning.

Malloch, K. (2010). Creating the organizational context for innovation. In T. Porter-O'Grady & K. Malloch (Eds.), *Innovation leadership: Creating the landscape of healthcare* (pp. 33–66). Sudbury, MA: Jones and Bartlett.

Malloch, K., & Porter-O'Grady, T. (2009a). *Introduction to evidence-based practice in nursing and healthcare*. Sudbury, MA: Jones and Bartlett.

Malloch, K., & Porter-O'Grady, T. (2009b). *The quantum leader: Applications for the new world of work*. Sudbury, MA: Jones and Bartlett.

Marshall, E. S. (2011). *Transformational leadership in nursing: From expert clinician to influential leader*. New York, NY: Springer.

Mazur, D. J. (2003). *The new medical conversation: Media, patients, doctors, and the ethics of scientific communication*. Lanham, MD: Rowman and Littlefield Education.

McClellan, M., McKethan, A., Lewis, J., Roski, J., & Fisher, E. (2010). A national strategy to put accountable care into practice. *Health Affairs, 29*(5), 982–990.

McStay, A. (2010). *Digital advertising*. Houndmills, Basingstoke, Hampshire; New York, NY: Palgrave Macmillan.

Miller, J. H., & Page, S. E. (2007). *Complex adaptive systems: An introduction to computational models of social life*. Princeton, NJ: Princeton University Press.

Miller, J., & Scott, P. (2007). *Complex adaptive systems: An introduction to computational models of social life*. Princeton, NJ: Princeton University Press.

Molter, N. (2007). *AAC and protocols for practice: Healing environments*. Sudbury, MA: Jones and Bartlett.

Nelson, R. (2006a). Protecting patients or turf?: The AMA aims to limit nonphysician healthcare professionals. *American Journal of Nursing, 106*(8), 25–26.

Nelson, R. (2006b). The politics of prescribing: In Georgia APRNs seek more authority. *American Journal of Nursing, 106*(3), 25–26.

Paley, J. (2007). Complex adaptive systems and nursing. *Nursing Inquiry, 14*(3), 233–242.

Parmelee, P. A., Bowen, S. E., Ross, A., Brown, H., & Huff, J. (2009). Sometimes people don't fit in boxes: Attitudes toward the minimum data set among clinical leadership in VA nursing homes. *Journal of the American Medical Directors Association, 10*(2), 98–106.

Patlak, M., Balogh, E., & Nass, S. (Eds.). (2011). *Patient-centered cancer treatment planning: Improving the quality of oncology care: Workshop summary*. Washington, DC: National Academies Press.

Pauly, M. V. (2010). *Health reform without side effects: Making markets work for individual health insurance.* Stanford, CA: Hoover Institution Press.

Porter-O'Grady, T. (2009). *Interdisciplinary shared governance: Integrating practice, transforming healthcare.* Sudbury, MA: Jones and Bartlett.

Porter-O'Grady, T., & Malloch, K. (2010). Leadership for innovation: From knowledge creation to health transformation. In K. Porter-O'Grady & T. Malloch (Eds.), *Innovation leadership: Creating the landscape of healthcare* (pp. 1–23). Sudbury, MA: Jones and Bartlett.

Rapp, C., Etzel-Wise, D., Marty, D., Coffman, M., Carlson, L., Asher, D., . . . Whitley, R. (2010). Barriers to evidence-based practice implementation: Results of a qualitative study. *Community Mental Health Journal, 46*(2), 112–118.

Resinicow, K., & Page, S. (2008). Embracing chaos and complexity: A quantum change for public health. *American Journal of Public Health, 98*(8), 1382–1390.

Rivington, W. (1879). *The medical profession.* Dublin, Ireland: Fannin.

Rouse, W. (2008). Healthcare is a complex adaptive system: Implications for design and management. *The Bridge, 38,* 1–2.

Shanine, K., Buchko, A., & Wheeler, A. R. (2011). International human resource management practices from a complex adaptive systems perspective. *International Journal of Business and Social Science, 2*(6), 6–11.

Shifflet, V., & Moyer, A. (2010). Staff nurse to nurse leader: Steps for success. *MedSurg Nursing, 19*(4), 248–252.

Solow, D., & Szmerekovsky, J. (2006). The role of leadership: What management science can give back to the study of complex systems. *Emergence: Complexity and Organizations, 8*(4), 52–60.

Styer, K. (2007). Development of a unit-based practice committee: A form of shared governance. *Association of Operating Room Nurses, 86*(1), 85.

Taylor, L. C. (1974). *The medical profession and social reform, 1885–1945.* New York, NY: St. Martin's Press.

Tolbert, P. S., & Hall, R. H. (2009). *Organizations: Structures, processes, and outcomes.* Upper Saddle River, NJ: Pearson Prentice Hall.

Waddington, I. (1984). *The medical profession in the Industrial Revolution.* Dublin, Ireland: Gill and Macmillan.

Wright, M. C., Phillips-Bute, B. G., Petrusa, E. R., Griffin, K. L., Hobbs, G. W., & Taekman, J. M. (2008). Assessing teamwork in medical education and practice: Relating behavioural teamwork ratings and clinical performance. *Medical Teacher, 30*(6), 1–9.

Zerwekh, J. G., & Garneau, A. Z. (2012). *Nursing today: Transition and trends.* St. Louis, MO: Elsevier Saunders.

Appendix A

Shared Decision-Making Requisites

- Shared decision making is point-of-service driven.

- Stakeholders are involved in their own decisions.

- Decisions are made where the work gets done.

- Staff focuses on population/patient care.

- Managers focus on empowering staff and creating a supportive work environment for staff decisions and practice accountability.

- The goal is to make the right decision as close to the point of service as possible.

- The structure of the organization is built to support point-of-service decision making and empower staff to decide and to act in a way that advances the exercise of their practice accountabilities.

21st Century Practice-Based Accountability of the Clinical Staff

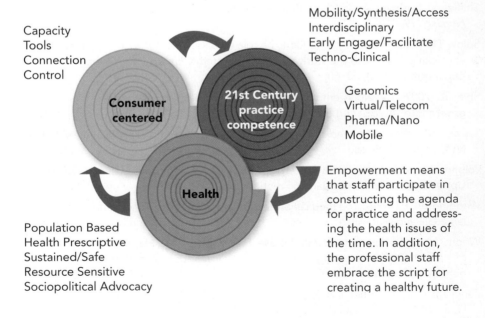

Capacity
Tools
Connection
Control

Mobility/Synthesis/Access
Interdisciplinary
Early Engage/Facilitate
Techno-Clinical

Consumer centered

21st Century practice competence

Genomics
Virtual/Telecom
Pharma/Nano
Mobile

Health

Population Based
Health Prescriptive
Sustained/Safe
Resource Sensitive
Sociopolitical Advocacy

Empowerment means that staff participate in constructing the agenda for practice and addressing the health issues of the time. In addition, the professional staff embrace the script for creating a healthy future.

Empowerment Values

- Confirm and commit to new values.
- Create a vision and enlist others.
- Role model management changes first.
- Promote and set expectations.
- Build skills along the way.
- Change structure and systems to support the new values.
- Define specifically the value of roles and link them to outcomes.

Values in Shared Decision Making

- Free-flowing information
- Mutual respect
- Diversity-infused collaboration
- Accountability for outcomes
- Empowered actions reflecting ownership
- Professional nursing model
- Shared decision making

Values are expressed through behavior and can often be elicited from observation. It is important to see values congruent with shared decision making, in the conduct of everyone, if it is to work. Strong leadership plays a key part in nurturing desired behaviors. Committed leaders work objectively on the road to change, model empowered behaviors, and encourage and praise mature behaviors that correspond to a professional practice environment. The norms, rules, and rituals of the past are scrutinized in order to filter out behaviors that do not match the envisioned environment. Initiating forums for discussion or an educational process may be needed to bring a level of awareness to the forefront about negative behavior ingrained in past practice and historic relationships.

The implementation of shared decision making changes organizational culture, which is defined by values. The organizational systems and structures assist in supporting the values and behaviors. Concurrently, values and behaviors shape development of empowerment. As the organization moves toward changing values, the structure and support systems are redesigned to meet the values.

Transformation of the culture involves diligence, careful planning, and time. Requisites for change include a firm, consistent set of values, long-term commitment, constant evaluation and reevaluation of each element in the system, and education of all parties to keep the vision alive. Role expectations impact behavior, as do skill and knowledge. Increasing knowledge and skill to affect changing values and behavior is helpful. Effective leadership guides behavioral changes that change culture.

The change leader recognizes that empowerment is a journey for both manager and staff. Clearly building change on a well-defined set of values with established parameters for behavior creates a firm foundation upon which to unfold new empowerment processes and actions.

Empowered Staff Behaviors

- Openness to new realities
- Sound practice standards
- Engagement of their issues
- Emerging curiosity
- Ability to express concerns
- Committed to competency
- Growing involvement
- Exhibiting creativity
- Willingness to change
- Clear sense of ethics
- Fundamental honesty
- Consensus seeking
- Structured risk taking
- Abide by consensus
- Increasing self-esteem
- Initiating partnerships

Changing Historic Culture

- Unclear or uncertain about quality
- Inhibits creative behaviors; values rituals and routines
- Diminishes the loftiest goals
- Challenges what is formally communicated in an organization
- Can create a powerful influence
- Requires laborious effort to alter

Influence of Culture

It is important to acknowledge the influence of environmental culture on employees and work because of the powerful force it exerts. Staff are not typically familiar with management skills and practices. Historically, managers have taken accountability for all the areas of the practice system, including many of the decisions regarding patient care. Structure and education are necessary in order to achieve the smooth transfer of accountability. In addition to the unfamiliarity with managing groups and systems, the staff have a level of fear related to change as an added element with which to cope. Many employees are afraid to ask questions and take positions. There often is an underlying culture that reinforces staff fear to initiate or act. It is obvious that this fear in a professional system severely hampers the organization's efforts to innovate and change.

Culture magnifies or ameliorates the trepidation of caregivers encountering new expectations for accountability. For example, an individual, hearing encouragement to participate, summons courage to speak in a meeting and is rebuffed. A discrepancy exists between the system's message of openness and the old culture of suppression. The culture sends a contradictory message that communicates that "this is not the way things work around here." Culture begins to change when peer pressure is brought to bear to extinguish unwanted behaviors. Trust, or lack of it, has enormous consequences for organizations. Consolidated and integrated actions are needed to counteract the effect of old culture until it is changed to reflect more professional behaviors. Leaders who develop strategies to address changing culture are more likely to obtain support because of their willingness to take risks and confront past habits and practices.

Changing Culture

- Is possible with a plan and creative and committed leadership
- Requires planned time for change to take hold; staff need to mourn losses, embrace the new
- Leaders create conditions for desired environment
- Immediate and continual feedback combats immature behaviors
- Key moments, celebration, evaluation of incremental changes

Context for Staff Work in Shared Governance

- Authority and responsibility for professional practice invested at the clinical point of service
- Individual accountabilities and expectations clearly delineated in role description
- Shared decision making embedded in relationships and structures that intersect role descriptions

- Knowledge workers' decisions and participation at point of service of prime importance to an organization's success

One of the roles of the manager is to conceive ways to help staff recognize how their work integrates into the whole and perpetuates the mission of the organization. Placing competence, authority, and **responsibility** for practice at the point of service is the purpose of shared decision making. The manager explains how it fits with the work of others in the organization. Authority and responsibility for professional practice are invested with the staff in shared decision making. The knowledge and skills staff bring to their roles are applied to the goals of the organization. Knowledge possessed by these workers is one of the major mediums of value and exchange in the workplace. Goals rarely get acted upon or fulfilled at the highest reaches of the organization. It is where the work is done, action is applied, and outcomes are achieved with the purposes and values of the organization that value is clearly exemplified. Managers recognize this context and work to build the infrastructure that supports it and create congruent leadership behaviors that advance and sustain it.

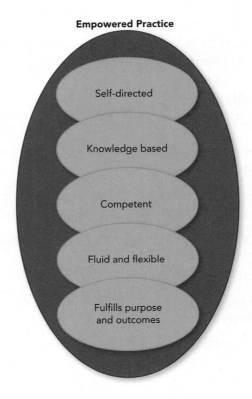

Empowered Practice

Self-directed

Knowledge based

Competent

Fluid and flexible

Fulfills purpose and outcomes

The Power of Empowerment

- System strengthened through integration
- Role of every player recognized
- System design ensures effective functioning
- Structure instills and sustains empowerment
- Flexibility key to cost-effective efficacy
- Order as a result of freedom to self-organize
- Delivery system supports all disciplines
- Optimum levels of performance and outcomes
- Ownership cultivates desire for excellence
- Depends on staff competence and judgment

Shared decision making facilitates the creation of an effective organization based on a new professional practice paradigm. When empowerment takes hold, the relationship between work and the result of work is better defined. This reduces the waste of human energy and other resources because a streamlined system focuses on integration, ownership, and outcomes. Structural characteristics that sustain the empowered processes of shared decision making and leadership also provide a frame for work and worker flexibility. This flexibility is key to the viability of an organization confronting change. Responsiveness to change comes from the successful integration and goodness of fit between environment and the willingness of staff to alter and adjust their work. Integration and interactions that are relationship based strengthen the clinical system and promote continual improvement. Successful adaptation in the organization is accomplished because of the competency-based framework supporting the shared decision-making process.

The structure and culture of an empowered environment enables individuals to combine autonomy and teamwork to fulfill expectations and roles and achieve clinical outcomes. Shared decision making represents the valuation of the profession and the professional, while creating a real partnership between the professional and the organization. Good shared decision making creates and maintains a structural format for facilitating staff participation in decision making and dialogue regarding decisions, requirements, and actions related to clinical practice. Additionally, interactions are relationship based, facilitating information flow and communication, a fundamental indicator of success. Shared decision making asserts the staff's right to control their practice and make decisions that influence practice, thus advancing the mission and work of the organization. The result is a more satisfying work environment, fulfilled professionals, and a more successful organization.

Appendix B
Shared Governance Staff Assessment Instrument

Instructions: This instrument provides you with the opportunity to assess your work roles and behaviors within the context of a shared governance organizational framework. This assessment provides you with an opportunity to determine the impact of shared governance on your work and role.

To use this instrument read the statements carefully. Choose your answer after consideration by selecting the response that best matches your personal feelings and the extent to which you agree with the statements below. Mark the corresponding space on your response sheet. Please complete all the statements and remember that you cannot be identified, so be frank in selecting the response that matches as closely as possible to your own view.

PART A: SURVEY

1. Shared governance is a system of management that allows staff participation.   1   2   3   4   5

2. Shared governance changes the way we relate to each other.   1   2   3   4   5

3. In shared governance, staff members make more decisions.   1   2   3   4   5

4. Our organization sincerely wants shared governance to work.   1   2   3   4   5

5. Staff will never let shared governance work here.   1   2   3   4   5

6. I believe in shared governance.   1   2   3   4   5

7. Shared governance is the key element in what keeps me working here.   1   2   3   4   5

8. Shared governance is just a fad that won't last long.   1   2   3   4   5

9. The processes associated with shared governance are consistent with my manager's style of management.   1   2   3   4   5

PART B: ATTITUDES

On a scale of 1 to 10, with 1 the lowest and 10 the highest, please rank the following:

1. I believe the overall commitment to shared governance in this organization ranks _____

2. I believe the quality of interpersonal relationships in this organization ranks _____

3. I believe the overall leadership ability in this organization ranks _____

4. I believe the emphasis on effective problem solving in this organization ranks _____

5. I believe the concern for the process of shared governance ranks _____

6. My level of satisfaction with this organization ranks _____

Any question you do not understand or do not have sufficient information to answer, please leave blank.

PART C: DEMOGRAPHICS

1. My current role here is:
   - ❏ Staff nurse
   - ❏ Specialist (not a manager)
   - ❏ First-line manager (responsible for one unit)
   - ❏ Other manager (responsible for more than one unit)
   - ❏ Senior manager (responsible for entire division)
   - ❏ Other _____ .

2. My regular unit is _____ .

3. My regular shift is _____ .

4. I have worked this shift for _____ years.

5. I have worked for this organization for _____ years.

6. I work here primarily because: (Select only one.)
   - ❏ It is convenient.
   - ❏ Pay and benefits are good.
   - ❏ Satisfying work environment and relationships.
   - ❏ I have to work and this is as good a place as any.
   - ❏ I do not like working here.
   - ❏ Other _____ .

7. If I left here, it would be primarily because: (Select only one.)
   - ❏ I was offered a better job.
   - ❏ I was unhappy working here.
   - ❏ Better pay and benefits.
   - ❏ Spousal transfer or domestic situation.
   - ❏ More work satisfaction.
   - ❏ I need a change.
   - ❏ Other _____ .

8. I typically work ___ hours per week.

9. My age is _____ years.

10. My highest level of formal education is: (Select only one.)
    - ❏ High school
    - ❏ Diploma program
    - ❏ Vocational or technical school
    - ❏ University degree
    - ❏ Community college program
    - ❏ Graduate degree

11. I am currently taking classes: (Select only one.)
    - ❏ yes
    - ❏ no

    If yes, then please answer the following questions: I am studying: _____ .

12. I have participated or been involved in shared governance in the following ways:

    _____

    _____ .

13. If my involvement in shared governance has been minimal or not at all, it is because:

    _____

    _____ .

14. Please comment about this questionnaire. Feel free to include anything you think will improve it or will address your issues more fully:

    _____

    _____ .

15. If you feel an important question was not asked, please write it for us so that we might assess it for future preparation.

    _____

    _____ .

Appendix C

Survey of Shared Leadership Practices

Instructions: This is a survey of your manager's practices and whether or not he or she engages in behaviors that allow you to do your best work in a shared leadership organization. You may also use this tool to evaluate your council or shared decision-making group leaders, as well as to facilitate the group to do its best work.

Managers and leaders in empowered organizations purposefully engage in behaviors that enable staff members to effectively meet their professional accountabilties. The items in this survey have been carefully selected as representative of these shared leadership practices. Please examine each scenario and reflect on how characteristic it is of your manager or group leader, by thinking about how frequently he or she engages in this behavior.

To the right of each scenario, you are asked to make two sets of ratings:

Actual: Your assessment of how frequently your manager is actually engaged in shared leadership behaviors.

Desired: Your assessment of how often, in order for you to meet your professional accountabilities, you would like your manager to be using a certain shared leadership practice.

Read each scenario and record both an actual and a desired assessment in the boxes located in the right margin of this survey.

Use the following scales in making your own assessments:

1. Always　　　　　　5. Sometimes

2. Nearly always　　　6. Hardly ever

3. Frequently　　　　　7. Rarely

4. Half the time

Actual	❏	❏	❏	❏	❏	❏	❏
Desired	❏	❏	❏	❏	❏	❏	❏

		1	2	3	4	5	6	7
1. Actively seeks opportunities to help staff groups who are trying to achieve a goal. Eases groups through a process to accomplish goals. Remains neutral and helps the group stay focused.	Actual	❑	❑	❑	❑	❑	❑	❑
	Desired	❑	❑	❑	❑	❑	❑	❑
2. Recognizes that the work of groups is based on each staff member's attitudes, commitment, values, and skills. Enthusiastically works to bring these into the problem-solving process.	Actual	❑	❑	❑	❑	❑	❑	❑
	Desired	❑	❑	❑	❑	❑	❑	❑
3. Clearly spells out his or her own facilitator roles and responsibilities to shared leadership groups.	Actual	❑	❑	❑	❑	❑	❑	❑
	Desired	❑	❑	❑	❑	❑	❑	❑
4. Observes the various roles that group members play in groups, the methods that they use in decision making, and their communication patterns. Freely shares this information with the group to help them work together better.	Actual	❑	❑	❑	❑	❑	❑	❑
	Desired	❑	❑	❑	❑	❑	❑	❑
5. Always protects individuals and their ideas from attack by other staff members. Through his or her own words and actions, communicates the dignity and the individual worth of each person and confidence in his or her ability to make a contribution.	Actual	❑	❑	❑	❑	❑	❑	❑
	Desired	❑	❑	❑	❑	❑	❑	❑
6. Assists staff to develop their skills but does not direct or take responsibility for people's skill development. Encourages staff to try new ways of working without fear of failure.	Actual	❑	❑	❑	❑	❑	❑	❑
	Desired	❑	❑	❑	❑	❑	❑	❑
7. Suggests to staff members the opportunities to expand their skills. Conveys to each person that his or her work is central to the success of the organization.	Actual	❑	❑	❑	❑	❑	❑	❑
	Desired	❑	❑	❑	❑	❑	❑	❑
8. When coaching people, the manager's conversation makes sense, follows logic, and communicates that the manager is giving the staff his or her undivided attention.	Actual	❑	❑	❑	❑	❑	❑	❑
	Desired	❑	❑	❑	❑	❑	❑	❑

		1	2	3	4	5	6	7

9. Sets time aside to assist staff members and work groups to develop their skills. Is approachable and available when needed. Does not remain aloof.

Actual   ❏ ❏ ❏ ❏ ❏ ❏ ❏
Desired   ❏ ❏ ❏ ❏ ❏ ❏ ❏

10. Clearly communicates to staff members any performance problems. Focuses on solutions rather than problems. Does not become emotional or critical when confronting staff. Protects people's self-esteem when discussing performance problems.

Actual   ❏ ❏ ❏ ❏ ❏ ❏ ❏
Desired   ❏ ❏ ❏ ❏ ❏ ❏ ❏

11. Really listens to staff. Asks questions to clarify understanding of other people's points of view. Does not interrupt or let mind wander during conversations.

Actual   ❏ ❏ ❏ ❏ ❏ ❏ ❏
Desired   ❏ ❏ ❏ ❏ ❏ ❏ ❏

12. Stimulates reluctant staff members to participate by drawing them out and engaging them in active dialogue.

Actual   ❏ ❏ ❏ ❏ ❏ ❏ ❏
Desired   ❏ ❏ ❏ ❏ ❏ ❏ ❏

Dimension I   ❏ **Total Score Actual**
               ❏ **Total Score Desired**

13. Works hard to gain support for his or her own ideas. Does not manipulate or withhold information to advance his or her own ideas.

Actual   ❏ ❏ ❏ ❏ ❏ ❏ ❏
Desired   ❏ ❏ ❏ ❏ ❏ ❏ ❏

14. Spends little time worrying about what the "higher-ups" are thinking. Bravely represents people and groups, even if the issue is unpopular with senior management.

Actual   ❏ ❏ ❏ ❏ ❏ ❏ ❏
Desired   ❏ ❏ ❏ ❏ ❏ ❏ ❏

15. Always puts people first. Is fair and consistent in treatment of others. Shows no favoritism. Helps people avoid conforming to social pressure at work.

Actual   ❏ ❏ ❏ ❏ ❏ ❏ ❏
Desired   ❏ ❏ ❏ ❏ ❏ ❏ ❏

16. Can be counted on to follow up. Keeps commitments and is respected for honesty. People know what he or she believes.

Actual   ❏ ❏ ❏ ❏ ❏ ❏ ❏
Desired   ❏ ❏ ❏ ❏ ❏ ❏ ❏

17. Solicits feedback about impact on others. Responds nondefensively to criticism about his or her actions.

Actual   ❏ ❏ ❏ ❏ ❏ ❏ ❏
Desired   ❏ ❏ ❏ ❏ ❏ ❏ ❏

		1	2	3	4	5	6	7
18. Communicates a leadership vision in a way that inspires others to act. Has a strong sense of purpose. Can describe how his or her own work and the work of others contributes to the achievement of the organization's mission.	Actual	❏	❏	❏	❏	❏	❏	❏
	Desired	❏	❏	❏	❏	❏	❏	❏
19. Communicates self-respect and personal commitment to doing the best job possible. Openly works to resolve staff difficulties with his or her leadership style.	Actual	❏	❏	❏	❏	❏	❏	❏
	Desired	❏	❏	❏	❏	❏	❏	❏
20. Sees power as available to everyone rather than a limited resource. Assumes that staff members are accountable, with the necessary freedom and authority to do their work. Affirms the personal power of each individual.	Actual	❏	❏	❏	❏	❏	❏	❏
	Desired	❏	❏	❏	❏	❏	❏	❏
21. Frees staff members to collaborate and share in decision making. Gets staff personally involved in the work to be done. Accepts staff's control of the content and pace of their own work.	Actual	❏	❏	❏	❏	❏	❏	❏
	Desired	❏	❏	❏	❏	❏	❏	❏
22. Works hard to eliminate policies, procedures, or systems that interfere with getting the job done.	Actual	❏	❏	❏	❏	❏	❏	❏
	Desired	❏	❏	❏	❏	❏	❏	❏
23. Translates the principles of empowerment to staff through role modeling and fulfilling expectations of staff decision-making groups.	Actual	❏	❏	❏	❏	❏	❏	❏
	Desired	❏	❏	❏	❏	❏	❏	❏
24. Questions staff members regularly regarding their understanding and participation in empowerment activities.	Actual	❏	❏	❏	❏	❏	❏	❏
	Desired	❏	❏	❏	❏	❏	❏	❏

Dimension II   ❏ **Total Score Actual**
    ❏ **Total Score Desired**

		1	2	3	4	5	6	7
25. Communicates to everyone well-defined and clear goals for change. Freely provides information for the duration of change.	Actual	❏	❏	❏	❏	❏	❏	❏
	Desired	❏	❏	❏	❏	❏	❏	❏
26. Establishes and then coaches staff work groups to manage the changes that affect their work.	Actual	❏	❏	❏	❏	❏	❏	❏
	Desired	❏	❏	❏	❏	❏	❏	❏

		1	2	3	4	5	6	7

27. Ensures that change is not disconnected
from organizational realities by obtaining the
necessary commitment, people, materials,
and financial support before embarking on
change.

Actual   ❑ ❑ ❑ ❑ ❑ ❑ ❑
Desired   ❑ ❑ ❑ ❑ ❑ ❑ ❑

28. Assists staff in using project management
processes to set time lines, allocate
resources, prioritize actions, and assign
responsibilities.

Actual   ❑ ❑ ❑ ❑ ❑ ❑ ❑
Desired   ❑ ❑ ❑ ❑ ❑ ❑ ❑

29. Helps staff identify specific and measurable
outcomes to track successes and failures.
Sees failures as opportunities for learning.
Facilitates staff's progress in evaluating
themselves and unit outcomes.

Actual   ❑ ❑ ❑ ❑ ❑ ❑ ❑
Desired   ❑ ❑ ❑ ❑ ❑ ❑ ❑

30. Acts consistently on the belief that every
person helps design his or her own work.
Instead of the manager informing people of
a better way to do their jobs, staff members
are coached by the manager to invent their
jobs themselves.

Actual   ❑ ❑ ❑ ❑ ❑ ❑ ❑
Desired   ❑ ❑ ❑ ❑ ❑ ❑ ❑

31. Rethinks work from the customer's focus.
Helps staff design systems of work that are
flexible, reflect what customers desire, and
provide meaningful work for each person that
is cost effective.

Actual   ❑ ❑ ❑ ❑ ❑ ❑ ❑
Desired   ❑ ❑ ❑ ❑ ❑ ❑ ❑

32. Encourages staff on different units, departments, or different shifts to organize their
work differently, depending on skill mix,
people availability, and so on. Recognizes that
there is more than one way to "skin a cat."

Actual   ❑ ❑ ❑ ❑ ❑ ❑ ❑
Desired   ❑ ❑ ❑ ❑ ❑ ❑ ❑

33. Avoids rigid or fixed ways of doing work. As
conditions change, helps the staff reinvent
the way work is performed as they learn and
as the world changes.

Actual   ❑ ❑ ❑ ❑ ❑ ❑ ❑
Desired   ❑ ❑ ❑ ❑ ❑ ❑ ❑

34. Confronts negative staff members with the
truth about changes in work expectations
and empowerment activities.

Actual   ❑ ❑ ❑ ❑ ❑ ❑ ❑
Desired   ❑ ❑ ❑ ❑ ❑ ❑ ❑

Dimension III   ❑ **Total Score Actual**
                ❑ **Total Score Desired**

		1	2	3	4	5	6	7
35. Directly addresses objections to participation in decision making, countering staff members' objections to participation in decision making.	Actual	❑	❑	❑	❑	❑	❑	❑
	Desired	❑	❑	❑	❑	❑	❑	❑
36. Staff decision-making meetings are held at least monthly to deal with staff accountability issues.	Actual	❑	❑	❑	❑	❑	❑	❑
	Desired	❑	❑	❑	❑	❑	❑	❑
37. Provides staff members access to information, resources, and time, at least weekly, regarding organizational changes. Asks for response and feedback from staff.	Actual	❑	❑	❑	❑	❑	❑	❑
	Desired	❑	❑	❑	❑	❑	❑	❑
38. Incorporates people from every staff role into discussions about patient care and staff work.	Actual	❑	❑	❑	❑	❑	❑	❑
	Desired	❑	❑	❑	❑	❑	❑	❑
39. Communicates budget and financial information regularly to the staff. Keeps them informed about changes in finance affecting their work and lives.	Actual	❑	❑	❑	❑	❑	❑	❑
	Desired	❑	❑	❑	❑	❑	❑	❑
40. Always helps the staff include financial or resource components in every decision.	Actual	❑	❑	❑	❑	❑	❑	❑
	Desired	❑	❑	❑	❑	❑	❑	❑
41. Provides staff members with the time to attend staff decision-making group meetings. Actively and enthusiastically embraces their participation in staff decisions.	Actual	❑	❑	❑	❑	❑	❑	❑
	Desired	❑	❑	❑	❑	❑	❑	❑
42. Shares with staff his or her own accountabilities and performance expectations as a manager. Seeks feedback regarding leadership performance.	Actual	❑	❑	❑	❑	❑	❑	❑
	Desired	❑	❑	❑	❑	❑	❑	❑
43. Communicates activities, concerns, manager's role, and issues with the medical staff. Has an ongoing and regular pattern of communication with doctors.	Actual	❑	❑	❑	❑	❑	❑	❑
	Desired	❑	❑	❑	❑	❑	❑	❑
44. Creates an environment where staff feel connected to their manager and feel great working and relating to him or her.	Actual	❑	❑	❑	❑	❑	❑	❑
	Desired	❑	❑	❑	❑	❑	❑	❑
45. Unit runs well. Staff and management generally relate well. Together, they confront change positively, with good results.	Actual	❑	❑	❑	❑	❑	❑	❑
	Desired	❑	❑	❑	❑	❑	❑	❑

Dimension IV　❑ **Total Score Actual**
　　　　　　　❑ **Total Score Desired**

Instructions for Scoring Your Self-Assessment of Shared Leadership Practices

PART I

The self-assessment of Shared Leadership Practices assesses your managerial or leadership practices along four core Dimensions, and whether or not they are productive. A total score for the survey can be computed as well as a separate score for each Dimension.

1. Please total the scores on your self-assessment for each component, and place them in the boxes below.

2. Add your Dimension scores together to get a total score.

❏ Dimension I
Facilitating and Coaching

❏ Dimension III
Change Management

❏ Dimension II
Empowerment

❏ Dimension IV
Shared Leadership Principles

❏ **TOTAL I-IV**

Instructions for Scoring Part II

PART II

1. Now total the performance scores from your staff survey.

2. Record your self-assessment scores in the appropriate boxes below.

3. For each Dimension, add together the staff actual scores for all of your staff surveys. Divide this number by the number of surveys returned. Enter the mean score in the appropriate box below. Repeat this exercise for the staff desired scores.

4. Record total scores by adding the Dimension scores you had recorded in the previous steps.

	My Self-Assessment	Staff Actual	Staff Desired
Dimension I Facilitating and Coaching	❏	❏	❏
Dimension II Empowerment	❏	❏	❏
Dimension III Change Management	❏	❏	❏
Dimension IV Shared Leadership	❏	❏	❏
MY TOTAL SCORES **Dimensions I–IV**	❏	❏	❏

How does my staff feedback compare with my self-assessment of my facilitation and my coaching skills?

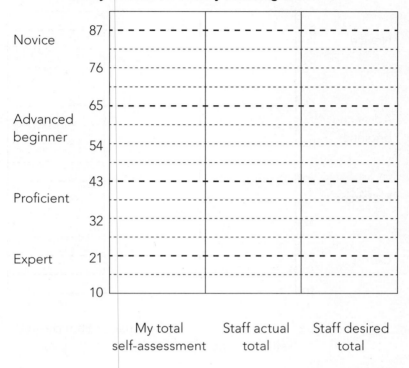

Instructions: Plot your Self-assessment, Staff actual, and Staff desired scores for Dimension I on the graph.

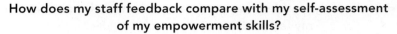

How does my staff feedback compare with my self-assessment of my empowerment skills?

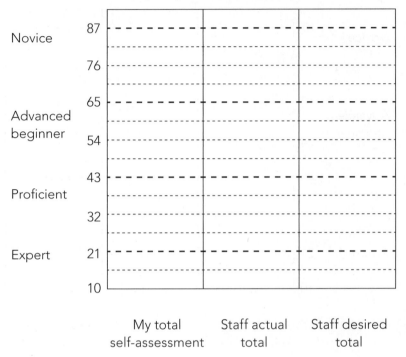

Instructions: Plot your Self-assessment, Staff actual, and Staff desired scores for Dimension II on the graph.

How does my staff feedback compare with my self-assessment of shared leadership principles?

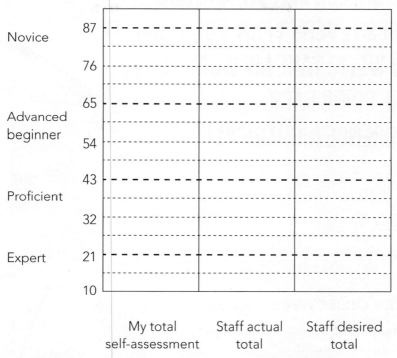

| | My total self-assessment | Staff actual total | Staff desired total |

Instructions: Plot your Self-assessment, Staff actual, and Staff desired scores on the graph.

FOR US WHO NURSE, OUR NURSING IS A THING, WHICH UNLESS IN IT WE ARE MAKING PROGRESS EVERY YEAR, EVERY MONTH, EVERY WEEK, TAKE MY WORD FOR IT, WE ARE GOING BACK.
—FLORENCE NIGHTINGALE

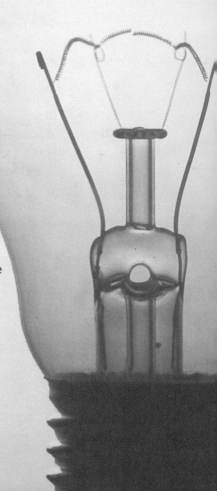

CHAPTER OBJECTIVES

Upon completion of this chapter, the reader will be able to do the following:

» Describe the essential components and responsibilities of the nursing professional role.

» List at least five options for career advancement.

» Outline the challenges and opportunities in creating effective continuing competence models for nursing.

» Understand the implications of violations of the nurse practice act and their relationship to continuing competence demonstration.

» Describe the challenges of integrating technology advancements into the role of the professional nurse.

Managing Your Career: A Lifetime of Opportunities and Obligations

Practice of Nursing. Nursing is a scientific process founded on a professional body of knowledge; it is a learned profession based on an understanding of the human condition across the lifespan and the relationship of a client with others and within the environment; and it is an art dedicated to caring for others. The practice of nursing means assisting clients to attain or maintain optimal health, implementing a strategy of care to accomplish defined goals within the context of a client centered health care plan and evaluating responses to nursing care and treatment. Nursing is a dynamic discipline that increasingly involves more sophisticated knowledge, technologies and client care activities (National Council of State Boards of Nursing [NCSBN], 2011).

Once a nurse, always a nurse! Nursing is a calling. The nature of the caregiver calling is about one's innate desire to offer comfort, to contribute to healing, and to alleviate suffering of another human. Once an individual has embraced the professional caregiving role of nurse with the completion of education and obtaining a license, one's DNA is genetically altered forever. The call to promote health and care for the sick is ever present in varying degrees. No matter how many hours you work, or even if you don't work, the public expects full engagement in your role. The public continues to see nursing as the most trusted profession in the country (Gallup, 2011).

The professional role and accountability of an individual who chooses nursing as a profession and a career can never be removed or used only in selected situations. The professional nurse is more than a technician with good communication skills. The professional nurse has knowledge of the mission and vision of the organization, an understanding of the culture in which patient care occurs, as well as the outcomes and cost of care provided.

> *I attribute my success to this—I never gave or took any excuse.*
> *—Florence Nightengale*

Understanding the dynamics of patient care services is essential for responsible use of resources. No one is better suited than the professional nurse caregiver to assess the effectiveness of patient care processes and to make recommendations for change when existing processes are no longer effective or when new evidence suggests better ways of providing patient care.

The purpose of this chapter is to discuss the role of the professional nurse, the challenges of transition from school to practice, the plethora of career opportunities available to nurses, options to demonstrate career progress, the importance of nurse licensure, and ideas on the achievement of work–life balance.

Transition to Practice

Supporting the transition from school to practice for newly graduated nurses has received significant attention, given the high levels of nurse turnover in the first two years of practice. The increasing complexity of the healthcare environment and the reality that a new nurse requires support to ensure a successful transition from school to practice have led to the creation of formalized transition programs. As shown in Table 10-1, the American Organization of Nurse Executives (AONE) has developed guiding principles for this process (2010). The principles clearly outline the importance of a team approach to transition into practice, effective leadership support, willing and competent preceptors, the use and integration of evidence-based processes, stress management, intolerance for lateral violence, and continuing collaboration with educational institutions. In addition, the NCSBN has developed a tool kit and research project to further advance the transition process (n.d.). This information provides several models or approaches to creating an effective, evidence-based transition plan that integrates the regulatory requirements of state nurse practice acts.

— **Table 10-1 AONE guiding principles for the newly licensed nurse's transition into practice**

1. Commitment for newly licensed nurse transition into practice occurs across all levels of the organization:
   - Senior leadership
   - Nursing leadership
   - Peers
   - Medical staff
   - Interdisciplinary colleagues

2. The nurse manager must achieve and is accountable for the leadership competencies that support the transition of the newly licensed nurse into his or her professional role.

3. Preceptors demonstrate professional competency and have a strong desire to teach, coach, and mentor.

4. Preceptors are prepared and supported by qualified nurse educators.

5. A structured transition into practice occurs in all settings and for all levels of academic preparation:
   - A continuous focus on evidence-based techniques and outcomes that foster patient safety and quality is evident throughout the transition process.
   - Widely diverse ages, ethnicities, backgrounds, and experiences of new graduates are taken into account when developing educational, social, and cultural supports.
   - The transition process is customized to the specific individual and practice area.

6. Social affiliation supports are in place to mitigate the emotional stressor role.

7. Organizations have in place policies and practices related to zero tolerance of lateral violence.

8. Posttransition support programs are in place to aid in the retention of newly licensed nurses.

9. Collaborative relationships exist with academic institutions that support dialogue to address preparation for practice gaps.

The implementation of a transition to practice model must be supported by the organizational culture not only in words but also in actions. In spite of the best intentions of a transition program, other practices within the organization may be obstructive to a wholly effective transition program. For example, it is important to be aware of the subtle hazing that may occur to new employees. While the intent may seem appropriate, further examination of other practices during the orientation process is needed. Consider the situation in which a new nurse is interviewed by the team and discussions focus on the importance of change and adopting the best evidence. The nurse is energized and believes his or her ideas are not only welcomed but needed by the organization. The subtle process of hazing (or reversing promises) begins when the new employee presents new ideas that are quickly dismissed and discouraged with feedback designed to support a smooth orientation. New employees are informed on the first day of employment that certain things did not work in the past and time shouldn't be wasted on them now, of the presence of current policies that prevent new ways of doing things, and of the importance of long-held traditions and not upsetting long-term employees who have been successful and are well respected. Seldom are the ideas of new nurses met with enthusiasm and support in figuring out how to examine and test new ideas in spite of the promises made during the interviews. It would be more appropriate to identify and discuss what could be done with the new employee's ideas rather than rationalizing with a new employee about why the current state of practice is what it is. Once a successful transition is made to professional practice, numerous opportunities are available to nurses.

Career Trajectories

Most nurses are unsure of what the future holds for them. One thing is certain, the opportunities for nurses are seemingly unlimited. Table 10-2 lists many of the partnership opportunities that are currently available to strengthen and advance the profession of nursing. These opportunities are found with healthcare organizations, community centers, and outpatient settings. It is hard to believe that the work of health care includes nearly every single professional discipline. Alliances with human factors researchers and ergonomic engineers are now essential to ensure effective work processes in an environment that is filled with personal computers, laptops, and wireless and mobile devices.

Table 10-2 Partnership opportunities

- Clinical medicine
- Cognitive psychology
- Human factors
- Ergonomics/biomechanics
- Safety experts
- Industrial engineers
- Mathematicians/statisticians
- Computer science/engineering
- Industrial design engineers
- Architects
- Fire science experts
- Interior designers
- Sociology experts
- Business experts
- Finance experts
- Communications
- Education
- Political science

There are several common career pathways that nurses regularly consider. These include advancements in clinical, educational, operational, technology, and research areas. In addition, opportunities also exist in legal support services, consulting, and entrepreneur roles for nurses to contribute to health care. New pathways can also be identified from published lists specific to challenges for health care in general and nursing specifically. Table 10-3 lists the top five challenges facing nursing as identified by *HealthLeaders Media*.

Table 10-3 Top five challenges facing nursing in 2012

1. Advanced degrees are no longer an option. The goal is for 80 percent of all RNs to have a baccalaureate degree by 2020.

2. Patient engagement is real. The patient experience specific to the nurse–patient relationship is now linked to system performance and reimbursement.

3. Patient safety must be owned by nurses.

4. Cost cutting continues to drive the work of caregivers. The goal is to apply evidence and embrace change and flexibility to increase effectiveness and efficiency and eliminate waste.

5. Retention of nursing staff continues to drive quality and effectiveness.

Source: Hendren (2011).

As one gains new knowledge and experiences, the world becomes larger. For example, the focus of the nurse shifts from surviving in the present to an orientation in which the future is envisioned, increasing capacity to see the whole picture, increasing ability to communicate persuasively, seeing change as an opportunity, and being proactive rather than reactive. In essence, as one grows professionally, the focus shifts from personal goals to larger system and professional goals. A framework to visually examine this progression is displayed in the novice to expert skill acquisition model (Benner, 2004; Dreyfus & Dreyfus, 2004).

Table 10-4, based on this model, describes in detail the areas of content focus for each phase from novice to expert and provides a discussion of the behaviors specific to relationship development that are consistent with the level of skill acquisition.

It is helpful to see the progression from an internal focus to an external focus and high levels of integration of information that seem to occur automatically at the proficient and expert levels. In some situations, it is important to note that individuals do not progress beyond the competent level. Some individuals are not able to see the bigger picture of organizational goals, embrace a proactive approach to situations, or envision a different and better future and thus never achieve the proficient or expert levels. Many nurses however, advance readily into the proficient and expert levels.

Table 10-4 The five stages: Coaching for professional relationships

Novice: Individual + Theory Content
The novice is a student of relationship development. The theory and information is context free, and the student or learning leader strictly relies on rules to form relationships or to manage relationship difficulties.

Advanced Beginner: Individual + Theory Content + Other Person
The advanced beginner has completed the workshop on relationships and is beginning to apply content to real-life situations following the maxims and rules learned in the workshop. A first-time manager can be considered an advanced beginner and will attempt some relationships and seek guidance in most employee situations.

Competent: Individual + Content + Other Person + Issue

With increasing experience, the number of features and maxims is now overwhelming, and the leader learns to adopt a hierarchal view of decision making, and skills of prioritization emerge. With additional experience and practice, the individual is able to form relationships with new employees and assist others in forming relationships based on maxims and rules with relative ease. The competent individual focuses on forming relationships as the means to achieve goals. An experienced manager can be considered a competent professional.

Proficient: Individual + Content + Other Person + Issue + Organization

An individual proficient in relationship skills is described as one who is able to both initiate, modify, and sustain basic relationships with only minimal assistance. The relationships are effective, predictable, and successful in most cases. Forming relationships is moving from reactive to proactive. The proficient leader knows the importance of relationships with employees and seeks out opportunities to strengthen the relationships. The focus of the competent individual is on completion of integrating the work of individuals into the larger picture and with others in the organization. An experienced director or leader can be considered a proficient professional.

Expert: Individual + Content + Other Person + Issue + Organization + Community

The expert is one who forms effective relationships in all areas impacting the work: the community, professional organizations, as well as internal teams and departments. The expert is able to address adversarial situations effectively, facilitate consensus building, and avoid unnecessary rumination about past events. The expert has fully integrated maxims and rules and uses them as references rather than road maps. The expert sees what needs to be done and then decides how to do it. The expert knows how to perform with calculating and comparing alternatives. The expert is able to form complex and competitive relationships in the most complex and challenging situations with successful outcomes. The expert routinely serves as a coach and mentor for those with less developed relationship skills.

Clinical Advancement

Specific career trajectories include development of expertise in specific patient care specialties such as women and children, critical care, or surgical services. Nurses interested in increasing their understanding of disease and health promotion processes for a specialty, increasing the use of evidence, and creating new evidence to practices are particularly suited for clinical advancement. This pathway requires additional education specific to the area of interest beginning with continuing education to formal educational programs at the master's and doctoral levels. Table 10-5 identifies graduate degrees in nursing.

Table 10-5 Graduate degrees in nursing

Masters:

- Clinical Nurse Leader
- Clinical Nurse Specialist

Doctorate:

- Doctor of Nursing Practice: Practice emphasis
  - Clinical practice
  - Leadership practice
- Doctor of Philosophy: Research emphasis

Leadership Advancement

Management and leadership opportunities are embraced by nurses seeking to be involved in the creation and modification for the infrastructure in which patient care occurs and the implementation of new processes to improve patient care and nurse satisfaction. The motivations for advancing to management and leadership positions vary widely; however, the underlying reasons are usually steeped in the desire to advance quality practices, advance excellence, and introduce new ideas for a better work environment. Moving to a management position also requires new knowledge specific to facilitating groups (nurses, therapists, assistive personnel, and support staff) of individuals to achieve shared goals, change and innovation leadership competence, oversight of safety and quality practices and behaviors, creating and managing fiscal resources for both operations and capital equipment, and course correcting when current practices do not meet desired goals (Cipriano, 2011).

Informatics

Informatics and related technology roles represent another career trajectory for nurses. The design and implementation of complex documentation and monitoring systems require computer specialists and nurses as well as nurse informaticists to bridge the disciplines and ensure that the intended goals of effectiveness, efficiency, and safety are enhanced. Electronic monitoring of patients from remote locations is also becoming more common and requires nurse clinical oversight. A nurse in these settings becomes a boundary spanner in ensuring team awareness of critical issues and facilitates effective hand-offs and transfers and overall relational coordination among team members (Gittell, 2009). Another extension of telemedicine and career trajectory includes school and child care centers as a means to not only assess child illness but also to allow parents to remain at work whenever possible.

Nursing Research

Nursing research is another career trajectory for nurses. In many ways, research is a natural for nurses who have been educated to make clinical observations and to evaluate patient progress and outcomes. Learning to become a scientist and nurse scholar requires education at the doctoral level. The National Institute of Nursing Research (NINR) provides an online course for nurses interested in the practical skills and strategies for preparation as a principal investigator (2010).

Interviewing for New Roles

As one moves through the skill acquisition and development processes, opportunities for new roles present themselves and require applications and interviews. At some point in most of their careers, nurses will take the risk and apply for a new position. These risks include social, political, financial, environmental, and personal risks as an individual chooses to leave a setting in which the policies and practices are known, the salary is fixed and reliable, the physical setting is familiar, and collegial relationships are understood. Moving to a new position will change the individuals with whom you socialize, your current abilities to manage policies and processes, salary and benefits, the specific location of the work, and personal position in an organization. The value of taking risks and applying for a new position necessarily stretches one's boundaries of current thinking and current practices and increases the potential for contributions to the nursing profession as well as to individual growth. Reducing fear in favor of seeing risk as an essential part of creativity and progress further increases nurse professional competence.

Several considerations are helpful to make this a positive and rewarding move. As previously noted, it is important to recognize that there is always some risk in leaving one position and moving to another. Individuals in the current setting may believe you are abandoning them and will leave an incredible void. Also, there is the possibility that you might not secure the desired position and experience rejection. To mediate or minimize the risks in applying for a new position, it is helpful for nurses to do an assessment of their motivations for a new position. Consider the following questions:

1. What are you best at doing? The goal should be to get even better at what you do best.

2. What do you like to do the most? This could be different from question 1. Doing what you like is as important as what you do best and should be the focus of your career.

3. What would you like to learn to do? Consider finding a mentor to assist in this new work.

4. What talents do you have that you haven't developed? Being able to develop new talents should be a reason to seek a new job.

5. What do others most often say are your greatest strengths? This helps you recognize talents that you might not see as significant.

6. What type of people do you work best with/worst with? Take time to define those behaviors that facilitate or obstruct your success: analytical, organized, creative, timely, social, etc.

7. What type of organizational culture brings out the best in you? Controlling and empowering cultures facilitate different work styles. Be sure to consider what works best for you.

8. How could your time be better used in your current organization? Identifying certain work that you believe could be valuable should be identified and included in a new position.

Continuing Competence

Maintaining one's competence as a professional nurse includes role, licensure, technology, and relationship competencies. Each of these competencies is essential for full demonstration of the nurse professional role (Table 10-6).

Table 10-6 Continued competence definitions

- **Competence:** Application of knowledge, interpersonal decision making, and psychomotor skills expected for the practice role; having the knowledge, skills, and ability to practice safely and effectively; the potential ability and /or capability to function in a given situation.

- **Competency:** One's actual performance in a situation. Competence is required before one can expect to achieve competency.

- **Competent clinical practice:** Situation-specific performance requiring an integration of skills including cognitive, psychomotor, interpersonal, and attitudinal.

- **Continued/continuing competence:** The ongoing synthesis of knowledge, skills, and abilities required to practice safely and effectively in accordance with the scope of nursing practice; the ongoing commitment of a registered nurse to integrate and apply the knowledge, skills, and judgment with the attitudes, values, and beliefs required to practice safely, effectively, and ethically in a designated role and setting.

- **Culture of nursing competence:** The shared beliefs, values, attitudes, and actions that promote lifelong learning and result in an environment of safe and effective patient care.

- **Remediation:** The process whereby identified deficiencies in core competencies are corrected.

Source: Statement on Continuing Competence for Nursing: A Call to Action, June 8, 2011. National Board for Certification of Hospice and Palliative Nurses; NCSBN; Retrieved from http://www.nbchpn.org/

Professional Nursing Role

The topic of continuing professional competency following initial licensure has been discussed for years. Experts have struggled with the content, the areas of focus, and the manner in which continuing competence is determined. As nurses move through different career trajectories, their work is more and more specialized and difficult to assess using an exam similar to the initial licensure exam. In addition, the ownership of continuing competency has also been discussed extensively. Leaders have been unable to determine who should be accountable for continuing competency, namely the state licensing agency, the licensee,

or a combination of the agency and licensee. While boards of nursing have the responsibility to ensure that licensees are safe to practice, experts believe that
→ continuing competence is a shared responsibility between the board and the individual nurse. Once licensed, the nurse is accountable for maintaining current skills and knowledge.

While several methods have been explored for determining and measuring competency, there is a still a lack of uniformity among state boards of nursing as to what should be required of licensees. To advance this dialogue, the NCSBN proposed principles to guide further development and initiation of pilot projects to identify methods and processes to determine and measure nurse competency (Table 10-7). These guidelines propose both regulatory and licensee accountability, define assessment frequency, and show integration of evidence.

Table 10-7 NCSBN continued competence guiding principles

1.	Nursing regulation is responsible for upholding licensure requirements, and competence is assessed at initial licensure and during the career life of licensees.
2.	The individual nurse in collaboration with the state board of nursing, nursing educators, employers, and the nursing profession has the responsibility to demonstrate continued competence through acquisition of new knowledge and appropriate application of knowledge and skills.
3.	A culture of continued competence is based on the premise that the competence of any nurse should be periodically assessed and validated.
4.	Requirements for continued competence should support nurses' accountability for lifelong learning and foster improved nursing practice and patient safety.
5.	A continued competence regulatory model for nursing is evidence based and offers a choice of options to address gaps in knowledge, skills, and abilities identified by a diagnostic assessment.
6.	The regulatory authority for establishing continued competence requirements should remain with the state board of nursing.

Source: www.ncsbn.org

Licensure Maintenance

In addition to nursing competence to practice, a current license is necessary. Most states require regular fees, a current address, and notification of any criminal convictions as minimal requirements. A summary of each state's requirements can be found on the NCSBN website at https://www.ncsbn.org/boards.htm. In addition to the single state licensure model, 24 states have entered into a multistate licensure agreement in which nurse licenses are recognized across state lines when certain requirements are met. This multistate model allows a nurse to have one license in a primary state of residence and be able to practice in other states with multistate statutes, subject to each state's nurse practice act regulations. The Nurse Licensure Compact (NLC) defines primary residence in the compact rules and regulations. Sources used to verify a nurse's primary residence for the NLC include at a minimum a driver's license, federal income tax return, or voter registration. In order to be designated a multistate participant, the state must enact legislation to authorize the NLC and adopt administrative rules and regulations to support the compact. The multistate model significantly increases nurse mobility across the country and decreases the cost of licensure fees when nurses practice in more than one state. The NLC also raises issues specific to different state requirements for criminal background checks and timely communication of discipline.

Technology

Another area of continuing competence for nurses is related to technology. The increasing numbers and types of available software and hardware creates issues specific to personal competence, selection of appropriate systems, boundaries between employer and personal systems, and the use of social media.

Ensuring that one is competent with emerging technology is essential as more and more organizations use electronic or digital systems for clinical patient monitoring and documentation. Indeed, the effective use of technologies is a core competency for contemporary professionals. What is equally challenging is the importance of differentiating which technology is appropriate to add and which technology does not offer additional value to one's ability to do work effectively. To be sure, not every new hardware and software product is necessary or affordable for patient care services. Professionals are now required to develop competence in determining which products will improve quality and safety and which are also affordable. Numerous frameworks for evaluation are available from both proprietary and state and federal agencies.

SOCIAL MEDIA

The term *social media* refers to the use of web-based and mobile technologies to turn communication into an interactive dialogue. Andreas Kaplan and Michael Haenlein define social media as "a group of Internet-based applications that build on the ideological and technological foundations of Web 2.0, and that allow the creation and exchange of user-generated content." Social media is media for social interaction as a superset beyond social communication. Enabled by ubiquitously accessible and scalable communication techniques, social media has substantially changed the way organizations, communities, and individuals communicate.

Source: Kaplan & Haenlein (2010).

Another technology challenge is the clear identification of the boundaries between employer and personal electronic products. The simplest approach is to fully segregate employer and patient information on one system and personal information and applications on personal computers or devices. Unfortunately, it is not always that simple and straightforward. In order to expedite patient care, providers often access patient records from personal computers. While this is not inherently a problem, the confidentiality of patient information by the nurse or user of the system must be fully safeguarded. The blurring of the boundaries between employer, patient, and personal data has received significant attention in light of recent violations of patient privacy.

In particular, the use of social media (Web 2.0) has become problematic. The use of interactive technology now requires principles for use that guide professionals in maintaining professional boundaries and protecting patient privacy. Table 10-8 identifies the most common do's and don'ts for social networking. Misuse of social media applications in which patient conditions were posted on the Internet and nursing unprofessional conduct was shared has resulted in the creation of guidelines to best use social media. It is the dark side of social networking that has raised issues of concern. In the digital world with boundary crossings between employer and personal technologies, the challenge to ensure patient privacy and personal professionalism becomes significant and requires purposeful actions.

Table 10-8 Social networking dos and don'ts

- Do use social networking as a tool to broaden your educational and professional horizons.
- Do use social networking to stay abreast of employer policies on social networking and Internet use.
- Do educate yourself about the privacy settings on websites you use.
- Do be aware that current and future employers may see what you post.
- Do know that your employer has the right to monitor your online activity on work computers.
- Don't use social networking sites at work.
- Don't reveal personal details such as your employer, your address, or your date of birth.
- Don't use your employer's e-mail address or handle.
- Don't upload images of videos of yourself in a clinical environment or uniform.
- Don't discuss patients, visitors, vendors, or organizational partners.
- Don't talk about coworkers, physicians, your supervisor, or your employer.
- Don't discuss clinical events or news stories about your employer.
- Don't friend patients, even after they are no longer patients.
- Don't give medical advice online.

Source: Prinz (2011).

The following websites provide additional resources for the application and use of social media:

- NCSBN social media guidelines: https://www.ncsbn.org/2930.htm
- American Nurses Association press release regarding social media and networking for nurses: http://www.nursingworld.org/FunctionalMenuCategories/MediaResources/PressReleases/2011-PR/ANA-NCSBN-Guidelines-Social-Media-Networking-for-Nurses.pdf
- American Nurses Association Social Networking Principles Toolkit: http://www.nursingworld.org/socialnetworkingtoolkit

- Chris Boudreaux's social media policy database: http://socialmediagovernance.com/policies.php?f=4#axzz1hZpGyzIU

To be sure, there are many positive aspects of social networking, such as career building and knowledge sharing. Social networking worldwide helps nurses to think more globally and network with colleagues who have similar interests. Most organizations and universities have created social media sites for sharing specific information to course work, marketing, and outreach tools. Specific policies have been developed for appropriate use of social media.

Performance Management

Demonstrating competence has traditionally been a supervisor-driven process in which the supervisor documents the employee's perceived performance for the year. Recently, nurse professional portfolios and professional demonstration evaluations by the individual nurse are proving to be more specific and comprehensive for the nurse's evaluation and overall career goals and accomplishments. Shifting from performance evaluation by a supervisor to performance demonstration by the nurse provides information that is more specific and more easily linked to documenting accomplishments and advancing career goals.

Some examples of elements of a professional nurse portfolio for the annual performance review include the following:

1. Contributions to the care and safety of patients
    a. Numbers, types, and outcomes of patients cared for during the year including particularly challenging and complex patients
    b. Interdisciplinary collaboration effectiveness identifying specific scenarios and the outcomes of the patient care event
    c. New practice behaviors based on evidence
2. Continuing education
    a. Internal and required
    b. External and voluntary
3. Contributions to colleagues
    a. Coaching situations and the outcomes
4. Contributions to the organization
    a. Internal committee contributions and outcomes
5. Contributions to the community

6. Challenges encountered; support received from supervisors and colleagues

7. Assessment of personal life and work balance

8. Required support and goals for the next year

Relationship Management

The second area of performance demonstration is relationship management. Relationships in the digital age require a new level of discretion in forming and sustaining connections. Professionals should regularly ask themselves which activities they should be involved in and to what degree they should be involved. The management of vast amounts of information and increasing expectations requires new approaches for work efficiency and time management. When time is limited, purposeful encounters become critical to enhancing and extending relationships and to get the work accomplished. Haphazard and unplanned encounters decrease productivity and delay goal achievement.

Be proactive. Professionals proactively develop relationships with colleagues in each discipline impacting the healthcare experience so that when the need is there the established relationship serves to facilitate efficient solution finding. To be sure, relationships are built one encounter at a time over time. When issues arise that need to be addressed by individuals from different perspectives, it is often too late to begin to build the necessary relationships. Such relationships need to be in place before they are needed to be effective in the accelerated technology world.

It is helpful to consider when to enhance, end, and avoid relationships. Individuals should consider enhancing and continuing relationships in the following scenarios:

- Supports the overall work of the organization and professional role
- Offers new ideas and information
- Is comfortable in engaging in discussions representing differing values
- Is able to challenge assumptions and beliefs
- Is able to see situations from another's point of view
- Portrays high personal integrity
- Accepts and incorporates feedback in a nonresistant and nondefensive manner
- Accepts responsibility for failure or errors

- Does not need reminders about responsibilities to patients or to other healthcare professionals in order to complete them
- Is available for professional responsibilities (i.e., required activities, available on clinical service, responds to pager)
- Takes on appropriate responsibilities willingly (not resistant or defensive)
- Takes on appropriate patient care activities (does not turf patients or responsibilities)

Not surprisingly, the goals and purposes of relationships change over time. Few relationships remain the same year after year. In one's work life, relationships that were once mutually beneficial and facilitative of the work are changed when an individual moves to another location or organization. Also, the values and interests of individuals change over time, thus decreasing the common bonds and goals once shared. This is not to say that the individual is not valued personally, but rather that the relationship as a means to effective work processes is no longer present. Consider ending relationships with individuals under the following circumstances:

- Values and goals are no longer congruent
- The individual is no longer in your area of work interest

Nurses are encouraged to avoid relationships in which individuals are known to have the following characteristics:

- Bully and harass others
- Engage in routine gossip
- Differ considerably in values/work processes specific to the respect of individuals and integrity
- Be unreliable and need constant reminders to complete work

Nurses should consider forming new relationships to accomplish the following:

- Reach out beyond traditional disciplines to disciplines outside of health care but within the community, such as school boards, legislators, and banking professionals to expand knowledge of the community.
- Gain greater insight into one's own discipline through university affiliation or membership in a national organization.

Course Correction: Life After Discipline

In the course of one's career, nurses may exceed their scope of practice or commit an error that violates the nurse practice act and be subsequently reported to the board of nursing for investigation. Boards of nursing review complaints and determine if a violation has occurred and what the appropriate actions should be, from dismissal, to letters of concern, to decrees of censure, to probation, to suspension, to revocation of the license. The reframing of errors to the concept of practice breakdown further enlightens the complexity of practice errors and the need for a more just approach. When a nurse is under investigation, it is highly stressful and emotional for the nurse. No nurse ever intends to practice beyond the licensure requirements; however, it does occur, and the sooner it is addressed, the sooner the nurse can refocus on acceptable practices. According to Marx (2001), practice errors may be one-time human errors for which discipline is inappropriate or a reflection of high-risk behaviors where the nurse practice needs to be assessed and remediated to ensure public safety.

Excellence Versus Perfection

It is important to note in our quest for patient quality and safety that the best goals are those focused on excellence, not perfection. Human fallibility is an unavoidable, predictable component of being human. When mistakes occur and harm results, we should give aid to those who are harmed and compassion toward the person who made the mistake (Marx, 2009). Further, Marx tells us that in the quandary we face when things go awry, there is a contradictory twofold challenge: hold those who caused the event appropriately accountable (perfection) and make fixes to prevent future events (excellence). The goal for any nurse following a report and sanction to the board is for course correction or remediation to occur quickly and effectively. Punishment should be considered when the nurse is willfully negligent and has a pattern of unprofessional conduct.

Personal Balance and Health

Nurses spend their work life taking care of others and too often forget or ignore the need for personal balance between work and personal life and don't make time for self-care. According to Shiparski, Richards, and Nelson (2011), it is dangerous to care for others before oneself. Such practices lead to unhealthy, deenergizing work environments. Also, the reality of compassion fatigue is experienced by those helping people in distress—an extreme state of tension and preoccupation with the suffering of those being helped to the degree that

NURSE SELF-CARE

1. Take time to think about yourself.

2. Get off the hamster wheel.

3. Say no without feeling guilty.

4. Avoid negative people and develop skills to extract yourself.

5. Eliminate appointments that are not necessary.

6. Create a space for mementos that trigger appreciation, gratitude, and joy.

7. Go on an e-mail diet. Answer e-mail no more than three times a day; text only on the hour.

8. Take time to plan rather than just diving in.

9. Stop watching mindless TV/negative news media, especially before bed.

Source: Richards, K., & Nelson, J. (2011). *Overcoming obstacles to create the optimal healing environment. Nurse Leader, 9*(2), 37.

it is traumatizing for the helper (Shiparski et al., 2011). Rest, tranquility, and stress management are essential for those working in the high-stress healthcare environment.

CRITICAL REFLECTIVE PRACTICE

"Being mindful of self within or after professional practice situations, i.e., processing the cognitive, behavioral, moral (ethical), socio-political, and affective components of professional practice situations, so as to continually grow, learn, develop personally, professionally and politically." (Lawrence, 2011)

Specific time for reflection and planning for the future can provide enormous support to thriving in a chaotic environment. According to Lawrence (2011), taking time for critical reflective practice positively impacts work engagement and decreases moral distress.

CRITICAL THOUGHT

Self-compassion is essentially extending compassion to the self for one's failings, inadequacies, and experiences of suffering (Stringer, 2011).

Minimizing negative thoughts is another strategy to enhance personal balance. Focusing on what could happen from a positive perspective rather than negative trajectories is more healthy and productive. According to Stringer (2011), when positive internal dialogue includes self-compassion, stress decreases. Nurses are typically hypercritical of their work, and in spite of the fact that the conditions for care and participation of patients in care is less than optimal, they blame themselves when the outcomes are not perfect.

CRITICAL THOUGHT

With all of the demands and expectations of nurses, maintaining focus is often difficult. Ask yourself the following questions to support focus on your work:

- Do your patient needs seem to blur across past and present patients? Keeping patients as distinct from one another is a continuous challenge.

- Are you focused on completing checklists before you complete patient care?

- Is it difficult to remember a day when you completed what you were able to do and hand off your patients to the next shift—and felt good about it?

Developing effective listening skills becomes more and more challenging in light of the increasing amount of information from both digital and print sources that is thrust upon us. Good listening requires preparation and concentration and includes sensitivity to both the context in which one is listening and the content of the conversations. Sensing both the location in which one is hearing information and what that information is about increases the richness of what one is hearing. Listening to dialogue from caregivers in a patient room may have a very different message than when listening to caregivers discuss patient care in a conference room without the patient. The purpose and goals of the communication can be quite different.

CRITICAL THOUGHT

Avoiding compassion fatigue is essential for all caregivers. Physical and emotional exhaustion can cause a decline in one's ability to feel compassion when taking care of others.

It is a cumulative result of internalizing the emotions of patients, coworkers, family, and friends. It is about focusing on caring for others and not providing care to yourself (Richards & Nelson, 2011).

Diet, Nutrition and Role Modeling

One area that is often challenging for nurses is diet, exercise, and nutrition. Given that nursing work pertains to health and healthy behaviors, the importance of role modeling takes on a new perspective. Specifically, nurses should not smoke, should manage their weight, and should participate in exercise on a regular basis. When a nurse is overweight and reeking of cigarette smoke, it is difficult for the patient and family to seriously consider education about smoking cessation and weight control. Health promotion is an ongoing career management activity that is important for not only role modeling, but also to minimize one's risk for cardiovascular and respiratory disease (Flannery, Resnick, Galik, & Lipscomb, 2011).

Contributing to the Profession

The role of a professional also includes contributing to the profession through membership in professional organizations, coaching, mentoring, sharing new ideas, scholarly writing, and recognizing the accomplishments of other nurses. Each of these activities serves to advance the profession and the practices of other nurses.

Professional Organization Membership

The work and oversight of professions necessarily needs to be accomplished by its members. Participation in professional associations has been traditionally low, including only small numbers of the profession. According to Reese (1999), the emerging workforce is not composed of joiners, and they do not become involved in professional organizations as members or leaders. Yet, the work of standards setting and expectations for outcomes for each discipline must still be accomplished. Models of engagement that integrate the values of the profession and the generational values of all members in new ways and include multiple types of communication, multiple media sources, and virtual collaboration and decision making will facilitate increased participation in professional issue discussion. The sophisticated electronic, audio, and video technology has diminished the value of many face-to-face meetings and large annual gatherings. This technology offers promise for rethinking professional organizations and the way in which the work is accomplished. Using discussion groups, chat rooms, and numerous other online tools can serve to involve all generations. This transformation will be especially important in sustaining the core values of each profession and at the same time linking professions in a virtual world.

Coaching and Mentoring

Coaching or **mentoring** colleagues in informal or formal ways is equally important in role development. No professional can ever expect to be fully self-sufficient as a single isolated individual. Feedback and counsel from trusted, competent colleagues specific to improving the quality of one's work life, learning to prioritize effectively, and advancing one's career are essential in the journey to leadership excellence. The role of the **coach** or **mentor** is designed to assist leaders in this work. The process provides the opportunity to continually seek open, honest, and timely feedback as well as an opportunity to share one's experiences and wisdom. Experts serve regularly in the role of both mentor and mentee; they are always giving of themselves to others and always learning from their interactions with others.

THE GOALS OF COACHING AND MENTORING

- Assist others to become more accomplished.
- Assist others to be the best they can be with their own knowledge, skills, and talents.
- Instill accountability and confidence in others so they can ultimately teach themselves.
- Assist others in using their own skills and knowledge to make decisions.

The need for coaching and mentoring is ever present. Initially, new nurses are best served with a more formalized relationship with a single mentor and commitment to a structured process. As the individual evolves, less formal and structured support is needed. New and different levels of mentorship with different emphases are identified. To be sure, the frequency and intensity of mentoring change throughout one's career based on the role and context of the work. Experienced nurses often have mentoring relationships that are not formal; rather the nurse seeks guidance from many mentors. When experienced nurses assume new roles or responsibilities, the need for more formal mentoring reemerges. At this point, mentoring focuses on enriching and accelerating the integration of the new work into the new role.

CRITICAL THOUGHT

The coach and mentor enable the mentee to find his or her own essence or presence of professionalism as a leader, to become a living vessel representing the character of a strong professional with vision, willingness, capacity, and commitment to the work of the organization.

Coaches and mentors have learned that all healthcare work is based on relationships and that individuals exist and become successful based on their relationships with others. Successful nurses have learned additionally that relationships can either enhance one's ability to get the work done or hinder it.

For example, relationships may advance the work of the nurse and the organization, invigorate and renew one's personal spirit and passion, stifle the work of the nurse and the organization, and/or do nothing to advance or stifle one's overall well-being. Day in and day out, the quality of those relationships serves to enhance or hinder one's effectiveness and can be considered the lifeblood of sustainable excellence. Coaches and mentors are well positioned to share experiences of both positive and negative relationships and most importantly to brainstorm with the mentee to identify future relationships that will support and enhance the work of leadership. Four types of activities around relationships and their impact are presented for discussion.

A coach or mentor begins with guiding the individual to develop skills in listening carefully, selecting reading materials, applying ideas, and observing. This work is always focused on supporting the individual as he or she progresses in the personal development journey to discover and live in the role that is the best fit for the individual, the role in which he or she is most successful.

> Coach: One who assists others to develop viable solutions, prioritize them, and then act on them. A coach works to assist healthy persons to achieve their goals, and when behaviors are unhealthy the coach refers the person to counseling. In this relationship, a partnership is being formed between the coach and the one being coached.
>
> Mentor: A mentor is a wise and trusted advisor who guides others on a particular journey. A mentor provides support, challenge, and vision.
>
> Mentoring: Mentoring is the process of a more accomplished person assisting others to develop expertise and learn new skills based on the mentor's personal, untapped wisdom, reinforcing their self-confidence, supporting real-life situations, and sharing personal experiences when appropriate.

Individuals approach the coaching experience in different ways. Not everyone is always ready for coaching or to be coached; however, sharing ideas, wisdom, and insights is important to advancement of individuals and the profession. Some individuals proactively seek out guidance and new ideas. They are adventuresome, visionary, and open to change and innovation. Others require more safety and security prior to a coaching experience. Some individuals remain quite skeptical and reluctant to seek or accept advice. Prior to formal or informal coaching, it is important to determine an individual's comfort level with new ideas and change. Working with this information will facilitate more successes than failures.

Coaches or mentors do not encourage individuals to adopt their own behaviors or to emulate their behaviors. Instead, effective coaches or mentors realize that the world is changing too fast to repeat their successful behaviors of the past, and they work with the individual to develop their own style of leadership based on principles and values. Coaches and mentors realize that the future is very different from the present or the past and requires new and creative behaviors for success—behaviors that the mentee is empowered to create.

In addition to professional role behaviors, mentors and coaches typically address the nuances of professionalism specific to appearance, **attitude**, and conflict management.

CRITICAL THOUGHT

- The mentor must always focus on avoiding the tendency to create a clone of him- or herself in the mentoring relationship.

- The mentor must avoid moving from a mentor to a therapist; the mentor focuses on guiding healthy behaviors, while the therapist focuses on correcting unhealthy behaviors.

- Communication between the mentor and mentee must be direct and honest, avoiding insincere and inaccurate messages.

- The mentee must be open to listen to new ideas but not to replicating ideas without careful consideration.

Attire

While there is always discussion as to who and what is professional, there are fundamental expectations specific to attire, communication, and attitude associated with the role of the leader. The professionalism of leaders is traditionally exemplified by the degree of presence of behaviors related to these three areas. Mentors can assist both emerging leaders and experienced leaders in ensuring the highest degree of professionalism through lifelong examination and reflection of these areas.

Much has been written about dressing for success and professional attire in the workplace. While each individual has developed his or her own understanding of what attire is or is not professional and appropriate for the workplace, the primary consideration must always be the customer, client, patient, or family to be served.

In healthcare organizations, the goal is to ensure cleanliness and support of the control of spread of infections. The goal must also be to minimize distractions to the patient to support a patient-family centered focus rather than attention to the dress of the caregiver. Clean, conservative attire best facilitates and supports an emphasis on the patient and family. Wild prints, exposed skin, excessive jewelry, and cologne shift the emphasis and attention to the caregiver rather than the patient.

The workplace should not be considered appropriate to make fashion statements or display new fashion styles, extensive jewelry, or strong colognes. The first impression made with patients and their families should be positive, one in which the organization is portrayed as competent, safe, and focused on the work of patient care.

In the mentoring dialogue, mentors and mentees should proactively examine their attire and be assured that personal appearance is not a hindrance to effective communication. Wise leaders ensure their personal presentation to team members continually exemplifies the highest level of professionalism as a mark of respect not only to one's individual reputation, but also as a mark of a good attitude.

Attitude

In addition to the physical presence of the leader, the attitude of the leader is important. Attitude, or the manner, disposition, or inclination as to how one approaches and reacts to situations, further defines one's level of professionalism. One of the simplest descriptions of positive or negative attitudes is often expressed from the perspective of a glass. Is the glass half full, indicating a positive, optimistic and hopeful attitude; or is the glass half empty, indicating a negative, pessimistic, and defeated attitude? A mentor can be helpful in assessing and reflecting with the mentee about attitude.

SCENARIO

Confronting internal negativity is an exercise that begins with identifying negative barriers to moving forward. In a small group, consider the following questions and statements:

- I've never been able to …
- It's too late for me to …
- I'm not very good with numbers …
- I never have enough time to …

Discussion Questions

1. Are these used routinely by any members in the team?

2. Are there other statements that are also used by team members?

3. Identify strategies to eliminate or at best minimize these statements both personally and in helping others eliminate internal negativity.

Discussion Question

Work with 2–3 team members. Using financial principles, value-driven outcomes, and multilevel measurements, build a convincing case to present formally to the supervisor.

Managing Conflict

Addressing difficult situations filled with conflict is another topic for coaching and mentoring. These are often referred to as the tough situations encountered in the provision of patient care—situations that are typically relational, recurring,

SCENARIO

Consider the following five categories of tough issues. Do any of these behaviors apply to you? Do you observe them in others? Use coaching and mentoring principles to address each of these areas of concern. Identify specific strategies and timelines to address each issue.

Lack of prioritizing:

- Fails to meet deadlines
- Repeatedly breaks appointments
- Continually extends beyond the planned time allocation
- Overloads schedules

Poor communication:

- Inappropriate interpersonal encounters
- Antagonistic and apologetic without results
- Rude, interrupts, and reacts before all the information is provided

Lack of collaboration:

- Manipulative, hard bargaining
- Avoids issues
- Tunnel vision

Lack of diversity:

- Avoids conflict at all costs
- Does not want to consider other viewpoints
- Limits team membership to selected similar colleagues

Lack of integrity:

- Fails to address the poor performance of a colleague who has become a friend
- Routinely offers insincere empathy
- Fails to identify the underlying issue before reacting

and deeply rooted in personal values issues. Learning to understand and address the trials and tribulations of organizational life requires persistence, commitment, integrity, and a trusted colleague! For some nurses, the ability to respond effectively to difficult situations is straightforward and only minimally stressful. For others, confronting difficult situations seldom comes easy and is usually filled with angst and trepidation.

Coaches and mentors who are competent in addressing these situations help the individual to avoid unnecessary missteps and additional stress. No strategy can ever fully remove the stress associated with such issues; however, strategies to increase the understanding of the issue, clarifying who really owns the problem, and reframing the situation can assist in more effective resolution of the issues. Seldom is a difficult situation limited to a single, specific event. Addressing difficult situations would be much easier to manage if there were no past history with an individual, one did not ruminate about the situation, and all recent experiences with the involved individuals had been positive.

The goal of the coach–mentor–individual relationship in managing tough situations is to transform difficult relationship problems into situations that are managed fairly and individuals are treated with decency in a timely manner. Coaches and mentors have experiences with what has worked for them in the past, the importance of timing, how to reframe difficult conversations from a personal event to addressing the situation directly and humanely, recognizing that individuals are not always positive and receptive, delivering the message in spite of resistance, and managing responses. These experiences should always be considered *informational* rather than *directional* for the individual. The individual needs to integrate the information into his or her personal style and comfort level in a way that is humane, focused, and goal oriented.

Professional Writing

Nurses are regularly involved in many patient care situations in which new and improved processes are identified, the application of new research works well, and, of course, certain practices do not work well. All of this information is needed by other nurses practicing across the country. Learning to write and sharing these experiences early in one's career will greatly enhance patient safety and quality.

Several resources are available to assist nurses in learning to write effectively. Textbooks, workshops, mentors, and online resources all provide guidance in the writing process. According to Sarver (2011), the following tips are helpful in becoming a successful writer:

- Narrow your topic.
- Ask first. Check with a journal or website to determine interest in the topic.
- Follow author guidelines.
- Make a writing appointment with a successful author for guidance.
- Be willing to revise.
- Ask at least two people to review the manuscript before submission.
- Never think you can't write; you can!

Appendix A contains additional information about writing for publication.

Additional Thoughts

It is important to note that information is dynamic and ever changing. Managing one's career requires thoughtful evaluation on a regular basis of career goals, interests, educational goals, and measurement of success as a professional. This chapter provides an overview of multiple areas for consideration in advancing one's reputation and contributions to the profession of nursing and to the health-care system.

CHAPTER TEST QUESTIONS

1. Nursing professionalism is determined by (a) the length of time in the profession, (b) the length of time the nurse has held a license in good standing, (c) the role identified by the American Nurses Association and the state nurse practice act, or (d) the AONE.

2. The transition from a competent nurse professional to a proficient nurse (a) requires time, experience, and knowledge, (b) occurs within the first 6 months of practice, (c) occurs in all nurses within 5 years, or (d) focuses on the integration of the community into critical thinking.

3. Performance demonstration differs from performance evaluation on the basis of (a) the time required for sharing performance goals, (b) the role of the unit-based team with whom the nurse works, (c) the amount of salary increase available, or (d) the creator of the performance document.

4. Nurse licensure (a) is not a requirement for continuing education credits, (b) is not affected when a nurse is involved in a system error, (c) is designed to inform the public that a nurse is safe to practice, or (d) is suspended when a nurse has multistate privileges.

5. Career trajectories (a) are limited by geographic regions, (b) are defined by local organizations, (c) are nearly unlimited for nurses, or (d) are highly overestimated for nursing professionals.

6. Continuing competence for professional nurses (a) includes integration of skills, including cognitive, psychomotor, interpersonal, and attitude, (b) is the accountability of the nursing board, (c) is the accountability of the individual licensed nurse, or (d) is not related to annual performance reviews.

7. Technology competence is (a) an emerging and essential requirement for competent nurses, (b) expected of all nurses providing patient care, (c) variable across organizations, or (d) not regulated by nurse practice acts.

8. Scholarly writing is (a) required for graduation from a bachelor of science degree in nursing program, (b) a challenge based on the required style formatting by the journal in which the article will be published, (c) an expectation in nurses' annual performance reviews, or (d) evidence of commitment to advancement of the profession.

9. Membership in a professional organization (a) is optional for a nurse professional in a rural setting, (b) is a reflection of commitment to support of professional standards review and development, (c) is seldom effective in supporting professional practice issues, or (d) can be expensive but worth the investment.

10. Discontinuing relationships (a) is appropriate in managing professional relationships, (b) is unprofessional conduct, (c) is best accomplished with a coach or mentor as intermediary, or (d) increases the amount of conflict a professional nurse must deal with.

www

> For a full suite of assignments and additional learning activities, use the access code located in the front of your book to visit the exclusive website: http://go.jblearning.com/leadership. If you do not have an access code, you can obtain one at the site.

References

American Organization of Nurse Executives. (2010). AONE guiding principles for the newly licensed nurse's transition into practice. Retrieved from http://www.aone.org/resources/PDFs/AONE_GP_Newly_Licensed_Nurses.pdf

Benner, P. (2004). Using the Dreyfus model of skill acquisition to describe and interpret skill acquisition and clinical judgment in nursing practice and education. *Bulletin of Science, Technology & Society, 24*(3), 188–199.

Cipriano, P. F. (2011). Move up to the role of nurse manager. *American Nurse Today, 6*(3), 61–62.

Dreyfus, H. L., & Dreyfus, S. E. (2004). The ethical implications of the five-stage skill-acquisition model. *Bulletin of Science, Technology and Society, 24*(3), 251–264.

Flannery, K., Resnick, B., Galik, E., & Lipscomb, J. (2011). Physical activity and diet-focused worksite health promotion for direct care workers. *Journal of Nursing Administration, 41*(6), 245–247.

Gallup. (2011). Honesty/ethics in professions. Retrieved from http://www.gallup.com/poll/1654/honesty-ethics-professions.aspx

Gittell, J. (2009). *High performance healthcare.* New York, NY: McGraw-Hill.

Hendren, R. (2011, November 15). Top 5 challenges facing nursing in 2012. *Health-Leaders Media.* Retrieved from http://www.healthleadersmedia.com/content/NRS-273338/Top-5-Challenges-Facing-Nursing-in-2012.html

Kaplan, A. M. & Haenlein, M. (2010). Users of the world unite! The challenges and opportunities of social media. *Business Horizons, 53*(1), 59–68.

Lawrence, L. A. (2011). Work engagement, moral distress, education level and critical reflective practice in intensive care nurses. *Nursing Forum, 46*(4), 256–268.

Marx, D. (2001). *Patient safety and the "just culture"; A primer for health care executives.* New York, NY: Columbia University.

Marx, D. (2009). *Whack a mole: The price we pay for expecting perfection.* Plano, TX: You Side Studios.

National Council of State Boards of Nursing. (n.d.). Transition to practice model toolkit. Retrieved from https://www.ncsbn.org/1603.htm

National Council of State Boards of Nursing. (2011). NCSBN model nursing practice act and model nursing administrative rules. Retrieved from https://www.ncsbn.org/Model_Nursing_Practice_Act_March2011.pdf

National Institute of Nursing Research. (2010). Online: Developing nurse scientists. Retrieved from http://www.ninr.nih.gov/Training/OnlineDevelopingNurseScientists/

Prinz, A. (2011). Professional social networking for nurses. *American Nurse Today, 6*(7), 30–31.

Reese, S. (1999). The new wave of gen X workers. *Business and Health, 17*(6), 19–23.

Richards, K., & Nelson, J. (2011). Overcoming obstacles to create the optimal healing environment. *Nurse Leader, 9*(2), 37.

Sarver, C. (2011). From practice to print: Creating a thriving culture of writing. *Nurse Leader, 9*(3), 23–25.

Shiparski, L., Richards, K., & Nelson, J. (2011). Self-care strategies to enhance caring. *Nurse Leader, 9*(3), 26–30.

Statement on Continuing Competence for Nursing: A Call to Action, June 8, 2011. National Board for Certification of Hospice and Palliative Nurses; NCSBN; http://www.nbchpn.org/

Stringer, H. (2011). Your own best friend. Nurse.com/Advanced Practice; 32–33.

Wasserman, S., & Faust, K. (1994). *Social network analysis.* Cambridge: Cambridge University Press.

Appendix A

Writing for Publication

Taking the leap and writing for publication requires content, courage, and resilience. Scholarly writing provides an opportunity to develop critical thinking skills and professionalism. Consider a recent patient care situation in which you believe there is information that other nurses would find useful. The situation could be a positive situation or a negative situation in which you want to warn other nurses to do or not do something.

1. Describe the specific situation in one or two paragraphs.

2. List the key points you are trying to make with your information. What problem are you trying to address or fix?

3. Review your situation and key points with another nurse in the class. Request constructive feedback to strengthen your article.

4. Complete a literature search in a major search engine (PubMed, CINAHL, ERIC, etc.) and summarize the information for inclusion in your article.

5. Identify at least two online and two paper publications that would be interested in your information.

6. Create one- to two-page submission for one online and one print publication using the specific author guidelines. (Note: Focus on content of the article, not the article length.)

7. Create a letter of inquiry to the editor for consideration of publication.

8. Describe your learning from this experience.

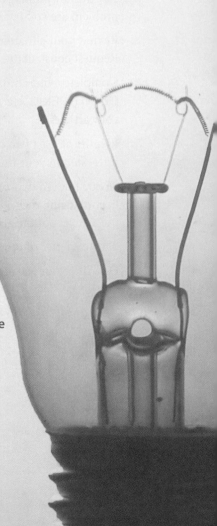

COMPROMISE MAKES A GOOD UMBRELLA, BUT A POOR ROOF; IT IS TEMPORARY EXPEDIENT, OFTEN WISE IN PARTY POLITICS, ALMOST SURE TO BE UNWISE IN STATESMANSHIP.
—JAMES RUSSELL LOWELL

CHAPTER OBJECTIVES

Upon completion of this chapter, the reader will be able to do the following:

» Define major concepts specific to healthcare policy.

» Develop an understanding of the challenges and nuances of policy development.

» Describe at least three major health initiatives and their impact on nursing.

» Identify future activities of the professional nurse to advance nursing from a policy perspective.

» List the desired competencies of the clinical expert nurse in advancing healthcare policy.

Policy, Legislation, Licensing, and Professional Nurse Roles

The area of healthcare policy is quite interesting and often focuses on national or state legislation initiatives and processes. For healthcare workers, there is much more to be considered from a policy perspective. Specifically, the study of healthcare policies can be expanded to include those organizational policies necessary for order and progress, external agency, and legislated policies adopted by varying levels of formal processes. Some policies hold the force of law with designated sanctions for noncompliance. Other policies hold the force of the organization's infrastructure and human resources requirements with designated disciplinary sanctions for noncompliance. In this chapter, the broader perspective of healthcare policy including internal and external policies will be presented along with the role of the professional nurse in policy management, discussion of both local and national policy issues, challenges in creating and sustaining effective policy, and thoughts about future healthcare policy.

To begin our discussion, it is interesting to consider why healthcare policy is needed. If everyone were equally gifted, equally educated, equally motivated, equally healthy, and equally wealthy—one wonders if national healthcare policy would be necessary. In spite of these equalities, one could wonder if there would still be issues when funding for health care exceeded certain targets. Or perhaps there would be no debate about how much funding would be needed for healthcare services because any allocation would benefit each individual equally. However, one could also wonder if there would still be access to care issues, given the wide geographic distribution of the population and location of providers for all geographic areas.

CRITICAL THOUGHT

Four stages of political development have been identified to describe nursing's evolutionary process in becoming savvy with policy processes. It is important to note that these stages are applicable to any types of policy development—organizational, public, social, or legislated health policies.

1. Buy-in: There is an emerging interest in policy issues and the relationship to individual nurse performance and ability to practice.

2. Self-interest: Nurses identify specific areas of interest to the profession and the need for formalization for action.

3. Political sophistication: Nurses are recognized by key stakeholders as knowledgeable and necessary for effective policies.

4. Leadership: Specific political agendas and identity are seen as legitimate.

Source: Adapted from Mason, Levitt, & Chaffee, 2007.

Regardless of this type of conjecture, the reality is that the playing field for health care is not level and effective policy processes that actively involve key stakeholders are essential. The unequal distribution of citizen knowledge, competence, skills, and physical and mental health in a society that values both proindividual and promarket perspectives requires sensitivity to both values in creating policy that meets the expectations of both. To be sure, the processes can be fragmented, incremental, and noncomprehensive, given the competing values (Shi & Singh, 2004). This work is never ending and continually changing as healthcare needs change and participants change. Embracing the work of health-care policy creation requires courage, time, persistence, and the ability to form effective and meaningful relationships. As the largest caregiver group in health care, the nursing community is positioned well to provide important input in these processes specific to quality, values, providers, outcomes, safety, patient care delivery systems, and funding.

CRITICAL THOUGHT

Caregiver competencies required in healthcare reform are as follows:

- Integrating between specialists and teams (chronic conditions, medically frail, and complex needs of seniors)
- Understanding financial management and getting value for the money
- Overcoming system inertia and moving the patient toward goals
- Clinical leaders innovating to improve the system
- Expertise in communicating and collaborating
- Information technology competence in documenting, monitoring, and mining data

It is also important to acknowledge the dark side of policy. Not all policy processes are perceived as open, honest, and collaborative. Some believe that the policy processes are quite negative and dishonest. In particular, the label of politician has often been associated with behaviors of controlling information, cajoling others to support issues, coercing others to support issues, being impatient while individuals consider information, being closed-minded to others' ideas, being confrontational and dishonest, and sharing only part of the information or partial truth telling. What is important to remember is that each one of us is part of the policy process whether or not we want to acknowledge it; there is no reason to engage in these negative behaviors. Further, when these negative behaviors are identified, calling others on these behaviors is equally important in the work of advancing effective healthcare policy.

Key Concepts

In this section a selected list of key concepts and their descriptions is presented to lay the foundation for future policy discussions. The list represents a wide range of concepts and is by no means inclusive of all of the healthcare policy concepts of importance to nurses.

Federal Register—The official daily publication for rules, proposed rules, and notices of the federal government and an unbiased source of information. It is an excellent source of current policy activity at the national level (GPO Access, 2004).

Health policy—Policy directed toward promoting the health of citizens (Mason et al., 2007); the aggregate of principles, stated or unstated, that characterize the distribution of resources, services, and political influences that impact the health of the population (Miller, 1987).

Institutional policies—Policies that refer to rules that govern the workplace (Mason et al., 2007).

Licensure—The process by which an agency of a state government grants permission to an individual to engage in a given occupation (Aiken, 2004).

Nursing certification—The provision of tangible recognition of professional achievement in a defined functional or clinical area of nursing (Aiken, 2004).

Organizational policies—Policies that pertain to positions taken by organizations to govern the workplace and behavior (Mason et al., 2007).

Policy—Encompasses the choices that a society, segment of society, or organization makes regarding its resources involving setting goals and priorities by a society or organization and the decisions about how and what resources should be used to achieve those goals. Policies reflect the values and beliefs of the leaders of society and/or organizations who make the policies (Mason et al., 2007).

Public policy—Policies that are authoritative rulings relating to those decisions made by government (Mason et al., 2007).

Social policy—Policy intended to enhance public welfare (Mason et al., 2007).

State nurse practice act—Regulates nursing practice, including requirements to enter into practice, licensure maintenance, scope of practice parameters, and disciplinary action (Aiken, 2004).

Statute—Laws passed by the legislature.

US Department of Health and Human Services—The overarching federal administrative agency concerned with monitoring the quality of health care in the United States (Shi & Singh, 2004).

The Policy Continuum: Local to National

While the emphasis of healthcare policy is typically on the national issues, healthcare policy is also required at the organizational levels. Specifically, organizations providing healthcare services are required to have policies specific to provider roles, patient care procedures, safety practices, equipment management, staffing and scheduling, and many others. Nurses are encouraged to become involved in these local policy processes in their organizations to better understand the organization and as a precursor to external policy processes at the state and national levels.

CRITICAL THOUGHT

The policy process is as follows:

1. Identify the policy or issue specific to a societal problem for a community, state, or nation.

2. Set the agenda and place it within other policy priorities.

3. Formulate a plan for gaining support and adoption of the policy.

4. Implement or adopt legislation.

5. Evaluate the impact of the legislation.

Policies are also generated from state legislatures, state agencies authorized by legislation, and state professional associations. These policies and processes are designed to serve the unique needs of the state. Examples include regulatory boards for licensure and state agencies for children, the elderly, and the mentally compromised.

At the federal level, policies are generated or enacted by the legislature, the designated agencies, and numerous professional associations. Generally, processes to achieve federal legislation or agency policy require more time and energy for consensus building and negotiation to ensure that the intent of the policy is understood and supported. In addition to the recently passed healthcare reform bill, other examples of federal legislation include the Health Insurance Portability and Accountability Act regulations and Patient Self-Determination Act.

Numerous national professional associations make recommendations for safe and effective practice; however, these do not hold the force of law. Examples include The Joint Commission, the American Nurses Association, the Institute of Medicine, and the Robert Wood Johnson Foundation. While the associations do not hold legislative authority, they are usually highly regarded and supported by both organizational and legislative processes.

Contemporary Healthcare Policy Issues and Initiatives

There are numerous healthcare policy issues facing states and the country. Common areas of focus include scope of provider services, provider competence, quality, safety, cost, access to care, timeliness, privacy, ethical issues, effectiveness, evidence, engagement of patients with providers, technology, coordination of care across the life span, waste, fraud, and abuse. In addition to the specific policy issues, there are numerous initiatives underway from a variety of sources to address selected policy issues.

The following initiatives are examples of both legislation and professional organization recommendations. These initiatives reflect the wide range of approaches to creating policies to advance health care in the United States. A brief discussion of each is presented.

Patient Protection and Affordable Care Act (PPACA)

This federal statute, enacted in March 2010, is designed to help replace a broken system with one that ensures all Americans have access to health care that is both affordable and driven by quality standards. The goal of this act is to deliver seamless (digital), high-quality, patient-centered care for Medicare beneficiaries instead of the fragmented care that now occurs. Two key components of the statute include meaningful use of technology and the implementation of **Accountability Care Organizations** (ACOs) to coordinate and integrate care services.

Meaningful use by users is intended to maximize the use of electronic health records to (1) improve quality, safety and efficiency and reduce health disparities, (2) engage patients and families, (3) improve care coordination, (4) improve public health, and (5) ensure adequate privacy and security protections for personal health information (Murphy & Alexander, 2010). Medicare incentives are linked to effective meaningful use, while reductions in Medicare payments will be realized by providers who fail to achieve meaningful use.

ACOs consist of networks of providers that are rewarded financially if they can slow the growth in their patients' healthcare spending while maintaining or improving the quality of the care they deliver. The Accountable Care Model emphasizes population care, value-driven outcomes, emphasis on the point of service at which patient care occurs, protocols for effective hand-offs, and inclusion of the family. An important distinction between health maintenance organizations and ACOs is that providers themselves, rather than an insurance company, control the diagnosis and treatment decisions. An overview of the components of an ACO is presented in Figure 11-1. It is important to note that the ACO rests on a firm technology foundation.

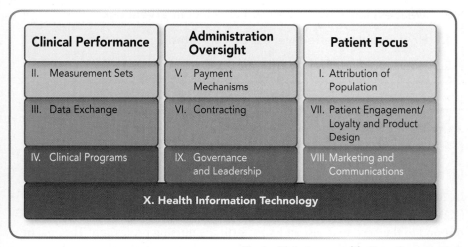

Figure 11-1 Accountable Care Organizations

Issues in the healthcare reform act that are of concern for nurses are related to advanced practice nurses. Certified nurse midwives were not included in the ACO professionals list. While nurse practitioners were included in the ACO professionals list, the method proposed for assigning beneficiaries to ACOs does not incorporate primary care services provided by nurse practitioners. Significant opportunities exist for nurses to engage both state and federal legislators specific to the exclusion of an active advanced practice nurse role in the reform efforts. This healthcare reform legislation continues to evolve in its implementation and will no doubt be modified many times before a stabilized model is created. Regardless of the turmoil, these changes are necessary to modify a very ineffective system.

SCENARIO

Pain management continues to be a problem. Patients continue to complain, particularly at the end of life, about inadequate pain relief. Providers vary widely in their skills and practices in the administration of medications and other nontraditional interventions.

Discussion Questions

Given the expectation of an effective ACO, consider the following:

1. Describe the policies that would be needed to correct this problem.
2. Which providers would be involved?
3. What evidence would be used to select interventions?
4. How would the effectiveness be evaluated?
5. How would interventions be documented?

The Future of Nursing: Leading Change, Advancing Health (Institute of Medicine Report)

In 2008, the Robert Wood Johnson Foundation and the Institute of Medicine (IOM), two national professional associations, launched a 2-year initiative to respond to the need to assess and transform the nursing profession. The goal of this work was to produce a report specific to the future of nursing, which was published on October 5, 2011. Four key messages were developed by the committee (Shalala & Vladeck, 2011):

- Nurses should practice to the full extent of their education and training.
- Nurses should achieve higher levels of education and training through an improved education system that promotes seamless academic progression.
- Nurses should be full partners, with physicians and other healthcare professionals, in redesigning health care in the United States.

- Effective workforce planning and policy making require better data collection and information infrastructure.

This report and recommendations from national professional associations do not hold the force of law; however, they are widely respected and supported by many in the healthcare community.

Transition of Care Program

Significant concern continues to exist specific to changing caregiver teams (hand-offs) and the nearly 20 percent readmission rates for several medical diagnoses. To address these challenges, the National Transitions of Care Coalition (www .ntocc.org) was formed in 2006, bringing together leaders, patient advocates, and healthcare providers from various care settings to focus on improving the quality of care coordination and communication. Transfers encompass moving a patient from primary care to specialty physicians; within the hospital they include moving patients from the emergency department to various departments, such as surgery or intensive care; they also occur when patients are discharged from the hospital and go home, to an assisted living setting, or to a skilled nursing facility.

This effort has resulted from a national professional association with the goal to decrease readmissions. Driven by research evidence, this group formed to address this significant quality problem. Oftentimes an initiative using this approach rather than a legislative approach is more expeditious.

Advanced Practice Registered Nurse (APRN) Consensus Model

Currently, there is no uniform model of regulation of APRNs across the states. Each state independently determines the APRN legal scope of practice, the roles that are recognized, the criteria for entry into advanced practice, and the certification examinations accepted for entry-level competence assessment. This has created a significant barrier for APRNs to easily move from state to state and has decreased access to care for patients. Because of the importance of APRNs in caring for the current and future health needs of patients, the education, accreditation, certification, and licensure of APRNs needs to be effectively aligned in order to continue to ensure patient safety while expanding patient access to APRNs. For these reasons, the APRN Consensus Model has been proposed by the APRN Consensus Work Group and the National Council of State Boards of Nursing APRN Advisory Committee (Figure 11-2).

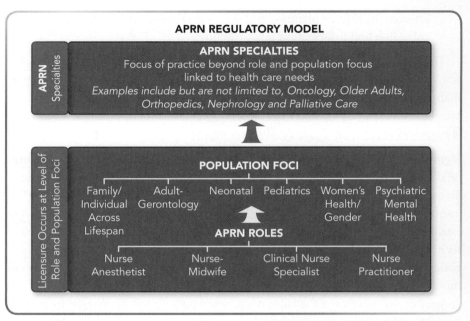

Figure 11-2 APRN regulatory model.
Source: Courtesy of the National Council of State Boards of Nursing.

In this document, The APRN Consensus Model at https://www.ncsbn.org/2276.htm requirements call for the board of nursing to be the regulatory body that issues licenses and provides oversight of APRNs. The requirements further specify that all APRNs will be educated, certified, and licensed in one of four roles and in at least one of six population foci. But all are given the protected licensing title of Advanced Practice Registered Nurse (APRN). Education, certification, and licensure of an individual must be congruent in terms of role and population foci. If all states adopt the regulatory requirements for licensure, accreditation, certification, and education for APRNs, as outlined in the Consensus Model, the benefits will be far reaching for healthcare professionals, regulators, and consumers (Figure 11-3).

According to the National Council of State Boards of Nursing, the following benefits are possible with the APRN Consensus Model:

- Consumers would clearly understand the role of advanced practice nurses and know there is a competent individual providing care who is consistently regulated across the country.

- Employers would understand the requirements for preparation, education, and scope of practice.

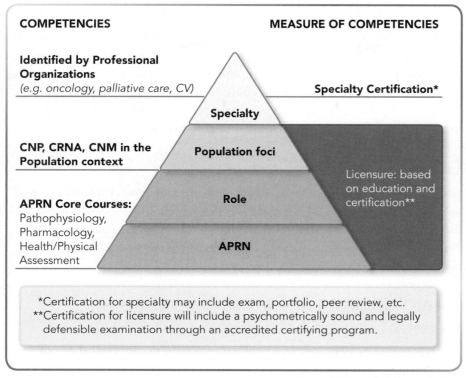

Figure 11-3 APRN competencies.
Source: Courtesy of the National Council of State Boards of Nursing.

- Future APRNs would have increased confidence in the quality and appropriateness of education programs.

- Boards of nursing would be able to fulfill the role of public protection and have confidence that APRNs entering the state meet uniform requirements.

- Legislators would be accountable to constituents, knowing that the APRN regulatory model consistently emphasizes public protection.

Informed Consent

Informed consent is an essential component of the healthcare process. Specifically, the individual provider performing healthcare services or procedures is required to explain the procedure to be performed, the risks involved, the expected outcomes, potential complications, and alternative treatments that are available (Barrett, 2005).

Patient Self-Determination Act

The Patient Self-Determination Act was enacted in 1991and requires organizations receiving federal funding to provide education for staff and patients on issues concerning treatment and end-of-life issues. Specifically, advance directives determined by competent individuals must be implemented if that individual becomes incapacitated in the future (Salmond & David, 2005). This act continues to be of great importance in upholding patient respect and autonomy.

Good Samaritan Laws

Good samaritan laws state that healthcare providers are protected from potential liability if they volunteer their nursing skills away from the workplace, provided that the actions taken are not grossly negligent. It is limited to emergencies and does not cover nonemergent care or advice given to others outside of the workplace (Brooke, 2004).

Health Insurance Portability and Accountability Act (HIPAA)

This law, passed in 1996, focuses on the patient's right to confidentiality and the improvement of the portability and continuity of health insurance coverage (Erickson & Millar, 2005). Both issues remain critical to quality healthcare services. Unauthorized release of information or photographs is not allowed. Written authorization by the patient is required for release of any information about the patient in writing, on the phone, or in person. The insurance portability requirement of this law has been more troublesome to implement; however, the efforts continue with revisions of rules to achieve the desired goals of simplifying the coding of health information to ease the digital exchange of information among healthcare providers.

Professional Nursing Role and Policy

It is important to remember that if you are not part of the solution, you are part of the problem! Thus ignoring issues steeped in political dialogue and conflict will not make them go away—neither will it bring about resolution. As nurses advance in their professional role competence, involvement in the profession becomes more realistic and interesting. The following four activities should be embraced by all nurses.

CRITICAL THOUGHT

The process of building competence as a political expert begins at the local organizational level and moves to external local, state, and national areas. It is a developmental process that requires time, reflection, and coaching from established policy experts. Components of the process are as follows:

- Build working relationships with policy committee members in your organization.
- Participate on committees focused on policy areas of interest, such as critical care or technology areas.
- Participate in professional organizations of interest.
- Develop relationships with local and state legislators.
- Develop relationships with state agency leaders, such as the state department of health services and the state board of nursing.
- Provide input to legislators specific to healthcare issues and other areas of interest.
- Participate on legislative lobby days with state nursing associations.
- Register to vote—and vote in every election.
- Develop relationships with US legislators.
- Get involved with a local political party.
- Share your ideas with leaders and elected officials involved in policy work.
- Run for office!

First, become competent in the processes of policy development and the differing approaches that are effective at the local, state, and national levels. Competencies begin with basic relationship development and participation on local committees. Recognizing the similarities to external political processes provides support and reassurance that this type of work is indeed possible and effective.

The second activity is to develop focused partnerships with stakeholders who know and understand the evidentiary support for policy making or changing. Learning to understand and integrate evidence into policies is desperately needed. In addition, working from an evidence-driven perspective further diminishes the tendency to create policy based on emotions and one-time events.

The third activity is to take a risk and propose a new policy that is of great interest to you. Consider virtual care, patient falls, medication errors, integrating workarounds, or some area of health care that you believe needs attention. Begin with local policy initiation and progress to the state agency level, such as the board of nursing or department of health services. It is seldom necessary to do this work alone. Engage in discussions in your organization or committees at the board or agency levels to determine interest.

CRITICAL THOUGHT

Specific topics for political influencing include the following:

- Funding for safety initiatives
- Technology implementation and standardization of applications and language
- Mandates for value-based health care and outcome evaluation
- National healthcare funding philosophy for patient care and education of providers
- Provider role clarity
- Healthcare research priorities

The fourth activity is to examine a current policy—either internal or external—and identify the effectiveness of the policy. This evaluation can often be a challenge; however, it is necessary to determine the pragmatic value of the policy. Some policies may be quite effective, while others may not have achieved their intent and may cost time and effort to continue to comply with the policy. Consider pain management or restraint policies for investigation. Many efforts to get to an ideal policy have failed to achieve the desired result of safety and respect.

The fifth activity is specific to integrating evidence into the policy processes whenever possible. The digital age has provided an increasing amount of information that can now be evaluated and integrated into policy when appropriate. The importance of integrating evidence into the policy process cannot be overemphasized. The need for compelling evidence for policy at any level is essential; however, this need is not always met given the multiple influences in the policy process. As more and more information becomes digital, the expectation for higher levels of evidence is appropriate.

Also, knowing that the values of independence and market forces often conflict in getting to the best healthcare policies, we must each be motivated to get involved to ensure that the balance between the marketplace and the individual is as good as it can be. Many relationships focus on influencing local, state, and national public policy as well as organizational policy, but there is not always appropriate evidence. The focus of political relationships, whether internal to the organization or in the public arena, must continue to evolve to ensure that healthcare work is evidence driven, occurs safely, and is affordable.

The sixth and final recommendation is about increasing nursing presence in healthcare policy discussions. According to Donelan, Buerhaus, DesRoches, and Burke (2011), nurses need to increase their presence at the national policy level with well-honed messages and participation in news media, research publications, and advertising to advance the issues of nursing supply, workplace safety, and funding for education.

Numerous resources are available for nurses to develop key messages specific to nursing's future. In addition, strategies to contact and communicate with local and national media are also encouraged from a proactive perspective. Being prepared for both internal and external inquiries about the challenges, needs, and expectations of the profession not only is proactive, but it is also stress reducing. The Farrah Consulting Group (2003) recommends several considerations in being "media ready":

- Know the position you want to take and articulate it clearly.
- Proactively reach out to the media whenever possible. Build on relationships so that reporters will contact you with questions or challenges when they are seeking information.
- Avoid reporters who tend to present biased stories with little objectivity.
- Stay on message. Repeat, if necessary!
- Practice your message and presentation with internal staff.
- Minimize off-the-record comments.
- Focus on proactive crisis management with a defined plan as to who the spokesperson will be, as well as preparing for the worst possible questions that someone could ask.
- Respond promptly

Final Thoughts on Policy

This is only the beginning of your work with healthcare policy as a registered nurse. There are so many needs and opportunities for nurses across the spectrum of key stakeholders who participate in making healthcare policy decisions. Oftentimes, these key stakeholders *and* legislators have very little, if any, background in healthcare issues. These stakeholders need your assistance and are usually very open to collaboration and discussion of emerging issues. For nurses, it is our day and time to be more known and more effective in advancing quality health care.

CHAPTER TEST QUESTIONS

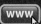

1. Healthcare policy is most effectively created (a) at the state level, (b) at the state and national levels, (c) at the national level, or (d) in a variety of legislative, association, state, and national levels.

2. Nurse practice acts (a) focus on discipline of nurses, (b) are state based, (c) require endorsement from the federal government to change any statutes, or (d) are consistent from state to state.

3. Nurse input into health policy is (a) essential because nurses are the largest caregiver group and are familiar with patient care issues, (b) seldom recognized or valued, (c) is best when done through a lobbyist, or (d) requires membership on a board of nursing committee.

4. The dark side of politics (a) is specific to certain types of legislation, (b) requires competence in negotiation, (c) is an unfortunate and negative result of negotiating in bad faith, or (d) is the result of extensive experiences in the political processes.

5. Policy is distinguished from politics in that (a) policy reflects the outcome while politics reflects the human processes to achieve a policy, (b) policy reflects the desired outcome while politics reflects the guidelines to achieve a policy, (c) policy reflects the intentions of elected officials while politics reflects political agenda required to achieve a policy, or (d) policy is the final result of negotiations while politics reflects the dark side of the negotiations to achieve the policy.

6. Institutional policies (a) are guidelines that do not have consequences if not followed, (b) are designed to serve the social needs of the community, (c) are created by state agencies to support healthcare organizations, or (d) are organizational policies designed for effective practices in the workplace.

7. The US Department of Health and Human Services (a) is a federal agency funded by the legislature, (b) includes funding for both federal and state initiatives, (c) does not include funding for Medicare, or (d) requires elected officials to participate on agency committees.

8. Healthcare reform as proposed in the 2010 legislation (a) is expected to be completed by 2013, (b) is designed to improve patient care outcomes and satisfaction at no increased cost, (c) is designed to reduce overall costs by 10 percent, or (d) is expected to completely overhaul the current healthcare delivery system.

9. Accountability Care Organizations (a) are expected to provide improved coordination and documentation of patient care, (b) are limited to urban areas near universities, (c) do not require initial funding to begin, or (d) are recommended in the HIPAA legislation.

10. Nurse licensure is (a) intended to provide a vehicle for continuing education documentation, (b) intended to provide evidence of safe practitioners and protect the public, (c) intended to inform healthcare facilities of those safe to practice, or (d) requires evidence of a negative criminal history.

References

Aiken, T. D. (2004). *Legal, ethical and political issues in nursing.* (2nd ed.). Philadelphia: F.A. Davis.

APRN Consensus Model. at https://www.ncsbn.org/2276.htm

Barrett, R. (2005). Quality of informed consent: Measuring understanding among participants in clinical trials. *Oncology Nursing Forum, 32*(4), 751–755.

Brooke, P. S. (2004). Stretching the good samaritan law. *Nursing, 34*(7), 22.

Donelan, K., Buerhaus, P. I., DesRoches, C., & Burke, S. P. (2011). Health policy thoughtleaders' views of the health workforce in an era of health reform. *Nursing Outlook, 58,* 175–180.

Erickson, J. L., & Millar, S. (2005). Caring for patients while respecting their privacy: Renewing our commitment. *Online Journal of Issues in Nursing, 10*(2), 1115.

Farrah Consulting Group. (2003). Polishing the pitch: A primer on effective media strategies. Boston, MA. Retrieved from http://farrahconsulting.com/

GPO Access. (2004). Federal Register: About. Retrieved from http://www.gpoaccess.gov/fr/about.html

Mason, D. J., Levitt, J. K., & Chaffee, M. W. (2007). *Policy and politics in nursing and health care* (4th ed.). Philadelphia, PA: Saunders.

Miller, C. A. (1987). Child health. In S. Levine & A. Lillienfeld (Eds.), *Epidemiology and health policy* (pp. 83–89). New York, NY: Tavistock.

Murphy, J., & Alexander, D. (2010). The journey to meaningful use and the impact on nursing. *Voice of Nursing Leadership, 6*(8), 6–9.

National Council of State Boards of Nursing. (2011). The consensus model for APRN regulation: Licensure, accreditation, certification, and education. Retrieved from https://www.ncsbn.org/aprn.htm

Reville, B., Miller, M., Toner, R. W., & Reisnyder, J. (2010). End of life care for hospitalized patients with lung cancer: Utilization of palliative care service. *Journal of Palliative Medicine, 13*(10), 1261–1265.

Salmond, S. W., & David, E. (2005). Attitudes toward advance directives and advance directives completion rates. *Orthopedic Nursing, 24*(2), 28–34.

Shalala, D., & Vladeck, B. (2011). Leading change: How nurses can attract political support for the IOM report on the future of nursing. *Nurse Leader, 9*(6), 38–39, 45.

Shi, L., & Singh, D. A. (2004). *Delivering health care in America: A systems approach.* Sudbury, MA: Jones and Bartlett.

Appendix A

Selected Resources for Healthcare Policy

This appendix contains a selected list of references and resources that are helpful in understanding national healthcare policy initiatives and issues. Many other resources can be added to your personalized list of resources as you become more familiar with healthcare policy specific to your particular area of interest.

Agency for Healthcare Research and Quality—The Agency for Healthcare Research and Quality's (AHRQ; www.ahrq.gov) mission is to improve the quality, safety, efficiency, and effectiveness of health care in the United States. AHRQ's research focuses on improving decision making as well as the quality of health care. AHRQ was formerly known as the Agency for Health Care Policy and Research.

American Nurses Association—The American Nurses Association (ANA) House of Delegates and the ANA Board of Directors work together to create policy for health care, the workplace, patient care, and many other areas where nurses are engaged. The House of Delegates and/or the Board of Directors often consider significant issues and address these concerns by way of a position statement or resolution (http://www.nursingworld.org/MainMenuCategories/Policy-Advocacy/Positions-and-Resolutions).

American Organization of Nurse Executives—The American Organization of Nurse Executives (AONE) is the national organization of nurses who design, facilitate, and manage care. Since 1967, AONE has served its members by providing leadership, professional development, advocacy, and research to advance nursing practice and patient care, promote nursing leadership excellence as well as shaping public policy for health care. AONE is a subsidiary of the American Hospital Association (http://www.aone.org/resources/future_of_nursing.shtml).

Commonwealth Fund—The Commonwealth Fund serves to promote health care that emphasizes improved access, quality, and greater efficiency, particularly for society's most vulnerable people (http://www.commonwealthfund.org/About-Us/Mission-Statement.aspx).

Health Affairs—*Health Affairs* is a monthly journal published by Project Hope and is a leading journal on health policy and research. The peer-reviewed journal, founded in 1981, explores health policy issues of current concern in both domestic and international spheres (www.healthaffairs.org).

Institute of Medicine—The Institute of Medicine (IOM) is the health arm of the National Academy of Sciences and is a nonprofit organization that works outside of government to provide unbiased and authoritative advice to decision makers and the public (http://www.iom.edu/).

Jefferson School of Population Health—The School of Health Policy and Population Health serves to foster health policies that contribute to the delivery of high-quality and cost-effective care through research and education for healthcare providers, policy makers, and consumers (http://www.jefferson.edu/population_health/).

US Department of Health and Human Services—The US Department of Health and Human Services is the US government's principal agency for protecting the health and well-being of all Americans through the provision of essential human services, especially for those who are most needy (www.hhs.gov).

Appendix B

Palliative Care Case Study

Option 1

According to the Jefferson School of Population Health, the provision of compassionate, quality care for individuals with chronic illness continues to be a challenge. Patients continue to suffer because pain is not adequately addressed during treatment, and patient preferences are neglected at the end of life. In particular, hospitalized patients with lung cancer, at the end of their lives, experienced barriers to palliative care access and were typical of patients in other parts of the United States (Reville, Miller, Toner, & Reifsnyder, 2010). There was confusion about the difference between palliative care and hospice care and when to initiate each type of care. Both doctors and nurses acknowledged lack of training in end-of-life communication and when to suggest a transition to palliative care. There was a delay in referral to palliative care until late in the disease trajectory, and the service was underutilized to address symptoms and psychosocial concerns. Palliative care professionals were consulted for only 8 percent of all hospital admissions among this patient population.

1. As an experienced nurse, identify and describe the specific opportunities at the institutional, organizational, public, social, and health policy levels specific to palliative, hospice, and end-of-life care.

2. What are the issues at each level that prevent adequate care?

3. Who are the key stakeholders that need to be involved in addressing this issue?

4. How will you evaluate progress at each policy level when changes are made?

5. Describe a plan specific to nursing interventions at each policy level, including the facilitators and barriers of the policy proposal.

Option 2

Given the significant challenges with patient readmissions within 30 days of discharge, there is a need for additional local analysis by nurses providing patient care. Substitute the problems associated with palliative care with patient readmissions and respond to the previous five questions.

THE BEST EXECUTIVE IS THE ONE WHO HAS SENSE ENOUGH TO PICK GOOD MEN TO DO WHAT HE WANTS DONE, AND SELF-RESTRAINT ENOUGH TO KEEP FROM MEDDLING WITH THEM WHILE THEY DO IT.
—THEODORE ROOSEVELT

BUT THEN AGAIN TO LOOK TO ALL THESE THINGS YOURSELF DOES NOT MEAN TO DO THEM YOURSELF . . . BUT CAN YOU NOT INSURE THAT IT IS DONE WHEN NOT DONE BY YOURSELF? —FLORENCE NIGHTINGALE

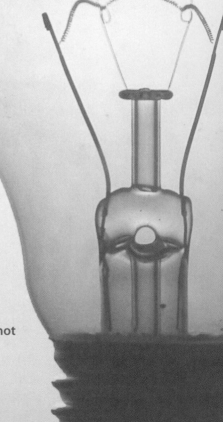

CHAPTER OBJECTIVES

Upon completion of this chapter, the reader will be able to do the following:

» Gain an appreciation of the complexities of management and clinical delegation.

» Describe the basic concepts of delegation and supervision as they relate to the delegation of nursing work.

» Identify inappropriate delegation processes and the implications for negatively impacting patient care.

» Develop strategies to address the common errors and breakdowns in delegation and supervision.

» Develop skills to manage situations when delegation does not proceed as planned.

Delegation and Supervision: Essential Foundations for Practice

It can be said that without effective delegation, an organization could come to a complete standstill. Each individual would do his or her work independent of others with no connections to any other individual. There would be multiple silos working hard and going nowhere! Delegation is required wherever there is a hierarchal order of individuals working together to accomplish goals. The importance of working with and through others has never been greater given the increased complexity, new technologies, and innovations in health care. The ability to delegate, assign, manage, and supervise is a critical competency for all healthcare workers, especially nurse leaders. Further compounding the challenges is the nursing shortage and increasing demands on those nurses in the system. In this chapter, an overview of the basic principles of delegation, key concepts related to delegation and supervision, the challenges of delegating effectively, and strategies to enhance delegation skills will be presented.

SCENARIO

Delegation is often misunderstood and not used as effectively as it could be—even though most nurses recognize that delegation is necessary to function effectively and efficiently as a nurse.

Discussion Questions

In a small group, complete responses to these three items. Share your responses with each other as well as suggestions to increase your competence in delegation.

1. My definition of delegation is:

2. I am reluctant to delegate because:

3. My delegation would be better if:

The **authority** for delegation is grounded in the organizational chart of the facility. Included within positional managerial authority are the right and duty to delegate authority. Just as the possession of authority is a required component of any managerial position, the process of delegating authority to lower levels within the hierarchy is required for an organization to have effective managers, supervisors, and employees.

DELEGATION

The transferring to a competent individual the authority to perform a selected nursing task in a selected situation. The nurse retains accountability for the delegation.

Delegation is both a management and a legal concept. As a management concept, delegation is discussed in terms of authority, responsibility, and accountability. Delegation begins with and occurs from the chief executive officer (CEO) throughout the organization. All work is driven by the oversight of the CEO leader. Formal or organizational authority may be obtained from specific roles. Other formal sources of authority may occur through a position in an organization or through an individual contract. An individual can delegate only the authority that he or she individually possesses. Delegation is about the giving of power, responsibility, and work to another qualified individual.

The legal concept of delegation is different from the management or organizational concept of delegation and is defined in terms of authority and liability. Legal sources of authority come from legislative, judicial, and administrative branches of government. Most frequently, legal delegation is derived from the authority of the nurse licensure or other professional licensure. To empower one to act for another requires one to possess legal authority; before delegation can occur there must be a source of that legal authority, which is licensure. It is important to remember that all decisions related to delegation of nursing tasks must be based on the fundamental principle of protection of the health, safety, and welfare of the public.

In order for effective delegation to occur, the following must be present:

- Autonomy: The power to do the job (a job description). An individual must have an organizational job description that identifies the expectation for specific work. For example, the registered nurse (RN) job description states the role of the nurse in providing patient care.

- Authority: The right to do the job (a license). The RN must also have a current and valid RN license to practice in the state in which patient care is being provided.

- Competence: The skill to do it. The nurse must demonstrate the knowledge and competence to effectively delegate.

If any one of these is missing, effective and legally defensible delegation cannot occur. The next section includes many of the key concepts and definitions specific to delegation.

CRITICAL THOUGHT

Nursing judgment is the essential element in every delegation decision.

Delegation: Definitions and Key Concepts

Accountability—Being answerable for actions or inactions of self or others; the obligation to account for or explain the events. There is both **individual accountability** and **organizational accountability** for delegation. Organizational accountability relates to providing sufficient resources, staffing, appropriate staff mix; implementing policies and role descriptions; providing opportunity for continuing staff development; and creating an environment conducive to teamwork, collaboration, and client-centered care. Individual accountability is about knowing the requirements and behaviors of effective delegation (Figure 12-1).

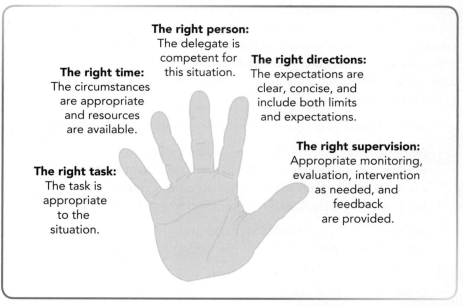

The right time:
The circumstances are appropriate and resources are available.

The right person:
The delegate is competent for this situation.

The right directions:
The expectations are clear, concise, and include both limits and expectations.

The right task:
The task is appropriate to the situation.

The right supervision:
Appropriate monitoring, evaluation, intervention as needed, and feedback are provided.

Figure 12-1 The five rights of delegation

Assignment—Describes the distribution of work that each staff member is to accomplish in a given time period. Assignment occurs when the authority to do a task already exists. Assignment means that a nurse designates another nurse to be responsible for specific patients or selected nursing functions for specifically identified patients.

Authority—The legal source of power; the right to act or command the actions of others and to have them followed. Authority is gained from licensure (law) or by virtue of such characteristics as intelligence, knowledge, moral worth, and leadership ability (personal authority). Authority is a key component in developing a clear understanding and definition of delegation. Through delegation, the **delegator** transfers a span of authority and responsibility to the delegate, while the delegate is accountable for accomplishment of what has been delegated. The delegator retains final accountability for the delegation decision and for his or her own authorities and responsibilities.

Critical thinking—Active, purposeful, organized thinking that takes into consideration focus, language, frame of reference, attitudes, assumptions, evidence, reasoning, conclusions, implications, and context when deciding what to believe or do.

Decision making—A complex cognitive process that involves choosing a particular course of action from among alternatives. Decision making is an essential component of the problem-solving process.

Delegate—The individual staff person receiving the delegated task.

Delegation—The transfer of responsibility for the performance of a selected nursing activity or task from a licensed nurse authorized to perform the activity or task to someone who does not have the authority. Delegation is the transfer of authority by one person to another; the act of transferring to a competent individual the authority to perform a selected nursing task in a selected situation, the process for doing the work. It is a skill requiring clinical judgment and final accountability for client care. Delegation is the transfer of responsibility of the performance of an activity from one individual to another, with the former retaining accountability of the outcome.

Delegator—The individual making the delegation.

Responsibility—Reliability, dependability, and obligation to accomplish work.

Supervision—The provision of guidance or direction, evaluation, and follow-up by the delegator for accomplishment of a task delegated to another; to watch over a particular activity or task being carried out by other people and ensure that it is carried out correctly. Supervision includes the initial and ongoing direction, procedural guidance, observation, and evaluation. It is the active practice of directing, guiding, and influencing the outcome of a person's performance of an activity, providing guidance for the accomplishment of a task or activity, with initial direction and periodic inspection of the actual accomplishment of the task or activity.

As noted in the definitions, while a licensed nurse must be actively involved in and be accountable for all managerial decisions, policy making, and practices related to the delegation of nursing care, there is both individual accountability and organizational accountability for delegation. Organizational accountability for delegation of licensed or legal functions of nursing requires that the organization provide the infrastructure for the delegation, supervision, and acceptance of delegated tasks by qualified individuals. The organization is accountable to ensure the individuals who accept delegated tasks are not only competent to perform the tasks but also are competent in their role in the delegation process.

Organizational accountability for delegation relates to doing the work of the organization based on the hierarchal positions and accountabilities in the organization. For example, it is the responsibility of the organization to ensure that delegators and delegates have received information specific to the principles of delegation and supervision, including age-specific training, and are qualified to care for the client population specific to the tasks being delegated.

Steps of the Delegation Process: Roles of the Delegator and Delegate

Learning to delegate effectively requires preparation and practice. To be sure, knowing the concepts as well as the basic roles and steps is an important start. Also, understanding the expectations of the delegator and delegate roles in delegation is essential. Basic principles for delegation guide the practice of nursing delegation.

The delegator is responsible for the following:

- Assessment of the situation
- Ascertaining the competence of the delegate (education, training, skills, and experience)
- Follow-up supervision
- Management of results

The delegate is responsible for the following:

- His or her own actions
- Accepting only those tasks or assignments for which he or she is qualified
- Providing feedback on tasks according to the guidelines specified by the delegator

Once the delegation process occurs, the delegate must ensure that the delegation is within his or her capability based on the following assessments:

1. Determine if the task is within his or her scope of ability, licensure, and job description.
2. Consider the current work assignment.
3. Consider the current situation, such as complexity or potential for harm.
4. Accept graciously and willingly identify concerns with delegator.

THE IDEAL DELEGATOR

- Delegates authority whenever possible in areas affecting his or her work
- Consults with employees before making decisions pertaining to their job responsibilities
- Gives employees the reasons for implementing decisions
- Does not play favorites
- Recognizes excellent work
- Counsels employees who fail to observe the proper chain of command relationships and delegation principles
- Never reprimands or disciplines in front of coworkers
- Encourages employees to offer their opinions and criticisms of supervisory policies
- Listens to employees' explanations before placing blame in disciplinary situations; accepts reasonable explanations, not excuses
- Role models all the rules that other employees are expected to follow

The following six steps present the basic actions in delegation processes.

Step 1

Assess the patient or client, the situation, and the appropriateness for delegation. It is important to know your personal delegation strengths and weaknesses as well as those of the members of your team. Decisions to delegate nursing tasks, functions, and activities are based on the needs of clients, the stability of client conditions, the complexity of the task, the predictability of the outcome, and the available resources to meet those needs and the judgment of the nurse (American Nurses Association, National Council of State Boards of Nursing, n.d.). Be sure to understand the importance and expectations of the state nurse practice act, practice limitations, and job requirements.

Step 2

Assess the patient's needs and appropriateness for delegation. Ensure that the delegate has the legal and organizational permissions or right to perform the delegated task. It is essential for the delegating nurse to have an understanding of what the assistive personnel's credentials are in terms of education and demonstration of skill.

BASIC DELEGATION PRINCIPLES

1. Delegation is considered a part of the nurse's role.

2. When the nurse delegates, the nurse assumes responsibility for supervision.

3. Each nurse is accountable to practice according to state law. Licensed persons are responsible for providing nursing care in circumstances that are consistent with their training, education, and experience.

4. The nurse delegator is accountable for the acts of delegation and may incur liability if found negligent in the process of delegating and supervising.

5. The person delegated to is accountable for accepting the delegation and for his or her own actions in carrying out the delegated tasks.

Note: It is the nurse manager's legal responsibility, in making assignments, to delegate appropriately and provide adequate supervision.

Making the Determination on What to Delegate

Based on nursing judgment, state law, and agency policies, a nurse must determine whether a task is delegable by relying on the criteria established in state nursing practice guidelines, the employing organization, and professional association recommendations. There are several guidelines to consider when determining what to delegate. The following list provides guidelines for determining what should be delegated:

- Routine or standardized tasks with predictable outcomes that are not threatening to the mental health of the patient

- The task requires no judgment based on nursing knowledge or expertise

- The results of the task are reasonably predictable

- The task can be performed safely, according to exact, unchanging directions, with no need to alter the standard procedures for performing the task

- The performance of the task does not require complex observations or critical decisions with respect to the task

- No repeated nursing assessments are needed

- The consequences of performing the nursing task improperly are minimal and not life threatening

In most states or jurisdictions, a licensed practical/vocational nurse (LP/VN) may delegate tasks to a trained, unlicensed person if authorized by the RN to delegate and if the task is within the LP/VN's scope of practice. An LP/VN may not supervise the practice of an RN because the RN scope of practice is outside the LP/VN scope of practice. An LP/VN may supervise employment activities of an RN that do not constitute the practice of nursing, such as human resource policies.

Examples of common tasks delegated by RNs to nursing assistants include most activities of daily living, bathing patients, feeding patients, ambulating patients, taking vital signs, and skin care.

Tasks That Should Not Be Delegated

Supervisory accountability cannot be delegated. Although a supervisor must delegate authority to employees to accomplish specific jobs, the supervisor's own personal accountability cannot be delegated. Assigning duties to employees does not relieve the supervisor of the responsibility for those duties. When delegating assignments to employees, the supervisor still remains accountable for the actions of the employees in carrying out these assignments.

Several other specific situations require mention:

- LP/VNs may delegate nursing tasks within the LP/VN's scope of practice, provided an RN first directs an LP/VN to do so.

- Assessment, evaluation, and nursing judgment cannot be delegated.

- Delegation is unnecessary if the particular activity or task is already within the legally recognized scope of practice of the individual who is to perform the activity or task.

If the activity or task is not within a nurse's scope of practice, it cannot be delegated by a nurse. You cannot delegate what you do not have! Note that physicians cannot delegate physician work to nurses.

Step 3

Planning for the work to occur. Determine with the delegate when the work is to occur and under what patient circumstances. The following five steps provide guidelines for preparing with the delegate:

1. Clearly identify the work that needs to be done.

2. Clearly identify the level of supervision and expected frequency of interactions between delegator and delegate.

3. Clearly identify the importance of requesting assistance when needed.

4. Create a plan for daily feedback between the delegator and delegate specific to delegation principle performance.

5. Discuss strategies to increase effectiveness of delegation and supervision activities, including frequency of supervision and potential for additional delegation.

CRITICAL THOUGHT

If a delegating nurse makes an acceptable delegation to a competent delegate and an error occurs, then the delegate is accountable for his or her actions in its performance, and the delegator is accountable for supervision, follow-up, intervention, and corrective action.

Step 4

Provide directions as to what is to be done. Always communicate in a positive, supportive manner. Maintain communication that is clear, complete, and constant. Ensure that the delegate understands what is to be done, when it is to be done, and what feedback is expected. Provide oversight and opportunity for communication during the task assignment time and as agreed upon.

Step 5

Evaluate the patient outcomes; compliance with standards of practice, policies, and procedures; and effectiveness of the delegation. Evaluate what happened and what the results were.

Step 6

Provide feedback to the delegate that includes recognition of work well done and areas of opportunity for improvement.

Protecting Your License: Nursing Liability for Delegation

Prior to learning the principles and processes of delegation, nurses are often concerned as to the potential professional liability specific to their RN or LP/VN license. Nurses initially believe they are responsible for the actual work of the delegate. The nurse is accountable for selection and delegation of tasks to the delegate. This includes ensuring that the conditions are appropriate for delegation and that the delegate is competent to perform the delegated work. The delegator nurse is *not* responsible for the actual work of the delegate. The delegate is fully responsible for his or her work. Thus, the delegator is accountable for the process; the delegate is responsible for the work.

The Challenges of Delegation

Not every delegation event is successful. There are several reasons why delegation may fail. Sometimes there is underdelegation in which not enough work is delegated. Sometimes there is overdelegation in which, although the work is appropriate to delegate, the workload is beyond what the delegate can reasonably do in the assigned time. Finally, the delegation can be improper in which any of the five rights are violated. The wrong task, the wrong patient, the wrong circumstances, the wrong directions, and/or the wrong supervision can all be involved in improper delegation.

Oversupervision

Unfair delegation occurs when the delegator is constantly looking over the shoulders of those asked to do the work. It is confining and restricting to the creativity and problem-solving potential that longs to come out of most people. It is also unfair to make decisions behind the backs of those to whom work is delegated. Oftentimes, the delegator begins to overmanage or add too many unnecessary check-ins, thus frustrating competent delegates.

Underdelegation

Too often, individuals fail to delegate for a variety of reasons. Some fear losing authority and recognition. It requires courage to turn important work over to others. Dictators never delegate; they just look for the weak willed to implement their every desire. Another reason for limited delegation is the fear of the work being done improperly or poorly. This is the most obvious reason why some just can't delegate. While there is always the fear of less than satisfactory results, often the reason is the lack of willingness to allow others to do the work their own way. In many cases, there is no perfect way to do the job.

There are numerous reasons why delegation does not occur as intended, including the following examples:

- Lack of training and positive experience specific to delegation. A failed experience in delegation requires refocusing on the basics of delegation and working with others to create effective delegation processes. It is a rational risk that is essential to take. There can also be a lack of supervisory skill or lack of ability to direct, or there can be uncertainty of how to develop subordinates through the delegation process.

- Not comfortable with risk-taking. Delegation inevitably involves risk—in nursing this translates into fear that if the work is not done by you, a patient could be harmed or there could be a lawsuit. Some people also have a desire to avoid conflict and confrontation and have a fear of being disliked.

- Unwillingness to take the necessary time to work with others. Task-oriented people want to just get the job done instead of waiting on others to do it through delegation. Some nurses prefer doing rather than managing.

- Fear of work being done better. Some leaders are paranoid about having others do a better job than they themselves could have done. Some also believe there is a lack of support for decisions.

- Sometimes, delegation is undermined from within. Individuals find it hard to let go of control and need to feel indispensable. They may have a fear of losing authority or personal satisfaction. Delegation requires trust.

- Fear of depending on others. Being independent reflects strength and competence. Shared leadership is quite different and requires learning and less aggressiveness to depend on others in a team environment where the whole task is not completed until each member does his or her part. Some leaders may have a lack of confidence in his or her subordinates.

- Preoccupation with negative fantasies about what could happen blocks working with others to develop effective delegation skills.

- A lack of skill in balancing workloads and disorganization may affect the delegation process.

CRITICAL THOUGHT

Thoughts on delegation, supervision, and oversight:

- The RN is accountable for delegation and supervision of assigned patients.
- Oversight is an expectation within the delegation and supervision process. There may be layers of oversight within the process; for example, RN → LP/VN → nursing assistant or RN → instructor → student.
- Hand-off activities are critical events in the delegation process to ensure continuity of oversight.
- Documentation of delegation and supervision/oversight should never eliminate the accountability or oversight of the work to be done.

Refusal by Delegate

Another challenge in effective delegation is the refusal by the delegate to agree to accept an assignment. Refusal of assignments poses a new challenge to the already overburdened clinical nurse. It is important to determine, as best as one can, the reason for the refusal to accept the assignment. While potential delegates may not freely offer the reasons for refusal, it is important to consider the following potential reasons:

- Lack of willingness to do the job (lazy, unmotivated)
- Lack of skill (not comfortable with skills)
- Perceptions of unfair assignments (feelings of overwork)
- Physical condition (not able to physically do the work)

Strategies to Support Effective Delegation

In light of the challenges, there are several strategies to address the challenges and improve delegation processes. The first is to gain an understanding of personal delegation competence.

Individuals can consider the following questions to assess their current status with delegation and supervision:

1. Why is it so hard to delegate? Is there something that blocks an individual from embracing delegation as a means to provide more effective and efficient patient care?

2. How does one know *what* to delegate?

3. How does one know to *whom* tasks can be delegated?

4. How does one know *when* to refuse an assignment?

5. Why don't I delegate? Again, what is blocking this behavior?

6. Why don't I willingly accept delegated tasks? Is it difficult to work on a team and be mutually accountable for team members?

7. What would help me improve my ability to delegate appropriately?

8. What should I do if I identify inappropriate delegation?

9. Should my performance be rated above average if I willingly accept appropriately delegated tasks? If I delegate appropriately?

10. Should I be rated below average if I routinely refuse and/or challenge the nurse when tasks are delegated? If I do not delegate appropriately?

In addition to these questions, Appendix B also includes scenarios specific to delegation. When considering the behaviors in the preceding list, also consider the tasks that are or could be involved in delegation of patient care work. Ask yourself the following questions:

1. Can someone else do the task?

2. Should someone else do the task?

3. Do I have to do the job?

CRITICAL THOUGHT

Delegation is an elementary act of managing.

Oftentimes, these types of challenging questions assist nurses in reevaluating situations and considering new approaches to patient care. These kinds of questions also provide insight into why individuals may be reluctant to accept delegated tasks as well as to delegate.

Another strategy is to access evidence-based resources for delegation and supervision. As the pressure increases for higher productivity without compromising quality, processes of delegation will become more and more important in health care.

The professional knowledge worker is always dealing with the translation of knowledge into action directed toward a positive impact. This discipline guides the action of the professional and informs the strategies and interactions necessary to advance the work of the profession. Because of the intensity of the professional work, the centrality of human relationships to professional action, and the profession's social obligation to positively impact society, complex interactions and relationships must be negotiated. It is the role of the clinical leader to facilitate and coordinate these interactions and through the use of good communication and negotiation skills to refine and advance the essential interactions and intersections necessary to translate knowledge and collective wisdom into meaningful action and purposeful impact.

Leaders cannot lead without a capacity to negotiate. However, negotiation is a learned skill and a journey more than an event. Negotiation is a continuously unfolding dynamic that matures and develops as the skills of the negotiators are advanced and refined and can be directed toward meaningful purpose and a positive outcome. It is not always easy to keep the focus of negotiation and the intent of the negotiators aligned with impact and outcome. This is where the skill, discipline, and attributes of the leader and the processes associated with negotiation become critical to the efficacy and effectiveness of knowledge work and the knowledge worker. Yet, consistency and faithfulness to the principles and practices of good negotiation yield the benefits of a positive context for knowledge work. The result is sound and purposeful relationships and interactions and effective deliberation and decision making that serve the interests and values of the community.

CHAPTER TEST QUESTIONS

1. Working toward achieving universally recognized and acceptable solutions is a discipline just as much as it is a process. True or false?

2. The negotiator must always be firm and resolute with regard to his or her bottom line throughout the negotiation in order to make sure personal objectives are met. True or false?

3. There must be a willingness to be open, available, and have a wide range of potential options and considerations that can provide creative and unique ways of satisfying needs and finding common ground. True or false?

4. When gathering data for negotiation, it is important that the individual focus on his or her own position, strengthening it with evidence strong enough to counter other parties' positions. True or false?

5. Positions should be broad based and open ended in order to provide room for alternative solutions. True or false?

6. Threats and challenges always arise during a negotiation. Each negotiator must be prepared to counter these with stronger challenges to point out the evidence and veracity of one's own position. True or false?

7. When leading questions are used to confuse, identify weaknesses, or force concessions, the leader delays answering a series of questions, breaks down the questions into single units, and seeks specific answers to each individual question as it relates to the originating issue. True or false?

7. Inappropriate delegation occurs when (a) effective supervision is on site, (b) medication administration is delegated by a licensed person to a nonlicensed person without medication administration authority, (c) an unlicensed person delegates to a licensed person, or (d) a licensed practical nurse delegates to a nonlicensed person.

8. The five rights of delegation include (a) the right nurse, the right task, the right circumstances, the right communication, and the right supervision; (b) the right task, to the right person, under the right circumstances, with the right supervision; (c) the right time, the right nurse, the right communication, the right supervision, and the right evaluation; or (d) the right task, to the right person, under the right circumstances, with the right supervision by the right person.

9. Accountability is different from responsibility because (a) accountability includes expectations to perform authorized work based on licensure or job description; (b) responsibility is about the provision of resources, policies, and staff development for delegates, while accountability is about using the resources effectively; (c) accountability is about ensuring adequate resources and staff development for delegation, while responsibility is about ensuring attendance at staff development workshops; or (d) accountability is about being able to answer for and explain actions and results, and responsibility is about doing the task.

10. Assignment is different from delegation because (a) neither delegation nor assignment making requires authority, (b) ownership of authority for the tasks belongs only to the RN, (c) delegation requires authority for tasks in delegation but not in assignment, or (d) delegation does not include authority for tasks, while assignment includes authority for tasks.

WWW For a full suite of assignments and additional learning activities, use the access code located in the front of your book to visit the exclusive website: http://go.jblearning.com/leadership. If you do not have an access code, you can obtain one at the site.

Reference

American Nurses Association, National Council of State Boards of Nursing. (n.d.). Joint statement on delegation. Retrieved from https://www.ncsbn.org/Joint_statement.pdf

Appendix A

Joint Statement on Delegation: American Nurses Association and National Council of State Boards of Nursing

Several years ago, the joint American Nurses Association (ANA) and National Council of State Boards of Nursing (NCSBN) issued a joint statement on delegation. There are nine principles that can be accessed that emphasize nine principles of delegations and they can be accessed on either the ANA or NCSBN website. These principles include:

1. The essence of professional responsibility and accountability.

2. Care coordination and the use of assistants in providing patient care.

3. Not delegating the nursing process, rather only parts of the process to assistive personnel.

4. The significance of nursing judgment.

5. Delegation to competent individuals.

6. The components of effective communication between the RN and the delegate.

7. The importance of two-way communication in the delegation process between the delegator and the delegate.

8. The importance of critical thinking, professional judgment, and the five rights of delegation.

   - The right task
   - Under the right circumstances
   - To the right person
   - With the right directions and communication
   - Under the right supervision and evaluation

9. The role of the chief nursing officer is ensuring adequate infrastructure for delegation and supervision (American Nurses Association, National Council of State Boards of Nursing (n.d.).

Appendix B

Delegation Assessment: Why Don't I Willingly Delegate or Accept Delegated Tasks?

In groups of three, develop your response(s) to each situation. Which principles of delegation were followed, and which principles were not followed?

1. Overdelegation
    - Would you pass my medications for me and sign off my orders? I'm really busy.

2. Underdelegation
    - I'll do it myself. The nursing assistant argues with me when I ask her to do something.
    - I'll do it myself. I always have to do it over.

3. Refusal to accept assignment—legitimate delegation
    - I don't have enough experience to perform that task.
    - I don't know how to do that very well (fear of criticism for mistakes—lack of self confidence).
    - I'd rather not risk the patient's life.
    - I have too much work already.
    - It's always me that gets the work; ask someone else.
    - I'm too busy, I won't be able to do a very good job, but if that's what you want …

Appendix C

Process of Delegation

1. Select a competent and capable person; consciously assess that person's skill, experience, and attitude.

2. Assign the task/duties to immediate subordinates.

3. Clearly and realistically define the goals, priorities, and outcomes for both the delegator and the delegate; give complete information.

4. Confer authority and the means to do the job; grant permission (authority) to take all the actions necessary to perform these duties.

5. Create an obligation (responsibility) on the part of each employee to perform the duties satisfactorily.

6. Keep in contact and give feedback during and after the completion of tasks.

THE GREAT QUESTION ABOUT POWER IS WHO SHOULD HAVE IT. —JOHN LOCKE

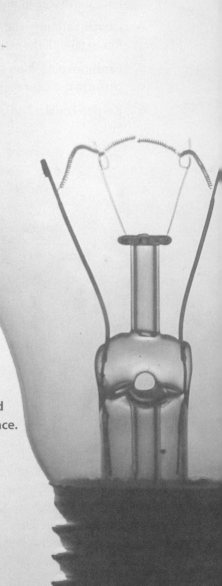

CHAPTER OBJECTIVES

Upon completion of this chapter, the reader will be able to do the following:

» Understand basic elements and characteristics of professional negotiation.

» Define the unique characteristics and obligation of the clinical leader in facilitating and coordinating negotiation and its processes.

» Delineate the elements and characteristics of dynamic negotiation and the stages necessary for successful negotiation processes.

» Outline the principles and characteristics of negotiation and problem solving as a part of the clinical leadership experience.

» List at least six components of negotiation and the characteristics of each.

» State at least three reasons why the clinical leader must use negotiation processes every day as a part of leadership expression.

Overcoming the Uneven Table: Negotiating the White Waters of the Profession

Negotiating skills are not optional for the clinical professional. At all levels of professional practice, the elements of negotiation will be continually used in the role of agent and acting in the best interests of persons and the public. The profession will continually negotiate with peers and patients, administrators and assistants, and a host of other professionals representing a wide variety of constituents in the professional workplace having an influence or impact on the work of the nurse.

Effective **negotiation** is entirely a learned skill. Although there may be some born with particular talents that reflect an easier capacity to negotiate, effective negotiation is learned through the process of discipline and application. In fact, much of the skill and talent necessary to negotiate well can be improved through continuous and effective use and refinements of skill development and learning. Those less naturally gifted with the basic negotiating skills can easily learn and adapt to the requisite of working with others to find common ground, agreement, or to move collectively within a diverse set of circumstances (Deleuran & Jarner, 2011).

Becoming an effective negotiator means learning some essential basic skills to help refine understanding and clarify the factual foundations for decision making and collective action. In all negotiation it is important to be able to develop and utilize good listening techniques, effective questioning methodologies, useful verbal and nonverbal communication approaches, and use creative mechanisms in advancing win–win solutions and shared values.

Chapter 4

CRITICAL THOUGHT

Negotiation does not result in a winner or loser. It leads to a mutually beneficial solution to a common issue in a way that engages the stakeholders and invests them in the deliberation process.

Principles and Basic Skills of Negotiating

Working toward achieving universally recognized and acceptable solutions is a discipline just as much as it is a process. Each party to a negotiation recognizes that the other parties have something that is important to each individual sufficient to require interaction, communication, and some level of argument. Basic processes of negotiation occur every day over things as small as deciding between the elements of a lunch menu to resolving the complex vagaries of a multinational contract. The principles that drive both of these levels of negotiation are generally consistent.

Negotiating is not about winning or losing. In fact, if winning and losing are a part of the negotiation or the result of the negotiation, the dialogue can be considered as having failed. Win–win is an essential characteristic of negotiation and forms one of its foundational principles. What negotiation attempts to do is to identify, enumerate, and undertake a process that clearly establishes needs and wants and where all parties work to reconcile their interests in a way that results in mutual advantage or value (Figure 13-1). In short, all parties must win something meaningful to them in order for positive negotiation to be satisfied. Because of the nature of win–win approaches to negotiation, developing effective skills and high levels of preparation are critical to successes between the parties to a negotiation (Heller & Hindle, 2008).

- Understand your own position.
- Collect data on the other's position.
- Concession is a strategy, not a loss.
- The solution must be mutual.
- Expect to be surprised by what emerges.
- The solution may be other than expected.
- The exchange must be thought fair by stakeholders.

Figure 13-1 Principles of positive exchange

Because negotiation is a skill, recognizing the principles and foundations that guide it is the first step to developing the essential insights and skills that ultimately make negotiation successful. There is a set of core skills that must be developed and refined in order to ensure successful negotiation:

- It is important that the individual can discern, identify, and declare specific goals for which the risk of negotiation is worth undertaking. These goals establish an entrée position but allow an approach with a level of flexibility that indicates a willingness for dialogue and negotiation.

- There must be a certain level of flexibility and fluidity with regard to wants and needs. Applying a firm and unyielding attachment to positions, demands, or needs eliminates the grounds for meaningful negotiation and polarizes the process before it even begins.

- There must be a willingness to be open, available, and have a wide range of potential options and considerations that can provide creative and unique ways of satisfying needs and finding common ground.

- Good negotiators are well informed, clearly prepared, and understand as much about the matter under negotiation as possible. It is important to know as much as possible of all points of view or positions to the concern at issue. A good negotiator knows how to argue on behalf of the other positions at the table almost as well as those who would make the arguments themselves. This means being well informed and well prepared.

- Negotiation is essentially the use of good communication skills and the discipline of positive interaction. Some level of competence in the discipline of communication is sound preparation for the meaningful dialogue of negotiation. All negotiation is a reflection of words and language combined with the communication capacity of body language, gestures, tone, and the use of the language. The better prepared and disciplined the individual is in negotiation skill sets, the more positively positioned he or she is for effective negotiation.

- Listening is perhaps one of the most essential foundational skills in effective negotiation. Strong negotiators are carefully listening to messages being delivered by others and observing the context as well as the content of the message. Here again, body language, gestures, tone, use of language, and the ability to discern supporting information or communication in a way that helps clarify true meaning all contribute to the effectiveness of the interaction.

- A good negotiator knows how to sort the extraneous from the valuable and the priority from the unimportant. The effective negotiator continually remembers the purposes and principles that bring individuals to the negotiation and the needs and wants that reflect how those purposes might be fulfilled. The more aware negotiators are about personal needs and wants, the more available they are for satisfying them with a wider range of options. There are a number of ways problems can be solved. Being available to alternative options that can address needs and wants provides a wider range of choices in getting issues appropriately addressed.

CRITICAL THOUGHT

The ability to listen carefully is one of the most important leadership skills associated with good negotiation. Hearing the real messages that are the basis for negotiation is critical to negotiating the right outcome.

Practicing negotiating skills in noncritical situations helps develop negotiating talent in a risk-free developmental environment. Negotiation is important enough as a skill that putting it into the continuing education developmental program for nursing staff could be an important way of making it a part of the effective tool set necessary for good clinical care. Refining these skills in the common and ordinary activities of daily life helps hone them for more specific and directed circumstances. The professional must know that just as negotiation occurs in personal life (for example, negotiating who takes the kids to school and who picks them up, negotiating a favorite restaurant, resolving a difference on child rearing, etc.), the process of negotiation occurs using the same principles and skills and just as frequently in the work arena.

Give and Take: The Principles of Exchange

Important to negotiation is the understanding that every party needs to gain from the interaction. Something of value must be exchanged. In order for individuals to feel as though they have accomplished something from the negotiation, they must feel that they are taking something meaningful away from the process. In negotiation, if one side wins and the other loses, the negotiation has essentially failed.

REFLECTIVE QUESTION

The most important issue for an individual involved in negotiating is what his or her precise bottom line is. When you think of a recent conflict with a coworker or family member, what was your essential bottom line beyond which you were not willing to go?

People must first be clear about what it is they most need or want from the negotiation process. This notion of an individual's **bottom line** helps establish the ground upon which the individual will negotiate. At the same time, individuals in the negotiation need to know that in order to get a satisfactory outcome for themselves there must be a fair exchange that results in a satisfactory outcome for other stakeholders to the negotiation. Individuals in negotiation must recognize that flexibility will be a vital element of the process if it is to be successful. The give and take, balance of power, and back and forth of the negotiation process provide a continual recalibration of the dynamic between the parties as each moves to obtain his or her needs and the chosen methods and mechanisms satisfy each stakeholder.

Stages of Negotiation

Like any formal process, negotiation has several phases or stages that participants move through as they advance to mutual solutions and satisfaction. There are generally five or six stages through which negotiation moves that must be satisfied in order for equitable negotiation to be advanced and satisfied. These six stages are: (1) readying for negotiation; (2) establishing the framework for the negotiation; (3) intensive interaction; (4) bargaining; and (5) closing the interaction, which sometimes includes a sixth step: performing the agreement (Figure 13-2).

- Getting ready for the negotiation.
- Establishing the framework for the negotiation.
- Intensive negotiation interaction.
- Bargaining toward solution.
- Bringing closure to the negotiation.
- Performing the agreement.

Figure 13-2 Stages of negotiation

Readying for Negotiation

Detailed and intense preparation for negotiation is the first secret of truly successful interaction. Information is always the source of power in the negotiation process. Those who are best prepared for negotiation will best benefit from it. It is not only important to be fully aware of one's own arguments and justifications in the negotiation process; it is also important to be able to argue with equal success the views of other participants. Understanding the issues at the table and fully engaging all of the facets that apply to them help participants better understand their own position and its relationship to the other potential positions at the table. This thorough understanding of the issues at the table requires some level of objectivity and broad-based assessment. Although emotion is clearly a legitimate element of the interaction process, preparation for the negotiation should be as free of the emotional component as is possible so the individual can be available to the information and data that are influencing his or her position and informing the negotiation process.

An honest interaction and confrontation with the data informing the negotiation provide an analytical perspective that helps participants avoid surprises and minimizes unplanned circumstances that directly affect the success of the negotiation. Here again, the individual bottom line, the essential nonnegotiable below which the participant cannot go, needs to be clear and specific. This is often called the individual's best alternative to a negotiated agreement. The individual establishes this as the absolute point of reference and the essential "get" necessary to make the negotiation successful for him or her. A "bad" negotiated agreement is generally worse than no agreement at all.

Establishing a personal bottom line raises the question about what happens when other parties to the negotiation cannot reach a satisfactory agreement with you. Each negotiator must place him- or herself in the context of the other negotiators and consider what might happen if an agreement is not reached. Remember, each participant to the negotiation has a bottom line. The more fully aware of what that bottom line might be and the individual's relationship to it advances a deeper understanding of the negotiating approach and method in a way that demonstrates mutual understanding of the variety of bottom lines in the negotiation.

Finally, after a bottom line has been established and the approach to supporting it has been enumerated, time should be taken to practice the individual's approach to the interaction. Individual participants are essentially choreographing their interaction in the negotiation and stepping through all the points at issue, arguments and counterarguments, positions, and interactions that might likely be a part of the negotiation. Much like a game of chess, the steps and stages in the approach to negotiation require that participants think through as many of the moves and positions in the interaction as possible. Each participant should recognize that other participants are likely as prepared and will have also done their homework for the negotiation (Figure 13-3).

- Be fully aware of one's own position.
- Know the arguments that support and oppose the position.
- Understand all of the issues at the table.
- Study the other parties' positions and issues.
- Be clear about personal emotional hooks.
- Establish the beginning personal bottom line.
- Discern best personal approach.

Figure 13-3 Preparing for the negotiation

Establishing the Framework for the Negotiation

Although preparation for the negotiation is an important first step, also important is establishing the terms of engagement for the negotiation encounter. Preparations for the negotiation are almost as important as the negotiation itself. Because of the anxieties, the nature of confrontation, and the stresses associated with opposing points of view, it is important for the negotiation leader to establish the rules of the negotiation and the terms of the engagement. The goal here is to provide a structured and positive environment as the negotiation requires. This allows the parties to more clearly establish expectations with regard to the process and to operate within the context of fairly formal rules of dialogue. Major elements of those roles of dialogue are as follows:

- Establish rules of speaking without interruption.
- Identify each other by first names, leaving titles and roles outside the negotiating table.
- Establish agreement to the behavioral parameters, refrain from attacking, eliminate put-down behavior, and ask clearly structured questions that can advance understanding and clarity.
- Refrain from coarse, crude, profane responses or negative use of language.

- Listen with respect and sincerity, attempting to fully understand the other party's communication and generation of interests.

- Respect differences and understand that each participant is entitled to his or her own perspective.

- Let go of failures and nonsolutions generated from past interaction; focus instead on decisions made from the current negotiated point forward.

- Agree to make an intentional effort to refrain from arguing, belaboring, venting, or comments of long duration. Each participant agrees to use negotiating time in a fair and equitable manner.

- Establish and respect needs for break time and time away from the negotiation.

- Establish regular times for rest and recuperation and breaks from the negotiation as a way of supporting individual needs and maintaining sufficient energy for the long-term negotiation process.

CRITICAL THOUGHT

Confrontation often creates anxiety. It is wise for the negotiator to understand which issues create anxiety, practice with a friend or colleague in objectively making an argument, and work with them in dealing with the emotional overlay. Practice diffuses emotional intensity and strengthens presentation skills.

Much of the preliminary work in establishing the terms of engagement provides a positive environment within which a generative solution-seeking approach to negotiation can unfold. Eliminating as many of the possibilities of negative energy and negative negotiating environment helps accelerate the likelihood of a successful negotiating process.

Intensive Interaction

Interaction with others is a reflection of the understanding that each participant has of the process as well as the role of each participant in the negotiation. Assessing the characteristics of the other parties helps the individual participant characterize the approach and the conditions influencing the interaction. Much of the case can be more fully understood in preparation for the negotiation as individual participants dig deeper into understanding the case of the other participants. Each argument should be reviewed with depth and detail to develop a specific counter to the argument presented. In addition, participants want to assess the strength of others' positions in an effort to find points of convergence or emergent elements of agreement. Sorting through others' basic arguments and starting points can give participants a clue as to the other predominant positions and the other participants' bottom line. Besides assessing the argument of the negotiation, participants should be reviewing others' skill in generating the argument, capacity for negotiation, and clarity with regard to presenting facts and expectations (Figure 13-4).

- Keep in mind that negotiation is a process, not an event.
- Remember your emotional hooks.
- Keep in mind that each session builds on previous sessions.
- Recalibrate your positions after gaining more data.
- Better articulate others' real positions at the table.
- Identify emerging points of convergence/agreement.
- Discern the best personal approach.
- Keep the intensity of negotiations level and consistent.
- Take breaks after tough issues or during lull moments.

Figure 13-4 Intensive negotiation

At the same time as the participants are assessing each others' arguments, elements related to lack of specificity, weaknesses of the argument, lack of clarity, or factors with which the other participants are unaware all serve to inform other participants about a particular argument or point of view. The product of this work is to provide points of comparison with one's own argument, utilizing this information to help strengthen, clarify, or reformat a particular position. Because negotiation is generally continued over a series of sessions, previous sessions provide exposure, background, prior information, and new data that informs subsequent sessions. However, it should be noted by the participants that previous sessions may not be a strong indicator of the action and interaction of the current round of negotiation. Each negotiation session stands on its own merits and reflects only the activities that occurred within that session even though they may be an aggregate of the work of previous sessions. While subsequent sessions always build on previous sessions, each session brings forth its own dynamics and generates conclusions as a result that may not have been as easily reached in previous sessions.

Important to the ongoing negotiation process is the opportunity for individuals to note and identify points of convergence or common ground. As the negotiation sessions unfold, clarity with regard to emerging arenas of common ground are generated more readily. Early agreements on particular issues of conflict can provide the floor for subsequent clarity and agreement on more difficult issues. This process is called "**chunking**." Instead of summarily reaching a point of broad generalized agreement, the final agreement may actually be the aggregation of smaller agreements that, when looked at comprehensively, satisfy the needs of the participants (Boulle, Colatrella, & Picchioni, 2008).

If you are the leader of the negotiation process, it is important that you create a safe space where the negotiation can unfold with a sense of balance and equity. Certainly, a neutral location that is comfortable, easy to access, and as informal as the negotiation requires is an important consideration. Comfort and attention to the supporting details related to the location itself will be important. The leader provides a good sense of control and facilitating environment for the negotiation situation. The leader completely orchestrates and manages the atmosphere, space, structure, and processes associated with the negotiation. Supplying supporting materials and information, as well as paper, pens, and other items that facilitate the process, is helpful. Attention to detail means ensuring that bathroom facilities are nearby, lighting is soft yet supportive, the room temperature is appropriate, and required audiovisual supports are available. It is also important to have a clock available so that everybody is aware of the time because it is important to various elements of the negotiation process. It may also be important for the leader to ensure that there are alternative places where individuals or groups can gather to do individual work in a private and uninterrupted environment (Figure 13-5).

- The environment of negotiation is as important as the negotiation.
- Soft balanced lighting reduces emotional intensity.
- The room temperature should be neutral, between 68 and 72 degrees.
- Water should be available at each position at the table.
- There should be alternative locations for party breaks or caucuses.
- Pens, papers, and flip charts should be available for the process.
- A box of tissues should be available at each position.
- The restrooms should be noted and should be nearby.
- The space should allow for parties to mingle informally.

Figure 13-5 Supportive environment

Leaders will frequently be conducting negotiations between two or more parties and must be aware of the dynamics related to the intensity of the interaction. Leaders should be able to assess the tone and mood of the participants related to the negotiation by reading body signs, which reflect levels of stress through the notation of nonverbal signals such as gestures, facial expressions, and body movements. The leader's preparation helps the individuals both anticipate and determine the best approach for initiating the negotiation. The levels of stress, the intensity of the issue, and the relatedness of the participants all help the leader predetermine what particular approaches may be essential to breaking through the stress, creating comfort, and reducing the intensity of the initiation of interaction. Here the leader's skills in reading nonverbal signs and body language, gestures, eye movements, and facial expressions help signal which particular approaches may be necessary to initiate the dialogue and sustain it. The leader should pay attention to even small gestures and movements, such as fidgeting, wringing of hands, raised eyebrows, crossed arms, sitting back in the chair, and eye contact; these are indicators of the mood and emotional intensity of the participants.

Participants of the negotiation should realize that negotiation is both an art and a science. The structural part of negotiation reflects more of the science of negotiation—the flow, dialogue, and interaction of the participants reflects more of the character of the art of negotiation. Some dos and don'ts related to the intensity of interaction at critical points in negotiation might be as follows:

- Do listen carefully to all parties.
- Don't make lots of concessions at the earliest stages of negotiation.
- Allow plenty of room for self-maneuvering in suggesting or proposing positions.
- Don't make opening statements or offers so polarized or extreme that the position is lost.
- Emphasize conditional offers that reflect what you will give based on what someone else offers.
- Never say "never."
- Familiarize and probe participants with regard to their feelings, insights, and attitudes.
- Avoid yes or no answers to questions; instead, expand for explanation or understanding.
- Stay away from demeaning, diminishing, alienating, and angering other parties.

In a negotiation, it is important that parties remain open for options and opportunities that may arise in the process of communicating and interacting in the negotiation. Avoid making thoughtless, quick, or brash statements that polarize the negotiation or make the process of movement impossible. Make sure that proposals are broad-based, open-ended, and exploratory, allowing all parties to expand and explore options and opportunities for consensus, convergence, or common ground. Parties to negotiation want to avoid forcing other parties into a corner, narrowing their opportunities for movement and reducing the chance that further negotiation can reveal concessions or consensus that will help move the parties to solution.

Seeking clarification of other participants' points or contributions is a critical element for ensuring clarity and specificity. The leader and participants to the negotiation want as much as possible to be clear about what is actually being negotiated and where participants are in relationship to the information and elements on the table for discussion. Remaining in questioning mode helps create a context for clarification and understanding and creates an environment that supports an open negotiation process. Although not all parties to the negotiation may be positively disposed, it is important to be able to pursue factual elements embedded in all responses in order to keep the negotiation balanced.

 CRITICAL THOUGHT

The leader periodically translates for the parties, enumerating points of convergence, issues, understanding, and opportunities for agreement. This restatement provides clarity and helps participants form language that clearly states their understanding.

At times in the negotiation, the leader will recognize tactics that delay, offset, stall, or place a negotiation off course. The leader has to manage threats, insults, intimidation, bluffing, dividing, emotional intensity, and boundary testing. Awareness of the potential of these behaviors in any human interaction is critical for facilitating the negotiation process.

With each of these, the leader must be willing to undertake strategies to offset the imbalance created by negative behaviors:

- If threats occur, the parties must be reminded that negotiation cannot occur with duress and that compromise and concession can be found only if the behavior that drives the threats can be offset by sound principles of communication.

- When insults occur, diffuse them with a balanced and calm reaction and a restatement of the principles that guide the dialogue and the interaction. Allow the participants to restate their position within the appropriate context and proceed with a more constructive dialogue.

- When intimidating language is used, identify and recognize it and its impact on reducing the positive context for negotiation and the negative connotation it implies. Restate the original contribution to the dialogue and ask for clarification and response with regard to its accuracy free of emotional intensity.

SCENARIO

You have two colleagues, Nancy and Jane, who express significantly different views on delegating patient care activities to nursing assistants. Each feels strongly about her position. Nancy feels that anything where nursing assistants demonstrate competence should be delegated to them. Jane, on the other hand, feels that delegation should be selective, ensuring that particular skills should be reserved for the registered nurse. They have maintained these conflicting positions for some time now, and it is becoming an issue with regard to the appropriate delegation standard on the unit.

You are a clinical leader on the unit and currently chair the unit's Practice Council. You would like to resolve this issue the most effective way possible and have set a meeting date with Nancy and Jane to address their differences.

Discussion Questions

1. How might you prepare them for this dialogue?
2. How will you prepare yourself as leader to facilitate their interaction?
3. What key data will you need to inform the discussion at the table?
4. Who else will need to be present at the table and what will their role be?
5. What conflicts do you anticipate and how will you prepare yourself for them?

- When a party evidences obtuse, nonspecific, dubious assertions (lying, for example) that represent bluffing, the leader should restate the original position in clear terms and wait for a factual response. Use question statements to advance clarification and avoid the obfuscation or the bluff.

- When exploitation of disagreements (using disagreement for personal advantage) by a participant occurs, restate the area of disagreement for clarification and enumerate the particular positions of participants as a mechanism for obtaining clarity with regard to participant positions.

- When leading questions are used to confuse, identify weakness, or force concessions, delay answering a series of questions, break down the questions into single units, and seek specific answers to each individual question as it relates to the originating issue. Any question that is not topically specific is eliminated from the clarification.

- When emotional extremes appear in an individual's response in the form of anger and accusations, blaming and pointing fingers, reactions, and polarization, affirm the commitment to fairness, equity, and balance. Refocus the conversation on specific issues and remind the participants of the terms of engagement. If necessary, a break in the process provides an opportunity for emotions to be addressed and balance to be reestablished.

- When participants infringe the terms of engagement, clearly enumerate and restate the terms in order to reemphasize their action in the negotiation process and to remind participants of the value they play in balancing negotiation. Here again, ensure that clarity is established, language is precise, and process is followed consistently.

CRITICAL THOUGHT

The leader is fully aware of the emotional content embedded in each participant's position. The leader should anticipate the potential for emotional reactions and outbursts with a strategy that honors the legitimacy of the emotional feelings, yet places them in context with the process at the table. The leader never stifles emotions. Instead, the leader ensures their expressions are appropriate and that they do not direct the negotiation.

Leading negotiation is a challenging and sometimes difficult experience, especially when there are a wide variety of personalities that must be dealt with in the effort to maintain balance at the negotiating table. Each participant brings his or her own cultural, social, and personal behavioral set that can facilitate and sometimes constrain a positive negotiating environment. Negative behaviors will invariably arise, and sometimes negative personalities will be present. Rather than ignore or ameliorate these conditions, it is important that the leader of the negotiation be able to identify patterns of response to negative negotiation behaviors. Some examples of common behaviors and the leader's responses to them are as follows:

- The perennially unclear negotiator: It may be helpful to be more visual with regard to establishing a higher level of clarity for this kind of negotiation. Putting thoughts in writing, using visual presentation, placing submissions in a bullet point format, or restating the participant's contribution as a way of clarifying it is helpful to supporting this kind of negotiator.

- Indecisive and uncertain negotiators: Careful and structured conversations are central to affirming positions and points. Periodically restating and reviewing the elements of the dialogue help confirm clarity and position. Staying in the question and exploring specific issues with the indecisive negotiator using new wording or language helps advance clarity and facilitate movement.

- The overly aggressive negotiator: Keep the discussion fact based and free of emotional content. Make sure language is clear and intent is clarified. Reinforce the terms of engagement and eliminate the acceptability of threatening or repressive behavior at the table. During times of high emotional content, allow for expression and use breaks for opportunities to spend time with personal negative emotions and diffuse their intensity.

- The overly emotional negotiator: Recognize and accept the feelings and expressions of the negotiator. Help the negotiator translate emotions into a language that clarifies and specifies their expression. Patiently allow for emotional moments but provide a context for them to prevent them from limiting the dialogue. Allow time for emotional expression during breaks and away from the negotiating table in order to provide less emotional intensity at the table. Balance emotional feelings with factual affirmations and translation of feelings into positions (Heller & Hindle, 2008).

Bargaining Positions

Bargaining is the phase of negotiation that emphasizes the give and take related to the variety of positions at the table (Figure 13-6). Bargaining is the work of exchange. There are a number of different bargaining approaches, most of which reflect positional bargaining. Here the negotiator attempts to bargain in a way that supports his or her position as the most correct position in a number of positions at the table. Positioned bargaining has some value in that it requires the development and support of a rationale for a particular position. A stated position reflects the appropriateness and logic of the position and helps clarify and justify its validity. Imbalanced or polarized positioned bargaining can provide the baseline for the consideration of additional approaches or positions that may spin off consideration of an original fixed position.

- Bargaining involves give and take.
- Positions often shift during the bargaining phase.
- Trade-offs are suggested and made during bargaining.
- At this time the legitimate positions are determined.
- Points of convergence and agreement emerge in this phase.
- The potential for conflict and shutdown accelerates.
- The potential for movement and agreement also accelerates.
- The essential skill of the leader is to keep bargaining on track.
- Positional restatement is frequently made to validate understanding.

Figure 13-6 Bargaining elements

In open and balanced negotiation, the bargaining process initiates the serious give and take necessary to determine which legitimate positions emerge and the degree of support for any particular position or view. If bargaining is open and equitable, and a positive goal is sought for the resolution of the negotiation, bargaining can begin to reveal points of convergence, areas of common ground, or particular positions that appear more legitimate and appropriate for resolution. In an absolute winner-take-all approach to negotiation, positions can become polarizing and limiting, providing a set of absolutes from which the position holder will not deviate. If this is the case, then the true bargaining process never unfolds; instead, people are holding to their position regardless of the nature of the dialogue or the potential for a mutual solution or satisfaction. This has the potential of shutting down the negotiation or, at least, limiting its effectiveness.

In clarifying positions and contributions to the bargaining process, it is important to compare proposals, positions, and suggestions from the negotiating parties to the original positions. The leader in the negotiation will often want to restate positions in light of subsequent information or discussion in order to illuminate movement, new information, the potential for new positions, or new decisions made about original positions (Lewicki, Saunders, & Barry, 2009). The leader tries to ensure the discussion and dialogue represent foundation in fact. In the process, particular bargaining positions may be strengthened, refined, or altered, forming a new floor for further dialogue and bargaining.

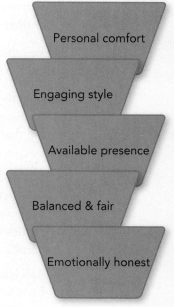

Figure 13-7 Negotiation facilitation

The most important skill of the facilitator/leader of negotiation is keeping the bargaining on track, ensuring that it does not move far afield into ever-widening issues that do not relate more specifically to the positions and issues at hand. Bargaining should be focused, detailed, and should move inexorably in a direction that suggests positive progress and some level of satisfaction from the participants. The facilitator/leader will have to keep a level head and bring all personal skills to the fore (Figure 13-7). Although positive bargaining should not necessarily reflect a win–lose scenario or positioning, the leader should be prepared to see particular positions or emergent positions accelerate in intensity and viability as more data and dialogue reveal a particular direction and more relevant choice making. Because bargaining is the predominant centerpiece of the negotiation process, the leader should ensure that good notes are taken, records are provided, and movement is recorded. As particular and seminal points of reference, decisions, or new positions emerge, so should they be documented, restated, and validated, and the general determination of support for the decision should be obtained from the parties to the negotiation (Garner & Lovering, 2004).

Because bargaining is the heart of the negotiation process, it demands the most skill and takes the most significant time commitment and attention to detail of all the phases. Here, all the skills associated with understanding dialogue, body language, language of expression, communication, styles of negotiation, and points of convergence will be very important to the leader/facilitator of the negotiation process. Like any significant skill, time and experience are the greatest moderators of competence and success. At the outset of learning the process of negotiation, novice leaders may want to associate with negotiating mentors or have such persons present in their own negotiating process in order to find support for their own negotiation learning and development.

Some critical elements of the bargaining process the negotiating leader may need to keep in mind throughout the interaction are as follows:

- Help the participants at the table separate relationship concerns and issues from the substance of the issue being negotiated. It's not that relationships and feelings are not important and shouldn't be considered; rather it is that the negotiation has a purpose and, ultimately, that purpose must be fulfilled.

- Constantly look for shared vision, issues, terms of reference, language, and goals. Remember that ultimately values define the solution, and parties to the negotiation must essentially value the solution they participated in obtaining.

- As a leader, use objective criteria, data, decisions, and progress as a basis for subsequent decision making. Decisions should be made on principles, not pressure, and reaffirming those principles is critical to the successful process of negotiation.

- Sort through the issues one at a time so that the table does not become crowded with a competing or complex array of issues and processes where the key point gets lost in the complexity.

- Avoid terms and language that are grounded in finality during the process of negotiating. As much as possible during the earlier stages of dialogue and interacting, emphasize open-ended approaches. Decisions should emerge, not be forced.

- Summarize the process to date frequently. This helps the parties remain clear about the progress, current positions, and the issues presently at hand.

- Help the participants avoid ultimatums, terminal language, and polarized positioning. Negotiation is a process, not a terminal event, and all of its elements should be used liberally.

- Take regular if not frequent breaks in a format that allows exposure of the participants to each other in an informal and friendly environment. Strengthening relationships always diminishes polarization.

CRITICAL THOUGHT

Bargaining is one of the more critical moments in the negotiation process. It is during this phase that the role of the leader/facilitator is critical to the success of the process. Participants are balancing on the edge of dissolution-resolution and need help in specifically refining understanding, potential for agreement, convergent and divergent positions, and renewed focus on real issues.

Bringing Closure to the Process and Implementing Agreement

As a process of negotiation unfolds successfully, a number of things should have occurred. New positions should be clarified and well defined, trade-offs noted, bargaining trades clearly articulated, specific consensus achieved, particular documented agreements available, and final understandings affirmed. These essential elements ensure the final stages of the negotiation process and indicate its point of closure. At this moment in the closure process, it is important for the negotiation leader to confirm the terms of the agreement and ascertain whether full understanding on the part of all of the parties has been obtained. Final form and language are important to the specificity and clarity of the agreement and must be sanctioned by all parties to the negotiation. All terms of agreement must be restated and documented in language clear enough for all parties to understand and to validate. All parties should have an opportunity to review, question, and clarify that they are satisfied before final language is created that will bring the negotiation process to closure. After agreement has been achieved, documented, and signed off by the parties, the process moves from closure to implementation. Therefore, it is important to address the following elements prior to expecting performance against the agreement:

- All of the facts of the agreement are in place. Documentation has been specific, clear, and focused, and all of the participants indicate they agree with the final documents.

- An action plan for implementing the agreements is identified by each of the participants in a way that demonstrates a consensus of understanding regarding role and action related to the agreement and commitment to implementing subsequent action.

- There exists a clear understanding between the parties of the contribution of each to the implementation of the agreement so that all parties understand the particular and specific role of the parties and the activities associated with their role in implementation.

- Particular and specific mechanisms of verifying and validating action and performance in fulfillment of the agreement are included in the action plan in a way that clearly demonstrates support of the agreement and the performance of its elements and expectations.

- Opportunities for regathering the parties to the negotiation to evaluate commitment, performance, progress, and further considerations are provided at regular intervals as a way of ensuring both progress and performance.

- A specific time line for satisfaction and completion of the work of the negotiation is clearly established as well as the persons most

SCENARIO

Building on the previous scenario in this chapter, assume that agreement has been reached and Nancy and Jane have converged to the point of resolution. As a nursing leader on the unit and chair of the Practice Council and now interested in establishing a standard for delegation, form a small team of colleagues to respond to the following questions.

Discussion Questions

1. Because you are attempting to establish a standard of delegation for practice on the unit, which critical elements about delegation are required to inform that standard?

2. Now that Nancy and Jane have agreed, who needs to be involved in the standards development process that reflects their agreement?

3. How will you obtain consensus around the standard once it is established as a protocol for practice?

4. What is the role of the Practice Council and how will the Council establish the expectations for performance with regard to the new standard on delegation?

5. What is the role of the unit manager in relationship to the established new standard for delegation?

accountable for determining performance and progress. A time line and accountability provide the definitive demarcation upon which success of the negotiation and its application and performance can be reflected.

Negotiation is a fundamental element of all human interaction. Negotiation reflects the constancy of the uniqueness and differences that each person and group brings to relationships, interactions, performance, and the satisfaction of wants and needs. The clinical leader will continuously confront situations that demand some level of negotiation and agreement. The elements of negotiation outlined in this chapter form a basic foundation upon which the skills of negotiation can be built. However, the clinical leader should be encouraged to read and study further the particulars of negotiation, especially those related to individual skills and needs as a part of the learning dynamic associated with developing and growing personal negotiation competence. Through learning, practice, and the discipline of the wisdom of time, the clinical leader can develop excellent skills and become a powerful resource in problem solving, relationship building, and effective decision making (Lewicki & Barry, 2010).

CRITICAL THOUGHT

In recent years, collective bargaining has shifted from an exclusive and more positional-based strategy to a format that represents stronger ownership of common interests and mutual advantage. Traditional, conflict-based collective bargaining often results in negative processes and long-term bargaining. Bargaining from the perspective of mutual interest establishes a stronger foundation for seeking common ground and helps to share responsibilities for problem resolution.

The Clinical Leader and the Unique Characteristics of Collective Bargaining

Collective bargaining is a formal process of negotiation defined and protected by the National Labor Relations Board (NLRB) in fulfillment of the National Labor Relations Act (NLRA) (Taft-Hartley Act) and the subsequent adaptations to health care in Public Law 93-360. These associated laws govern collective bargaining activities specifically in unionized hospitals but also have implications for supervisory roles in nonunionized environments, providing opportunities for professional workers to file unfair labor practices in any healthcare environment. The details of labor–management relationships that operate under the auspices of these various labor laws are usually found in management texts or union information resources at a level of specificity and detail beyond the scope of this clinical leadership text. It is important, however, for the clinical leader to be aware of the specific characteristics and processes associated with collective bargaining in those hospitals and healthcare settings that are unionized and have collective bargaining agreements (Carrell & Heavrin, 2009).

From the collective bargaining negotiation perspective, unionized health-care institutions operate under formally negotiated agreements between staff and management known as collective bargaining agreements. These agreements focus predominantly on salaries, benefits, and working conditions as specifically negoti-ated between employers and their employees' union. Usually these agreements are renegotiated over defined periods of time and cover a specific number of years. In addition, these negotiated union agreements clearly define the rights of manage-ment as distinct from those of employees. Historically, these agreements operate as an outflow of positional bargaining, as the collective bargaining process often demonstrates. Often this model of negotiation has resulted in contentious, polar-ized, and negative relationships between the parties. As a result, in recent years broader and more engaging collective bargaining negotiating processes have been generated in a way that facilitates and strengthens the relationship between healthcare organizations and their staff. These negotiations focus more on the principles and relationships than simply the facts or factors around which a nego-tiation is often based. These more principled approaches help the parties to the negotiation focus on mutual challenges, problems, issues, interests, values, and in finding common ground. Many of the principles of negotiation discussed in this chapter apply to the formal process of collective bargaining (Blanpain, Bamber, & Pochet, 2010).

As a clinical leader, it is important to understand the fundamentals associ-ated with leading in a unionized environment and operating within a collective bargaining agreement (Figure 13-8). If the staff seek union representation, sec-tions of the NLRA are triggered as a formal petition for representation is filed, initiating a complex series of events that lead to aggressively campaigning for signed and dated authorization cards from employees that must accompany the petition for representation within a specified time frame. During this time the employer cannot interfere or impede upon the rights of the employees to advan-tage themselves of the opportunity of collective bargaining. Although a minimum of 30 percent of employees must demonstrate interest, union members typically seek 50 to 60 percent in order to ensure the highest level of support that can be demonstrated. Subsequent to this determination of level of interest, staff members vote in a formal NLRB supervised union election. Prior to the selection, the employees, the union, and the employer all have the opportunity to engage in representing their interests with regard to their desired outcome in the forthcoming election. Through a secret ballot, nonmanagerial staff vote under the observation and supervision of the NLRB. A simple majority of votes cast determines the outcome of the vote. If the NLRB determines that the vote was valid, it supports the outcome, the union is certified, and the formal process of collective bargaining between the union and the organization is established (Carrell & Heavrin, 2012).

- Employees are represented by a union.
- All employees covered by the union agreement must abide by its requirements.
- Union members elect union representatives to negotiate on their behalf and represent their interests.
- After negotiation, a collective agreement is arrived at by employer and union.
- Union contracts set out the obligations and requirements of both the employer and the union.
- Time limits exist for the union contract after which the agreement must be renegotiated.
- Union members must pay dues to the union to which they belong.

Figure 13-8 Critical elements of collective bargaining

In the United States, petitioning for union representation and collective bargaining is essentially considered an employee right. Under the NLRA, employees are determined to have a right to self-organization and to become members of labor organizations resulting in their right to bargain collectively through representatives of their own choosing for the purpose of advancing their own mutual interests. These rights are protected by law, and both union and employer must uphold the agreed-upon contents of the formal bargaining agreement between them. As a clinical leader, the individual's bargaining environment will be subject to the agreement between the union and the employer and the leader will often be required to address its elements, represent its principles in his or her own behavior, and advance the interests of the agreement when there are potential and real conflicts between the agreement and the behavior of staff and management. It is important that the clinical leader be aware of the requirements of the collective bargaining agreement and his or her role as a staff leader in adherence to its requirements and in resolving issues and concerns related to the agreement. Some common areas of reference in the collective bargaining agreement affecting staff relationships and negotiation can sometimes relate to the following:

- Limiting the possibility of compromising any component of the collective bargaining agreement by either management or staff in a way that compromises the agreement or places people at threat in relationship to it.

- Effectively minimizing the questioning of staff with regard to their union activities or collective bargaining related activities that may constrain or coerce them in ways not permitted by the NLRA or the specific collective bargaining agreement.

- Limiting employer, management, or clinical leader suggestion of benefits or favors that are not contained within the collective bargaining agreement and have not been formally agreed to by the employer or the union.

- The clinical leader should not act as an agent of either the employer or the union in issues or content related specifically to the collective bargaining agreement in a way that would jeopardize the agreement or marginalize behavior covered by the agreement.

- Clinical leaders should avoid rumor, gossip, unsubstantiated dialogue, or inappropriate discussion regarding the employer, the union, or the collective bargaining agreement in a way that diminishes, polarizes, or in any manner subverts the agreement or the relationship between the employer and the union.

- Clinical leaders must avoid personal discussion of opinions and feelings with regard to the employer, the union, or the collective bargaining agreement in any way that is not consistent with the content of the collective bargaining agreement.

- Just as the clinical leader expresses support for the management and organizational leadership of the institution, the leader should also extend respect and support to union leadership especially as it relates to the elements of the union obligations in fulfilling the requisites of the collective bargaining agreement.

Collective bargaining creates equity in the workplace by giving workers a voice through collective action in a way they otherwise would not and serves as a counter to the equally powerful collective voice of organizational management. Generally, the desire to unionize in an organization represents the employees' sense that their collective self-interest and benefits have been challenged or there has been a failure by organizational management to directly and positively support employees. Usually, when management adheres to sound principles of professional shared governance, contemporary leadership principles and practices, and relates to professional knowledge workers as partners in the workplace, and when equity is the driving force of relationships between them, unionization is frequently deemed unnecessary. Failure to adhere to strong evidence-based principles of leadership, shared governance, empowerment, equity, and engagement creates the landscape that advances the potential for employee interest in unionization.

CRITICAL THOUGHT

Usually, when management adheres to sound principles of professional shared governance, contemporary leadership principles and practices, and relates to professional knowledge workers as partners in the workplace, and when equity is the driving force of relationships between them, unionization is frequently deemed unnecessary.

Collective Action, Collective Bargaining, and Employee Strikes

Every collective bargaining agreement has a particular tenure that ends the agreement and calls the parties back to the negotiating table to renegotiate a new contract and time line. This is generally a tenuous period of time where issuing of positions and counterpositions by the employer and the union determine the subsequent content of the collective bargaining negotiation at the bargaining table. Representatives from the union and the employer establish a process and time frame for negotiating positions, interests, and proposals representing the interests of each in pursuit of mutual agreement, which will result in a contract supported by both management and union membership.

Negotiations can operate for an extended period of time depending on the distance of the positions from each other, the intensity of the negotiations, and the number of items at issue. If much work has been done by the employer and the union ahead of time, the collective bargaining process can often be simple and straightforward. However, if difficult positions require a great deal of negotiation, dialogue, and member contribution, the negotiation process can be quite extended. If the parties can reach a satisfactory agreement and both employer and union membership certify that agreement (the union has its members vote their support), the contract is completed and signed. However, if there is dispute and disagreement and a solution cannot be satisfactorily sought at the bargaining table, the union exercises its right to strike upon vote of its members to do so. In health care, strike preparations usually involve altering the workload of management to ensure patient care is not threatened and to address the critical needs of the healthcare facility. While union member employees strike, other staff and management usually fulfill the limited obligations of patient service during the extent of the strike period. For the clinical leader, it is important to keep in touch with the human resource department information sources and directives as a guide for professional behavior, action priorities, personal roles, and approved conversations acceptable during an employee strike period (Figure 13-9).

- A strike is a mass refusal of employees to work.
- Picketing occurs to discourage employees from working or others from conducting business with the employer.
- A strike occurs in response to employee grievance or lack of agreement on a contract.
- Strikes are used to pressure employers to reach an agreement with the union.
- Accommodations to the strike regarding patient care must be made by the employer.
- Union or nonunion workers may cross strike lines to provide patient care on behalf of the employer.
- Strikes are stopped when settled by agreement by the union and employer or by court action.

Figure 13-9 Strike action

Negotiations usually continue during the strike. The pressure of the strike process and the slowdown of normal healthcare organization work and patient care activities usually create additional pressure on the employer and the union. Often emotions are high during the strike process and can create challenges for the clinical leader both inside and outside the organization. Traditional liaisons and friendships between the clinical leader and other members of the staff can frequently be challenged and stretched during emotionally intensive times, especially over the strike period. At these times, the leader must stay faithful to the principles of the contract, good leadership expression, and personal emotional balance. The clinical leader must remember that collective bargaining is an exercise of basic American rights but is also fraught with all the human emotional vagaries that intensive and complex interaction frequently entails. Patience, consistency, adherence to the letter of the law and collective bargaining agreement should positively guide the clinical leader in maintaining a balanced work environment and positive relationships with peers and managers.

Negotiating the Profession

The clinical leader should find that much of a professional relationship is a continuous and dynamic negotiation. Negotiating skills and capacity are essential foundational characteristics of the leader. Developing and enhancing negotiation skills will expand the capacity and viability of the leader in a wide variety of leadership scenarios and circumstances.

CRITICAL THOUGHT

Usually, negotiation is not just a formal process in the organization. It's a basic constituent of all human communication and incorporates values, exchange, problem solving, and seeking common ground as a fundamental relational dynamic. One cannot live in a community without refining good skills of negotiation.

Negotiation is not simply a formal process. It is an element of human communication and interaction that deals with values, exchanges, and problem solving. Critical thinking and problem-solving skills serve as a fundamental part of the negotiation process and help to discipline the process so that it yields positive results and advances the interests of those involved. Negotiation is simply disciplined communication. Furthermore, negotiation is communication that reflects purpose, value, and outcome. None of these elements take precedence over the other and all essentially work in concert to advance relationships, improve conditions, and have an impact on people and work.

For the clinical leader there are critical elements of communication and negotiation that should be constants that drive the role and relationships in all processes of interaction and engagement. Those basic elements include the following:

- The clinical leader applies translational capacity to delivering messages and communicating with others. This leader always uses language and images that can be understood and effectively repeated by the listener.

- Listening for tone and context is as important as listening for message. The clinical leader is always aware of what is going on between the lines in the message by reading other indicators (body language, gestures, movements, attitudes, facial features, etc.) that operate as corollary to the language and often represent additional matters of significance to the communication.

- The clinical leader recognizes that every individual deserves the respect to be heard and to have a voice. Sometimes the voice needs to be clarified and focused, and the clinical leader provides the tools to ensure an accurate and correct representation of the message and its meaning.

- Messaging always needs to have focus, specificity, and clarity in order to have value. The clinical leader establishes a high standard of clarity and works to provide supports necessary to help individuals and teams achieve it.

- Knowing when it's time to move the message forward is a central communication skill for the clinical leader. Often points get stuck in the morass of repetition and at a time when people are eager for clarification, agreement, and forward movement. The leader knows when the point has been made and times the movement of the message to represent its understanding, timeliness, and the need to move on.

- Keeping the discussion focused and iterative (one issue at a time) helps people to resolve problems and keep the discussion away from confusion, confabulation, obfuscation, and too much complexity. Too many issues on the table actually facilitate conflict; staging and singling out issues help sort and align them in a format that can accurately address them.

- The clinical leader needs to be aware that issues have personal meaning and are accompanied by feelings of ownership and emotional attachment. Although it is important to separate fact from emotion, it is important to support people's feelings, providing opportunities for their expression as a part of the exploration and problem-solving process.

- Solution, resolution, and achievement are all the products of good negotiation, communication, and problem solving. The clinical leader knows that there are processes and solutions for dealing with all human activity, interactions, and relationships. Patience, consideration, the discipline of good process, and the effective use of collective wisdom all act in concert to solve problems with integrity, equity, honesty, and effectiveness.

The professional knowledge worker is always dealing with the translation of knowledge into action directed toward a positive impact. This discipline guides the action of the professional and informs the strategies and interactions necessary to advance the work of the profession. Because of the intensity of the professional work, the centrality of human relationships to professional action, and the profession's social obligation to positively impact society, complex interactions and relationships must be negotiated. It is the role of the clinical leader to facilitate and coordinate these interactions and through the use of good communication and negotiation skills to refine and advance the essential interactions and intersections necessary to translate knowledge and collective wisdom into meaningful action and purposeful impact.

Leaders cannot lead without a capacity to negotiate. However, negotiation is a learned skill and a journey more than an event. Negotiation is a continuously unfolding dynamic that matures and develops as the skills of the negotiators are advanced and refined and can be directed toward meaningful purpose and a positive outcome. It is not always easy to keep the focus of negotiation and the intent of the negotiators aligned with impact and outcome. This is where the skill, discipline, and attributes of the leader and the processes associated with negotiation become critical to the efficacy and effectiveness of knowledge work and the knowledge worker. Yet, consistency and faithfulness to the principles and practices of good negotiation yield the benefits of a positive context for knowledge work. The result is sound and purposeful relationships and interactions and effective deliberation and decision making that serve the interests and values of the community.

CHAPTER TEST QUESTIONS

1. Working toward achieving universally recognized and acceptable solutions is a discipline just as much as it is a process. True or false?

2. The negotiator must always be firm and resolute with regard to his or her bottom line throughout the negotiation in order to make sure personal objectives are met. True or false?

3. There must be a willingness to be open, available, and have a wide range of potential options and considerations that can provide creative and unique ways of satisfying needs and finding common ground. True or false?

4. When gathering data for negotiation, it is important that the individual focus on his or her own position, strengthening it with evidence strong enough to counter other parties' positions. True or false?

5. Positions should be broad based and open ended in order to provide room for alternative solutions. True or false?

6. Threats and challenges always arise during a negotiation. Each negotiator must be prepared to counter these with stronger challenges to point out the evidence and veracity of one's own position. True or false?

7. When leading questions are used to confuse, identify weaknesses, or force concessions, the leader delays answering a series of questions, breaks down the questions into single units, and seeks specific answers to each individual question as it relates to the originating issue. True or false?

8. Employees seek union membership when management isn't listening to them and employees can't get what they want from the system. True or false?

9. Collective bargaining is governed by law. These laws prescribe how employees can form a union, collectively organize, negotiate, and strike. True or false?

10. Negotiation is not a leadership skill; it is instead a learned skill that anybody can apply to any situation that demands negotiation. True or false?

www For a full suite of assignments and additional learning activities, use the access code located in the front of your book to visit the exclusive website: http://go.jblearning.com/leadership. If you do not have an access code, you can obtain one at the site.

References

Blanpain, R., Bamber, G., & Pochet, P. (2010). *Regulating employment relations, work and labour laws.* Frederick, MD: Kluwer Law International.

Boulle, L., Colatrella, M. T., & Picchioni, A. P. (2008). *Mediation: Skills and techniques.* Newark, NJ: LexisNexis Matthew Bender.

Carrell, M., & Heavrin, C. (2009). *Labor relations and collective bargaining.* New York, NY: McGraw-Hill.

Carrell, M., & Heavrin, C. (2012). *Labor relations and collective bargaining: Private and public sectors.* New York, NY: Prentice Hall.

Deleuran, P., & Jarner, S. (2011). *Conflict management in the family field and in other close relationships: Mediation as a way forward.* Portland, OR: DJØF International Specialized Book Services.

Garner, S., & Lovering, M. (2004). *Conflict resolution.* Princeton, NJ: Films for the Humanities and Sciences.

Heller, R., & Hindle, T. (2008). *Essential manager's manual.* New York, NY: DK.

Lewicki, R., & Barry, B. (2010). *The essentials of negotiation.* New York, NY: McGraw-Hill.

Lewicki, R., Saunders, D., & Barry, B. (2009). *Negotiation.* New York, NY: McGraw-Hill.

Appendix A

Negotiation Skills Assessment

In order to undertake successful negotiation, the leader must have specific skills. This is a simple and basic inventory of negotiation skills. For each of the points made, select the appropriate answer. The higher your score, the greater your negotiation skills value. This assessment should be looked at as a developmental tool, not a test.

1. Almost never

2. Sometimes

3. Often

4. Regularly

I collect relevant data in preparation for a negotiation.

1	2	3	4

I understand my own position in the negotiation.

1	2	3	4

I understand and use an appropriate range of negotiation strategies.

1	2	3	4

I recognize that all parties must take something of value from the negotiation.

1	2	3	4

I remain positive and persistent in the negotiation process.

1	2	3	4

I am determined to reach a mutually satisfying agreement.

I find I consistently negotiate win–win situations.

1	2	3	4

I work to understand the other parties' positions.

1	2	3	4

I am able to state my position in clear and precise language.

1	2	3	4

I know what my bottom line is, and I negotiate to support it.

1	2	3	4

My body language is consistent with my meaning and message.

1	2	3	4

I recognize opportunities for compromise and consensus when I see them.

1	2	3	4

I respect and honor all differences and seek to learn from them.

Scoring:

1–13   Need more learning/skills

14–27   Learning and growing

28–40   Building skills well

41–52   Growing into a negotiator

IF WE WANT UNITY, WE MUST ALL BE UNIFIERS. IF WE WANT ACCOUNTABILITY, EACH OF US MUST BE ACCOUNTABLE FOR EVERYTHING WE DO. —CHRISTINE GREGOIRE

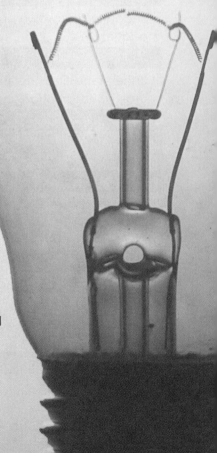

CHAPTER OBJECTIVES

Upon completion of this chapter, the reader will be able to do the following:

» Understand basic elements and characteristics of professional accountability.

» Define the unique characteristics of an obligation of ownership and its relationship to accountability.

» Delineate team and interdisciplinary characteristics of accountability and the need for discipline-specific clarity in directing purposeful teamwork.

» Outline the unique characteristics of professional accountability and its role in fulfilling a profession's social mandate.

» List at least five elements of the role and relationship of accountability and undertaking risk in clinical practice.

» State essential relationship between performance and accountability and impact of the leadership role in the clinical service environment.

Accountability and Ownership: The Centerpiece of Professional Practice

All professions are grounded in principles of accountability (Tilley, 2008). Professions have a social obligation to the society that empowers them. That accountability is invested in the profession as a whole and envisioned in the individual practices of each member of the profession. This obligation for social accountability represents the social contract between the society that licenses the professional and the persons who act in the best interests of the society that empowers them. This social contract forms the centerpiece of the profession's role in society and sets the framework for the role and performance obligation of the profession and each of its members within the context of the social contract.

Each individual brings to her or his role a specific accountability representing the full commitment of the characteristics, skills, competencies, and capacities to contribute to and advance the interests of the society the profession serves. Vital to undertaking professional work is a precise and clear understanding of the nature of the profession, its accountability for performance, the contribution that it makes in fulfilling its work, and its relationship between its members and with its members together with the people it serves.

CRITICAL THOUGHT

Perhaps one of the most challenging elements of accountability is the lack of clarity with regard to what it means in the context of work. Furthermore, there are many challenges with regard to how it is evidenced in the work of the team and how it influences the outcomes of work. There is no other concept in work that is used as much as accountability yet is so little understood.

Accountability most simply reflects the achievement of sustainable outcomes. Responsibility, on the other hand, is the effective performance of actions in the exercise of doing work. One (accountability) is about the achievement of results and the other (responsibility) is about the quality of the work effort. Once can be responsible without being accountable. In fact, responsibility without accountability is one of the work crises of the current age. Many people do good work and work very hard on processes or activities that have a questionable relationship to the achievement of sustainable outcomes.

Because of the traditional business fixation on process and action, short-term and interactive products are evaluated as signs of performance effectiveness and progress. However, sustainable results can be achieved only over much longer periods of time. To achieve them means to better tie the actions of work to their products. Good research relates to creating a very tight goodness of fit between the effort of work and its results. Effectiveness is best indicated by the directness of the work effort to the expectations for results and the actual results. The better the relationship, the more sustainable the outcome and the more valuable the relationship between the two. It is this set of circumstances that creates the ideal work relationship in that it directly connects responsibility and accountability.

To achieve this direct connection between responsibility and accountability requires a clear understanding of the elements of accountability and the expectations for performance of each of the parties. Without it, there exists no foundation for defining or delivering accountability.

There has been extensive debate with regard to whether the structural, functional, and behavioral characteristics of nursing and nurses truly represent the character of professional practice (Moanojovich, 2005). On the face of it, many of the elements that characterize professional practice are present in nursing—a foundation in a specific body of knowledge, a disciplined educational pathway, a rigorous code of ethics, clearly articulated standards of practice, and the licensing body that ensures the appropriate rigors of regulation. If these were the only arbiters of the character and content of a profession, nursing would meet those conditions. However, much of the debate with regard to the professional character of nursing relates to the predominant level of minimum education of the majority of its practitioners, its dependency role in relationship to other disciplines, its lack of clarity with regard to its specific contribution to the health of society, and an ongoing lack of a disciplined professional self evidenced by the many other broad constituencies that claim to represent nursing's interests. In addition, nursing demonstrates a continual lack of political clout, locus of power, policy influence, and presence at the decision-making tables where health policy is set, strategic decisions are made, and health resources are allocated.

Many in health leadership would assume that lacking a place at the table would be a problem in key roles related to policy, politics, strategy, and decisional power, is a clear indicator of the limited role that nursing plays in critical health decision making, and prescribes the limited independent parameters that the nursing role represents in the broader social landscape. This subordinating social condition and lack of primary ascendancy of role on the broader societal stage serve to indicate to some that nursing is a subsequent or dependent work group that fails to meet critical indices of truly professional behavior.

This challenge seems generally to be supported by the evidence. In comparison to the fact that nursing is the single largest professional healthcare body in the nation, its representation in those forums that set direction and make decisions for the healthcare system fails to proportionately represent nursing as a key player at the healthcare decision table nationally, regionally, locally, and in health organizations. While this level of representation is undergoing significant change currently, it has presented the clearest testament of nursing's historic lack of place, position, power, and role in societal decision making related to health policy, strategy, resource allocation, and provider roles (Jameson, 2009).

CRITICAL THOUGHT

Expectations are the foundation for performance. Every worker has the right to know what is expected and what skills are necessary to meet those expectations; otherwise, the worker should not be in the role.

The Professionalization of Nursing in the 20th Century: The Path to Accountability

Nursing's journey to professional equity has been long and somewhat torturous. The history of the maturation of the nursing profession closely matches the tenure and circumstances of the journey of women to social and political equity (Buhler-Wilkerson, 2001; Goodnow, 1938; Hein, 2001; Lagemann & Rockefeller Archive Center, 1983). Much of the character, content, and role of the nurse mirrors the unfolding of the role of women over the centuries. Women's long foundation in subsequent, subordinating, passive, and secondary roles in a historically paternalistic equation serves as the contextual framework for the same subsequent, subordinating, passive, and secondary roles of nursing. Finding legitimacy, obtaining a voice, establishing theoretical and practice foundations, building a legitimate body of knowledge, and claiming "space" for the value and roles of nursing practice in health care has characterized the long and arduous journey to establish legitimacy, value, impact, and equity for the professional practice of nursing (Group & Roberts, 2001). A number of historical texts detail the account of this journey and serve to exemplify and to validate the content and character of this long process (Bonvillain, 2007).

CRITICAL THOUGHT

Accountability for excellence rests with those who do the work!

The whole of the 20th century has served to provide a concentrated representation of the formalization and structuring of the profession of nursing. Nursing is clearly one of the oldest practices in history, yet it is one of history's youngest professions. It is only since the time of Florence Nightingale that nursing as a profession and practice has been codified and formalized in a manner that disciplines its framework and content, grounding it in science, evidence, precedence, standards, and ethics (Dossey, 2005; Fitzpatrick & Whall, 2005; McDonald, 2010).

Much of the social characteristics of the masculine professions at the time (law, medicine, architecture, engineering, etc.) served as the exemplar nurses used to translate and morph within the parameters of the emerging nursing discipline (Cope, 1958). Because nearly 100 percent of nurses were women, many contemporary feminine modifications and adaptations were created to accommodate contemporary reality, which served to set the limits of the portability to

SCENARIO

Florence Nightingale was the original accountability-based nurse leader. In her time she confronted many of the vagaries of transformation and change as society moved out of the Victorian age into the industrial age. She confronted many challenges related to beliefs, social attitudes, gender, science and technology, women's roles, and a host of other cultural and contextual barriers.

In our time many new challenges have arisen to create a landscape for transformation and change. In small groups of four or five colleagues, discuss the parallels between the change confrontations in the time of Florence Nightingale and the challenges of contemporary change. Focus your discussion on the similarities that Florence Nightingale confronted on the cusp of a new age with those that you as leaders will confront on the cusp of this new sociotechnical age. Enumerate how she addressed those challenges and how her example may serve as an exemplar for confronting leadership challenges in the contemporary age.

the nursing role, position, authority, and power structure (Pollard, 1911). Much of the regimented, formalized, hierarchical, militaristic, and religious overlay to the structuring of the nursing profession strongly reflected the social requisite requiring the establishment of limited parameters and containment of the nursing function within prevailing perceptions of appropriateness for women (Group & Roberts, 2001). Clearly, over the contemporary history of nursing, this emerging equity during the latter half of the 20th century changes the parameters and patterns of nursing roles and relationships from regulation to practice and clearly exemplifies the corollary changing roles and characteristics of women in contemporary society. As equity has become more apparent in women's role expectations, education, opportunities, performance factors, pay, and position in society, these changes have also been reflected in the nurse's role (Cowen & Moorhead, 2011).

As a result, the contemporary nurse is a reflection of this journey to equity of women in society and serves also as a clear example of the impact of this change on nursing role and function. Today there are a large number of graduate-educated nurses at the masters and PhD level, researchers and practice leaders, and advanced practitioners who now practice both independently and interdependently to provide clearly value-based health services to specific populations (Cowen & Moorhead, 2011). While the noise of the products of equity have not yet subsided, their relevance and value can no longer be legitimately argued. The road to professional clarity and social equity has, however, not yet ended. While much has been done and the foundations of the profession have been established beyond question, many of the historic insights, notions, and attitudes with regard to the role and its legitimacy and equity are still subject to question. These will continue to require concerted action on the part of nursing professionals and their partners in asserting the legitimacy, value, and contribution of nursing to advancing social health. It is because of this arrival that the appointed equity and the obligations and demands of equity-based accountability become important cornerstones of the role of the profession and are now the requisites of the behavior and practices of every professional.

CRITICAL THOUGHT

Much of the history of nursing parallels the history of the women's movement. Much of the experiences that nurses have in the workplace reflect the same experiences that women share in a wide variety of work settings. The challenges associated with achieving equity in nursing match those same challenges in seeing equity for women in our larger society and many of the requisites to do so are precisely the same.

Maturing the Profession: The Age of Accountability

For professionals, responsibility is not the definitive foundation for work—accountability is. Historically, the nurse as worker was judged to be acceptable if this worker simply did what he or she was supposed to do and was told to do and what was characteristic of the function. For this employed worker to be evaluated as competent, the individual needed only to focus on the work and do it well. This focus on the function of work and how well it was done forms the foundation for demonstrating the exercise of effective responsibility (Oliver, 2004). One can be responsible without being accountable; they are fundamentally different concepts. Responsibility is embedded in the work, its processes, how well they were done, and how effectively they were completed. This focus on responsibility represents and characterizes the individual's performance as a reflection of process, action, task, function, and job. Responsibility sees the individual from the perspective of the work and values that individual as a reflection of what work was done and how well it was completed. This focus on responsibility creates a task frame—a job orientation. In fact, it describes job-driven work and creates the conditions that enumerate the characteristics of jobs and job categorization of work. This can be evidenced quite clearly in most historic workplaces in a number of different ways. Notably, job descriptions are often laundry lists of functions and activities ascribed to a role. These functions and activities zero in on the elements of work rather than the results that demonstrate the impact of work. In addition, performance evaluations review the worker within the context of the capacity to function and the ability of the individual to do or perform the work. The responsible person's behavior and ability to do the work, get the job done, and get along with others who are also doing their jobs are all included in the list of functional competencies that represent responsible behavior reflecting how well a person does the work, how much of that work gets done, and how effective the person is in doing that work. This evaluation of work tends to concentrate on the quality of the work processes, the character of the effort, and the content of the functions of work, and less on the value of the work, the meaning of the work, and the impact the work had on making a difference; these are not the characteristics of responsibility. What has resulted in this focus has been a slavish attachment to process and function and the heavy creation of job orientation. Even as the nursing profession is fundamentally driven by value and meaning, much of the character of the profession's work is delineated in job functionalism, process, activity, and task performance. It is not unusual to hear a nursing professional speaking of his or her work essentially as a job, a laundry list of tasks, functions, actions, processes, and effort. As a result, a stronger *employee work group syndrome* operates to frame the work of nursing as perceived from the position of *job*. The job characterization of the work of the nurse leads to an entirely different assumption than can be obtained through the lens of professional practice and behavior. Nurses can do jobs responsibly, but they cannot act accountably and operate only within the frame of job performance. Regardless of how much activity is identified as professional in most job categories, one thing we can be assured of is that

CRITICAL THOUGHT

The primary focus of accountability is on the achievement of results and the effect of those results over the long term. Sustainable organizations do not simply look at the next increment of time with regard to sustainability. Instead, they establish a long-term vision and tie their work processes to all of the efforts necessary to achieve it. Ultimately, individuals and teams must define their accountabilities as a reflection of this long-term viability. This focus on accountability instead of process responsibility calls for rethinking of a unilateral focus on job elements and processes.

every profession should be able to demonstrate professional behavior and create a frame of reference within which particular work activities can be characterized. In short, if the nurse wishes or seeks to be treated as a professional, he or she must be able to demonstrate behaviors consistent with professional delineations.

Accountability and Ownership

There can be no accountability without ownership. Accountability assumes some level of intensity of the individual and any investment and ownership of the role, tasks, and activities as they represent the characteristics and demands of the profession (Malloch & Porter-O'Grady, 2009a). In the professions, preparation for work occurs in the academic setting and incorporates prerequisites, examinations, regulation, and often licensure as a prerequisite for entry into the profession (Gebbie, Rosenstock, & Hernandez, L. M. (Eds.). 2003).

CRITICAL THOUGHT

Ownership is commitment to the following:

- Fully applying one's own skills
- Growing and learning to enhance talents
- Development of others
- Evaluating effectiveness of contribution
- Continual lifelong learning

Professions are knowledge dependent. Professional knowledge workers operate in the workplace with the assumption that they have been adequately prepared in the principles and practices of the profession sufficient to generate trust in their efforts and to ensure competence in the application of their work. Membership in the profession is a requisite to role performance at work. However, in many organizations the notion of membership as a part of the script and relationship between the organization and the professional worker is not fully or adequately addressed. In fact, participation in job categorization overcomes delineation of membership in the profession. As a result, the relationship between the individual and the workplace unfolds through the lens of job categorization. As a result, the job becomes the contextual framework for the relationship between the individual and the workplace, subsequently establishing job parameters that get clearly reflected in functionalism, task focus, process orientation, action over reflection, and measures of productivity embedded in action (Werhane, 2007).

Ultimately, the professional worker becomes divorced from the drivers embedded in professional membership and, instead, becomes more strongly attached to job requisites and the action and functionally based drivers embedded in job performance. For the leader, it must be clear that creating a job context for work cannot produce professional outcomes. When the job predominates, the obligations of professional membership and its accountability dissipate, and the expectations for performance at that level simply never come to fruition.

This calls the leader to be able to revise and recalibrate the role of the relationship of the professional worker to the organization. This calls leadership to create an organizational context that doesn't impede membership and ownership of the work (as job categorization of the work does); instead, the structural context for professional work becomes a framework within which work expectations unfold. In order for that to happen, the following circumstances and conditions need to be present in the role of the leader and the structure of the organization:

- Professional ownership implies that the ownership of the work belongs to the profession, not to the workplace. The relationship of the workplace to the profession is one of partnership, not dependency, creating a strong framework for horizontal rather than vertical interaction.

- Contemporary research on the orientation of the professional/ knowledge worker suggests that traditional incentives often seen in employee-driven models do not succeed to motivate the action of this worker. In fact, the use of these traditional incentives actually impedes or diminishes the commitment and motivation of the professional/ knowledge worker to the work and the workplace.

- Clear indicators of performance expectation and deliverables must be a part of the professional role charter or contract at the outset and in a way that clarifies the expectation of professional membership, specifics regarding obligations of ownership, peer-based expectations, and an agreement to participate fully in the life of the profession in the workplace.

- Employee work group models, job descriptions, job performance, job measures, job satisfaction, job orientation—indeed all job categorizations—must be separated from the delineations that identify professional characteristics, roles, expectations, and performance factors if professional behaviors are ever to be exemplified as normative factors in the workplace.

- Leaders must on-board new professionals through the use of well-identified professional processes, such as granting privileges instead of hiring, peer-based selection of incoming members instead of management hiring practices, credentialing processes, clinical/career advancement mechanisms, and continuous professional development as foundational to the onboarding process.

- As with most professional bodies, the development of terms of behavior, operating rules and regulations for professional members, professional bylaws, and professional decision-making councils should become the framework within which the discipline makes decisions about its character, content, ethics, contribution, and mechanisms for advancing the interests of the organization and its users.

- Normative shared leadership practices and professional shared governance structures create the behavioral and operating frame of reference for the professions and establish a milieu where both the organization and the profession work collaboratively, collaterally, and seamlessly to advance the health interests of the community and the particular health needs of people.

The critical element of understanding and value in creating effectiveness for the profession of nursing in the healthcare workplace is the recognition that professional outcomes cannot be advanced, demanded, strategized, or expected in the presence of an employee work group organizational structure and operational arrangement. It is simply impossible to obtain professional behaviors when the prevailing infrastructure of the organization is designed to achieve job behaviors. Congruence between professional structure and professional ownership is an essential correlate to sustaining professional behaviors (Figure 14-1). In the absence of a structure that operates in a way that reflects commitment to professional membership, ownership, and partnership, expecting performance that reflects that commitment becomes an effort in futility.

At the same time, the individual professional must come into the professional organization with a clear understanding of the obligations of membership in the professional community and ownership of the profession's work. A strong part of the preparation of the professional is deepening his or her understanding of the terms of membership in the profession and the obligations that membership incurs. Often, new members of the nursing profession share an equal burden of responsibility for job categorization, fixed, finite, and functional work patterns, and an addiction to the safety of ritual and routine. If individuals have an attachment to these patterns of behaviors, they should not become members of a

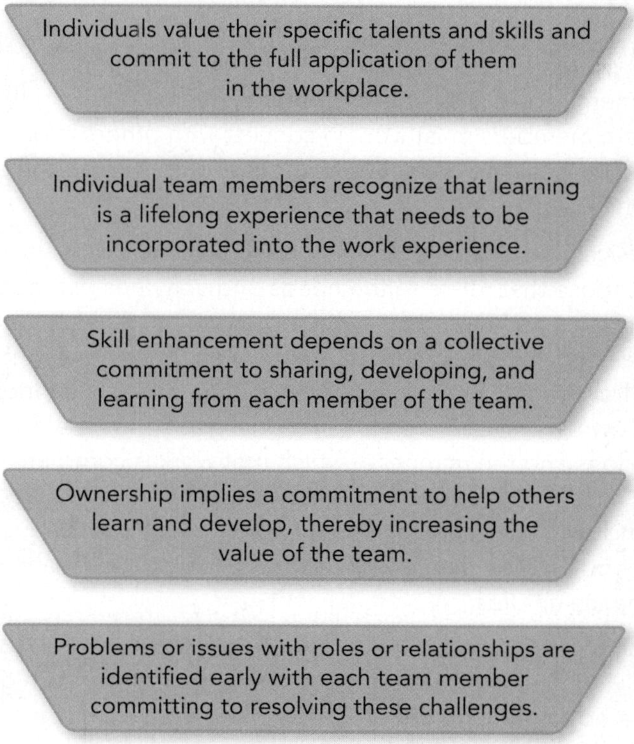

Individuals value their specific talents and skills and commit to the full application of them in the workplace.

Individual team members recognize that learning is a lifelong experience that needs to be incorporated into the work experience.

Skill enhancement depends on a collective commitment to sharing, developing, and learning from each member of the team.

Ownership implies a commitment to help others learn and develop, thereby increasing the value of the team.

Problems or issues with roles or relationships are identified early with each team member committing to resolving these challenges.

Figure 14-1 The critical elements of ownership

profession. Professional membership is a significant obligation, a demand for full engagement, ownership, and investment in the life of the profession. Playing roles that advance the ethics, standards, evidence, and best practices of a profession are equally, if not more, important to the profession and the quality of patient care than is the functional action of the nurse. Frequently nurses can be heard saying, "I'm too busy with my patients" to participate in deliberations and decisions about standards of care, protocols, evidentiary dynamics, and best practices. One is simply left to wonder, if the nurse is too busy to participate in those things that define the foundations of his or her practice to inform its action, what is the source of that busyness and how legitimately does it represent best practices and the state of the art and science of nursing? For the professional nurse, accountability and ownership are not options.

CRITICAL THOUGHT

Every team member has a specific accountability for achieving the team's goals. All team members must work in concert with others in order to ensure that individual and collective effort is contributing to the achievement of team goals.

There are basically two kinds of team goals to which individuals contribute. First are those that relate to the needs and activities of the team that fulfill the purposes and direction of the organization of which the team is a part. These goals and objectives are the work priorities of teams and provide the framework within which team action unfolds. Secondly, the team has its own specific service or functional goals that relate to the work that it does and the manner in which that work is completed. Here the team focuses on the application of standards, protocols, processes, pathways, and plans. These goals identify the frame for individual and team action and provide the context within which individual and collective performance unfolds.

Team members recognize that if effectiveness is to be achieved, the effort of individual team members must converge around team goals. All activities related to the function of the team should coalesce in a way that advances performance against the anticipated goal achievement. It is in failing to recognize this fundamental reality for all teams that infrastructure and relationship begin to break down. When any one member's performance operates out of concert with the team, the integrity of the team begins to disintegrate. It is important for team members to recognize that although individual work is unique and important, it must ultimately advance the team's work effort as well as fulfill the organization purposes for that work. Good teams assess the relationship between the work of individuals and the collective work of the team and its effect on achieving outcomes.

The Cycle of Personal Accountability

At a very personal level, the individual professional must draw specific conclusions and certain references to his or her personal ownership of membership in the profession, contribution to its work, and fulfilling the obligations of the social trust that membership in the profession implies. This means that at a very personal level the individual understands the nature of the relationship of the person to the profession.

One of the unique characteristics of a professional, as mentioned previously in this text, is the recognition of the intensity of the fit between the person as individual and the person as professional. In the professions, these unique elements converge to create in the person the unity between professional identity and personal identity. This means that the individual must continually reflect on the value of that connection, how that connection gets best represented in the life and action of the person, and what that convergence between person and professional means in terms of sense of self, values, self-expression, and the broader role of the person in society.

This personal deliberation on accountability is a fundamental part of role identification with a profession. There are several functional characteristics that this represents, which calls the professional and personal level to assess who and where the individual is in relationship to his or her profession and how that gets expressed as a part of personal commitment.

CRITICAL THOUGHT

In the professions, the identity of the person and the professional are one. The work (practice) of a professional is not a separate part of his or her life. The practice and the person are so linked that they are one and the same thing.

Some of the issues and elements that relate to this self-assessment are as follows:

- Action is driven by principle. The question for the professional relates to whether action and principle in personal expression are coherent and consistently linked in such a way that the expression of the work of the discipline represents the principles that drive it.

- Personal action is informed by commitment to learning and knowing. The professional seeks to ensure that clinical action is informed by knowledge and evidence that the choices made by the most rational and best fit with the needs to which they are directed. In so doing, the professional affirms personal commitment to continuous learning, growing, and adapting as a part of ensuring that practices are meaningful and relevant.

- In the interests of reflective practice, there is a level of personal self-reflection that the professional undertakes as a part of his or her personal assessment evidencing a goodness of fit among values, decisions, actions, and outcomes. This personal reflection attempts to more deeply assess the intensity and effectiveness of the personal work of the professional and the difference that work makes in the lives this person touches.

- The accountable professional is able to identify incongruence, brokenness, or inadequacies and make effective judgments with regard to changing his or her role and practice to become more effective. This corrective and adaptive capacity provides for the individual professional opportunity to be flexible, innovative, and better align work with the evidence that both justifies and validates it.

- In the interests of personal ownership of the profession, the individual recognizes his or her role in relationship to other members and works to join with them in the effort to advance and improve the profession and its work. The individual professional recognizes that the profession is not an objective entity but rather the collective wisdom of each member that comprises it. The profession can do nothing for the individual if the individual is not acting on behalf of the profession. The profession has no life except that of the collective energies of the members that comprise it. It can do nothing without the concerted action of its individual members. Members move a profession; a profession cannot move its members without their engagement.

Accountability in Action

There are critical elements of ownership that should be evidenced in the practice of each professional nurse. As with all professions, this ownership comes with membership as a part of the set of individual obligations that each nurse must bring to his or her practice. These are demonstrated in a way that can best exemplify the contribution the nurse makes to the profession, to the organization, and to the patients. Critical elements of professional ownership include the following:

- The individual nurse values his or her specific gifts, talents, and skills and agrees to commit to the full application of them in undertaking the work of the profession in a way that positively impacts the patient's experience.

- The individual professional member of the staff recognizes that his or her competence depends on continuous and dynamic lifelong learning and practice that is a fundamental commitment of membership and is evidenced by continuous advancement of his or her learning experience.

- Competency and skill enhancement depends on the individual's commitment to membership and contribution to the collective activity of deliberating, sharing, developing, learning, and deciding on standards and protocols of practice that are required as a part of a collegial agreement.

- Individual ownership implies the commitment to engage with others in their learning and development and in mentoring and sharing in the learning process in a way that evidences and advances the value of the profession's work and its impact on the patient's health experience.

- Each individual professional member recognizes and understands the inherent challenges and issues in professional relationships and collegial action. This individual acknowledges and accepts the obligation to fully engage those differences and deliberate common ground with others in a way that demonstrates the profession's capacity to problem solve in concert.

Each individual member of the professional community recognizes that he or she has an inherent obligation to make a contribution to that community in a way that benefits both the individual and the community (Porter-O'Grady, 2004). The life of the individual professional cannot be advanced or improved if the life of the discipline isn't addressed as a whole. Team performance is simply the aggregation and synthesis of individual performance. The success of the performance is a reflection on the agreement and understanding regarding the principles and standards of practice and the common action that represents the consensus of professional members. In complex responsive processes, there exists a deep understanding of the goodness of fit between the action of each individual of the profession and the collective impact the profession has in making a collective difference in the lives of those they serve. The more unilateral and nonaligned the action of the individual is, the less significance or value the impact has on advancing the work of the profession. On the other hand, the more aligned, collaborative, and integrated the actions of individual members are, the more impact these actions have on the profession and the more likely the profession can sustain its promise of quality and effectiveness.

REFLECTIVE QUESTIONS

- Does the work I do relate well to the purposes of the team?
- Do my work efforts integrate well with the efforts of others on the team?
- Am I clear on the essential value of each of the elements of my work?
- Do the efforts of all team members link and integrate well around expectation?
- Do I reassess my functions and activities regularly to determine their relevance?
- Do I join with the team in evaluating effectiveness of work effort?
- Is there clear evidence that my work and the outcomes directly relate well?
- Am I willing to adjust my work activity when a change is clearly indicated?
- Do I actively problem solve with team members to resolve critical issues?
- Am I flexible in adjusting my work activities when the team needs to change?
- Do I join actively with team members in identifying specific work changes?
- Do I initiate discussions and dialogue when problems in work processes emerge?
- Is there a willingness on the part of all team members to confront each other?
- Do I join with the team in celebrating successes and accomplishments?

Individual Role Accountability and Team Performance

Clearly identifying the elements and characteristics of the individual professional's role is a critical first step in relating it to the collective work of the profession. Each individual professional member must know the unique contribution he or she makes as a member of the profession and recognize with clarity that individual contribution has a direct impact on team effectiveness. Teams are effective to the extent that their members coalesce their unique and individual contributions around a common aggregated contribution that cannot be achieved without the synthesis that emerges between each member's efforts (Stacey, 2009). Before team effectiveness can be delineated, the basic foundations of individual contribution and the unique character of that contribution as it integrates with team effort is critical to ensuring a lasting positive impact.

CRITICAL THOUGHT

Focusing on team goals includes the following:

- Incorporating team goals and individual work
- Defining the fit between individual and team
- Clarifying organizational work expectations
- Identifying team performance factors
- Specifying individual needs related to work
- Supporting each other in the collective work
- Removing impediments to team effectiveness
- Ending incongruent individual performance
- Evaluating progress regularly and often

There are several elements of individual accountability that affect the collective or team effort of any discipline. Each individual professional member must realize that one of the primary arenas of accountability is the extent to which he or she owes the professional colleagues on the team. Here again, the individual member of the team contributes to the team to the extent of his or her unique gifts and role. Each of the critical elements of ownership previously identified has a specific and direct impact on the life of the team, its viability, and, ultimately, its clinical outcomes. Some of those relationships can be best described as follows:

- Individual member skills, when connected to the unique skill set of every other member, create the frame for the collective team contribution. It is the aggregate of the individual skills when synthesized collectively that evidences the value of the work of the clinical team. The diversity of contribution and the clarity regarding the unique character of that contribution are critical to ascertaining the value of the team and the impact of its collective efforts.

- Teams can't be constructed simply because people want to meet or work together. Teams are purposeful. Therefore, the construction of the team is a critical first step in team performance. There must be a goodness of fit between members of the team and the work of the team. This goodness of fit is not an accidental achievement. The leader must do intentional work in assessing the unique and specific characteristics of team members to ensure that their fit coalesces across the team to make the contribution to which the team is directed.

- Accountable teams are relational bodies. Members must be able to act synergistically with each other, reflecting an agreement with regard to their contribution and the activities of their collective effort. In short, they must be able to work well together. This relationship competence and integrity of team members is a critical element of team effectiveness and should be considered a fundamental part of the work.

- Individual and collective accountability calls both the person and the team to understand that the relationships in the team and the functions of the team demand a continuous openness and availability to learning. Therefore, learning is embedded in the individual and collective action of the team as the team continues to unfold its work, and in doing so discover new facets, insights, and approaches refining that work that makes a difference.

- Purpose-driven teams are formulated as a primary mechanism for fulfilling that purpose. Teams do not exist just to exist. Leaders must therefore assume that a constant reference back to purpose, meaning, and goals serves as a critical reminder to the team of its reason for being and the driver for its work. Achieving outcomes means fulfilling purpose and staying focused on this connection. This is critical to the sustainable effectiveness of the team.

Individual accountability is represented in the person's commitment to the team effort that represents the profession's collective obligation to have an impact on the health of those served and to make a difference through that collective effort. It is important, however, for each individual professional to remember that the team cannot be effective if the questions of individual accountability and ownership are not addressed and resolved by each member as a part of understanding his or her contribution to the efforts of the team. In fact, accountability is the centerpiece of every meaningful professional action.

Delineating Professional Work and Accountability

Historically, job descriptions have been used as a vehicle for delineating role functions, tasks, and activities of the nurse (Zedeck & American Psychological Association, 2011). Organizations have historically placed a great deal of stock in these job descriptions as a justifiable and legitimate framework for defining functional performance expectations. The problem with this approach is that the dynamic nature of professional work, the significant dependence on individual relationships and critical judgments, and the highly variable nature of the user professional service seriously belie the validity and value of work defined as a fixed, finite, functional, and incremental set of activities (Malloch & Porter-O'Grady, 2009b). The only product of this framework or approach to defining work is a continual fixed notion that results in static ritual and routine. In fact, standardized, static, ritual, and routine mechanisms become the product of these environments. Job descriptions simply codify this pattern of behaviors and create an incorrect notion that work elements for the professional can be codified and fixed in a set of activities that are essentially nonvariable and rarely change. Of course, this is simply not true.

For the professional to be effective, professional performance must be tied to role (Figure 14-2). This is a reflection of the relationship between action and outcome moderated by the needs of the user in an interaction that reflects a dynamic mosaic that is fluid, flexible, focused, portable, and mobile. The professional must be intuitive, incisive, responsive, and adaptive in relationship to the needs of the patient. Although standards form the floor of practice and the ground of good judgment, they do not fully encompass the judgment and adaptability necessary to accommodate the specific and unique needs of each person served. Principles, standards, and practices must be adapted and adjusted to reflect the very real and powerful influences of the user's resources, experience, behaviors, culture, and responsive capacity. Established and fixed functional delineations of this work simply do not adequately address nor do they appropriately codify personal demand in a way that legitimately meets patient needs. The more the role is embedded in ritual and routine and fixed practice, the less capability the individual has for rendering the kind of critical judgment necessary to be appropriately adaptive and responsive in a way that advances quality and outcome and adequately addresses the unique needs of the user. Without embedding this reality into practice, any vehicles or measures of quality, impact, and outcome suffer from diminishing returns and ultimately cease to sustain. Describing and codifying the role of the professional requires a different configuration than job descriptions can provide.

This does not, however, abrogate the responsibility of the professions to codify and frame practice in a way that can be effectively delineated and delivered with excellence, demonstrating positive impact. Evidence-based practice and the evidentiary dynamics that are reflected call for the professions to establish a true cause-and-effect relationship between the principles of practice and their application. This evidence-based approach to defining practice changes practice delineations in a way that requires real-time, just-in-time, and readily accessible

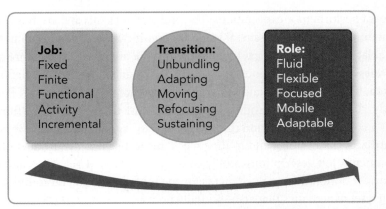

Figure 14-2 From job descriptions to accountability

information resources that serve to inform practice in-process in a way that can create the conditions to alter, adjust, or change practice in a way that demonstrates congruence with the evidence (Figure 14-3).

- The ability to generate the right information
- The quality of the information gathered
- The willingness and ability to share the right information
- The technology and hardware supporting the use of information
- The accuracy with which the information is translated
- The applicability of the information to the work
- The competence of the worker in using information
- The ability to evaluate the effectiveness of information

Figure 14-3 Information factors affecting accountable performance

This new demand for asserting the foundations of practice reflects how professional roles and functions must now adjust to the use of more high-tech tools and approaches to defining, delivering, and evaluating care in-process. Because of the just-in-time nature of digitally related clinical delivery and of user-driven service structures, professional work must be fluid and flexible and demonstrate responsiveness to the evidence in a way that indicates how and when it needs to change. Role descriptions, performance charters, and professional accountability call the individual to be accountable for reflecting transitioning and higher standards of practice as they are applied, using digital tools of practice and documentation. Clinicians have no choice but to become adaptable in configuring practice to the emerging evidence for changing it, effective use of the technical tools that provide momentary data informing practice, make immediate changes within the process of practice, and demonstrate a highly refined willingness to own the outcomes of practice rather than simply manage the tools of practice. The tools of practice—technology hardware, data, information, evidence, and past practice—continuously change and shift clinical work in a high-level sociotechnical clinical environment. Rigorously defining and codifying these tools does nothing to advance the meaning and work of the profession (Figure 14-4). However, molding and shaping these highly adaptive work sets to better match user need and demand are the work of the professional and require defining and advancing an adaptive and predictive capacity and establishing role protocols that state the requisite for these skill sets rather than provide a laundry list of tasks and actions. Clinical leaders should be aware of the need to transition and adapt away from traditional job descriptions to these more accurate professional role delineations in a way that more effectively supports the professional role, defines the requisite capacities for effective professional judgment, and better delineates the interface between the technology that supports just-in-time clinical practice and advances the viability of the professional nurse.

- The competence of the individual to do the work
- Staffing and scheduling arrangements supporting the work
- The goodness of fit of individual work effort with collective effort
- The team's ability to understand the contribution of each member
- The work tools affecting the ability to do the work
- The utility of managing and applying information
- The clarity of expectations with regard to performance
- Time or workload affecting the ability to accomplish the work

Figure 14-4 Work factors affecting accountable performance

From Process to Outcome Focus

The primary point of accountability is to be able to demonstrate impact, results, and affect in the service relationship, sustained over a longer-term continuum of health (Kleinpell, 2009). Effective and sustainable organizations and the professions that practice in them do not always simply look at incremental and action steps in isolation of impact and effect. Instead, in the interest of sustainability, the clinical organization and its professionals work to establish a longer-term vision of the clinical role and its impact on patients and populations and tie work processes to the collective effort to make a difference in the lives of those they serve. Ultimately, the professional individual and the teams within which they work must define their unique and collective accountabilities as a reflection of their commitment to achieving long-term impact and viability. This represents a focus on accountability instead of simply process responsibility. It calls for rethinking and recalibration from the unilateral compartmental late stage engagement of work to a much more integrated, collective, interdisciplinary team frame for delineating the elements of process as they relate to creating meaningful impact on patients and populations.

CRITICAL THOUGHT

Accountability points to remember:

- Accountability must always be experienced within the role.
- Accountability cannot be externally directed or controlled.
- Accountability must be owned by those who do the work.
- Accountability must be directed to outcome, not process.
- Accountability is represented by team commitment to goals.

SCENARIO

Michael, the clinical nurse leader on the medical–surgical unit, has been experiencing significant staffing problems for the past year. What was difficult for Michael has been trying to find a match between the needs of patients and the availability of professional nursing staff. The problem wasn't so much a shortage of nursing resources; instead, it was that a wide variability in patient acuity and census created difficulty in scheduling and staffing.

Michael recognized the need to blend financial, administrative, and clinical realities and create a framework for appropriate staffing at a level that would meet the needs of the patients but still operate within specified financial constraints. Furthermore, he wanted to engage the professional staff in a way that would help bring ownership to the processes

(continues)

Scenario (*cont.*)

developed and to the standards created in designing and organizing an evidence-based approach to resource use. Michael discussed these issues with Nancy, the manager for the unit. They have laid out a grid related to labor productivity, clinical nursing work, productivity measures, workload issues, patient and staff variances, and value and quality issues related to the delivery of nursing care. They realized that all of these elements would need to be included in a systematic plan directed to meeting patients' needs and defining specific nurse staffing and patient care delivery relationships.

Michael and Nancy were challenged with clarifying the next steps in initiating an evidence-based approach to nursing-staff-driven patient care. They both recognized that each of the elements would need to be explored with regard to existing information, best practices, research-based information resources, and experiential data generated out of the practice environment. They have called on you as their practice consultant to help them organize a systematic process for patient care using evidence-based approaches. They formulated the following questions to initiate this process.

Discussion Questions

1. How does the unit create a model that integrates the elements identified above and establishes a framework for planning evidence-driven care?

2. How can we engage the staff in the process of planning and implementing an evidence-based model so that there are higher levels of ownership from each of the practitioners?

3. Can we link patient needs, workload measurement, staffing skills and competencies, acuity needs, and resource parameters in an ongoing dynamic application that adjusts to the reality of a highly variable census?

4. As the consultant to this process, your obligation is to help gather information necessary to address these questions and help management and clinical staff develop a partnership around building an evidence-based format to address practice, resource, and quality issues on the nursing unit. Where might you begin, and how can you help them through these initial steps based on information already covered in this chapter?

In the contemporary healthcare environment where value is the driver, it becomes imperative that clinical organizations and their professionals reflect the focus of their work on advancing sustainable and meaningful health for populations and communities. Individual providers serve the population one patient at a time. However, that service should reflect the intent on the part of the providers that each patient represents the whole of his or her population, and these populations represent the community. Nurses demonstrate in their service that the individual and collective action of the professional and their clinical teams results in a positive health impact on populations and communities. This principle drives and informs individual accountability and collective action in a way that represents the value, sustainability, and continuing viability of clinical practice. The following elements, therefore, are critical to understanding accountability within the context of impact:

- Accountable organizations and the professionals that comprise them clearly identify who they serve and how they serve them in a way that demonstrates a meaningful positive impact on the health of that population or community. These professionals are continuously committed to redefining, refining, and advancing their processes and mechanisms to ensure this impact is positive and sustainable.

 REFLECTIVE QUESTION

How many of the following can you check off that demonstrate accountable self-management?

- Personal sense of ownership
- Role self-confidence
- Good role fit with others
- Clarifies ambiguity
- Good problem-solving skills
- Relates well with others

- Strong communication skills
- Doesn't seek permission
- Tolerates differences
- Easily explores alternatives
- Questions rituals for relevance
- Good self-evaluation skills

- Professionals who fully understand personal accountability continually join their efforts with each other to recalibrate, redefine, and accelerate the value of their work effort as a reflection of the goal of achieving population and community health. All clinical work recalibrates goals as service effectiveness advances in light of continuing the positive impact on the health of populations and advancing the health status of communities.

- Professional organizations committed to impacting the health of those they serve understand the essential character and needs of accountability and create structures and infrastructures that support individual and collective autonomy. They delineate accountability and action in a way that best reflects economic utilization of resources and effective application of evidence and knowledge in positively impacting populations and communities.

- Emphasis on effective clinical systems doesn't just reflect on processes or outcomes. Instead, the focus of effectiveness is on establishing a tight goodness of fit between processes and outcomes that demonstrates effective interactions, actions, relationships, and interfaces between the work of the professions, the needs of the user, and the health of the community.

- Accountable partnerships do not simply exist among professionals, their disciplines, and each other. Individual members of the community also share in the accountability for advancing the health of that community. The contract for effective health is between the provider and user, the organization, and the community. This occurs in a way that demonstrates an effective convergence of accountability and action that exhibits a mutual commitment and effort to advancing the conditions, circumstances, and actions that best evidence healthy patterns of behavior.

Accountability Is About Adding Value

Accountability is not simply about doing a job well. In fact, as previously established, accountability has nothing to do with job orientation. Therefore, job models should be avoided at all costs when dealing with professional workers. In the past leaders would often acknowledge individuals for having done a good job. What evidence suggests with regard to work is simply doing a good job does not necessarily mean that the right job was done (Bowles & Candela, 2005). Value is about doing the right work rather than doing a good job. Creating a strong configuration between the activities of the professional and the right work is a critical and fundamental part of the contemporary leadership role. Today, the value of one's work depends on how strong a goodness of fit exists between the work of the professional and the impact that work has in making a difference in those to whom the work is directed.

Work is not inherently valuable. Simply doing work and being busy is not a point of value. Work is valuable to the extent that it is informed by purpose; if its purposes are not fulfilled, the work does not demonstrate real value. Value is evidence of how directly the work relates to its contribution, to the intentional fulfillment of its purposes, to the achievement of its ends, and to its sustainability. This value notion of work is critical to a deeper understanding of its application and the increasing willingness of the professional to validate the sustainable value of the outcomes of the work and the dynamic processes that best obtain them.

This notion of value is the product of a measured and defined relationship between effective process (cause) and meaningful outcome (effect). Value demonstrates the convergence of the number of variables that make up the complex elements of good decisions and actions necessary to good practice. Generating from purpose, meaning, expectation, performance, and outcome, the visible expression of value serves as a reflection of how these dynamic factors operate in concert to ultimately impact patient outcomes. This notion of the achievement of value causes both individual professionals and their teams to fully apply their energies and talents to configuring work in a way that will lead to producing the desirable impact and outcome. Even while work and action may be highly variable, it does not diminish the importance of their fit between selected clinical actions and particular related health impacts achieved. For the professional, the continuous dynamic of creating this "fit" is the central constituent of clinical work. In this case, it is the role of the clinical leader to create the conditions and the environment that supports assessment of the evidence, adjustment of clinical action, management of clinical information (documentation), and evaluation of impact. In looking at the role of the professional, these attributes and behaviors articulate a stronger set of skills and performance factors than historic functional or task-based delineation for the role. This continuous dance among the individual professional, the clinical team, the user, and these care attributes and behaviors creates the essential conditions for the continuous living expression of value in a way that drives toward positive health impacts and outcomes.

The Individual, Creativity, and Accountability

Professional practice implies a close relationship with personal innovation and creativity in practice. Clinical leaders should encourage and advance the creativity and innovation embedded in practice as a part of the adaptive capacity of each nurse to ensure that the most relevant and appropriate practices and behaviors unfold in a way that can make the most difference in the lives of those they serve (Figure 14-5). Everyone is born creative. However, life's circumstances can often bring out the creative or diminish creative efforts and expression. Often, in job-based organizational arrangements, the need for uniformity, similarity, and standardized performance mediates against the action of innovation and creativity. Life experience, challenges to personal growth, continuous threats to dynamic self-image, and the social structural limitations that create the rigid parameters that impede creativity all work in concert to limit innovative expression.

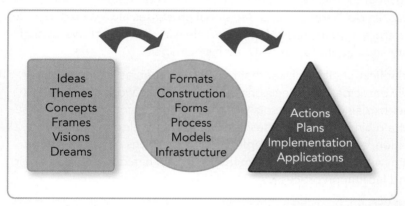

Figure 14-5 Generating the creative urge

Although organizations must carefully manage the creative effort and carefully construct the infrastructure of innovation, they can ensure that it thrives in the system. This means, of course, that the system's design values and generates the conditions amenable to innovation and creativity. This is a continuously active and dynamic process that requires good leaders to be both aware of the requisites of innovation and creativity and clear about the disciplines necessary to focus it on the purpose and values of the system.

Innovation and creativity demand infrastructure and leadership behaviors that exhibit openness, trust, free expression, and availability to ideas in a way that moves the organization beyond habit, rote, ritual, and routine. Creative leadership and organization reflect the leader's capacity to embrace the different and the creative, to challenge existing patterns and practices, to push the walls, and to reflect in new ways, generating new patterns of response. The most significant leadership deficit is the failure to create an effective and safe context or environment where creative and innovative practitioners can safely emerge and positively change patterns and practices in a way that advances the science and art of practice, the experience of the user, and the impacts and outcomes of patient care.

SCENARIO

Stephen was the newly elected chair of his unit-based practice council. He was not familiar with the demands of the role but wanted to respond with his best effort. He looked at the rules of engagement for the council and reviewed the terms of reference for its actions on the unit. Stephen was a little concerned when he saw the statement "the practice council has the accountability for the practice decisions on the unit; since the council represents the clinical staff and reflects its accountability for practice decisions, its deliberations and decisional processes always lead to action and therefore require staff compliance." He was unaware of this level of authority and sought to clarify it with his manager.

Upon clarification, it was clear that his role was seen as a clinical leader who fully participated in decisions that affected the work of others. His manager explained that her role was to support the council's decisions and to help him in the processes associated with dialogue, discussion, negotiation, and making and implementing decisions. She also encouraged him with her personal commitment to help him develop leadership skills and facilitation processes.

Stephen was encouraged by this support but a little intimidated that he would be responsible for the staff making decisions that could affect practice and patient care in a direct way. This was a powerful break from the past when the manager was the prime mover and controller of decisions. Now accountability means that clinical decisions are placed with the staff, where they have the best chance of being implemented and evaluated. This clearly increases staff engagement and extends their role in having an effect on the work of the organization.

Discussion Questions

1. Knowing what you know about accountability, what advice would you give Stephen in helping him get started in building and expanding the notion of accountability for all of the staff?

2. How do you change the staff participation terms of engagement from invitation to expectation?

3. What might be one of the first arenas for building the expectation of accountability?

CRITICAL THOUGHT

The leader is the role model for safe risk taking and appropriately engaging the innovative or different. Colleagues won't take risks if the leader does not make it safe to do so.

True accountability assumes that openness and availability to creativity and innovation are fundamental parts of a meaningful and appropriate clinical environment. Out of this clinical context, the impulse and the urge that is present in each nurse to create, to improve, and to advance is continually expected and supported. Professionals have a right to expect that practice creativity will respond to changes in the evidence, new technology, environmental shifts, and newer insights regarding practice; indeed, nurses are accountable for adjusting their work to such shifts.

Leaders who create an environment that supports creativity and innovation in their practitioners provide a context for excitement, generativity, and a high-level engagement that enthuses the team, converges positive forces, and generates a deeper accountability as well as a broader desire for involvement. This clearly calls leaders to embrace their own self-creativity and to recognize, even in their own leadership, the urge to innovate. The leader who is limited in his or her leadership of clinical creativity ultimately fails to recognize in others the creative urge and the value of tapping that innovation in a collective effort to make positive change and to personally embrace the intentional construction of the future.

There is no doubt that in most workplaces it is often difficult to live in a creative and innovative way. Certainly, the routines and normative expectations of work that emerge in the day-to-day effort can submerge the creative urge in ritual and routine. However, the leader must recognize that the effort for innovation and creativity involves systematically addressing risk. This effort must be intentional, not accidental, and that unless it is well served and purposeful, the creative and innovative urge gets submerged and sublimated in a way that guarantees nonexpression. Although there is always some regulatory, procedural, policy, or performance requisite that could serve to impede the capacity to bring an expressive or experimental response, it is the leader's obligation to place these parameters in context and define mechanisms that raise the standard of practice and its impact on patients in a way that belies the limitation of past practice, policy, and regulation. This is accountability in action (Figure 14-6).

Accountable organizations clearly identify who they are and their relationship to those they serve. They are continually committed to redefining their processes to fit their identity.

Individuals who understand accountability continually redefine their work effort as a reflection of their work goals. They also redefine goals as their work landscape and customers change.

Organizations understand accountability in light of fulfilling the real needs of those they serve, not just their wants. The ability to sort through and distinguish need from want is key to success.

Processes always lead to define outcomes. As the outcomes adjust or advance (or are enhanced), work processes are adaptable and redesigned to create a better fit.

Figure 14-6 Accountability in action

Regulatory socialization has historically been well entrenched in the organization, resulting in a demonstration of the values of sameness, consistency, policy, and routine all serving at the expense of the potential of innovation. The presence of these constraints often reflects the uncertainty in applying innovative practices that are necessary to create the stimulus for creativity and transformation. Also, the limitations of time spent in meeting the sometimes mindless requisites of regulation, policy, ritual, and routine limit the leader's ability to explore outside the box within the work environment, to find opportunities to move above and beyond the regulatory "floor" of organizational life. Often missing from the role is the capacity that creates an opportunity to explore differently and provide unique incentives for innovation and contribution. The leader's focus on creativity and innovation in a highly changing social construct is absolutely essential in order to advance sustainability, life, and meaningful impact on the work of the organization and the life of the community. The wise and effective leader acknowledges that creativity is not an option but a necessary condition to growing and adapting.

This leader continuously seeks opportunities in his or her own self-expression to validate and value the innovative and creative and to create a context that provides a safe space for that same urge to be expressed and fulfilled by every member of the professional community. This is not an addendum to leader accountability; it is, instead, its centerpiece.

Accountability and the Engagement of Risk

The only truly effective work that leaders do is to create a context for the efforts of others. Leaders become ineffective when they leave the obligations associated with creating the context for work and become deeply involved in the machinations related to the content of work. In professional organizations, the content of work is the obligation of the profession, not the manager. In every professional organization that operates consistently with professional values, the discipline protects its right and obligation to own the activities of its practice and control those activities in the hands of those who do the profession's work. When leaders move out of the work of creating a context that enables the professional practitioners' ability to own and manage the content of the work, effectiveness and accountability diminish and, over time, dissipate.

CRITICAL THOUGHT

There is risk embedded in all human action. It is not possible to eliminate risk. If there were no risk, life would be flat, indeed, lifeless. Risk is a sign of reaching out in new ways or in new directions without a compass or ability to absolutely predict what will happen. Risk can be only accommodated and managed. The more the leader understands the nature and occurrence of risk, the better able he or she is in predicting it and designing responses that accommodate it or manage it well. In fact, the good leader is able to anticipate the degree of risk inherent in a change and to predict it with a level of accuracy. In this way, the leader can help the staff grapple with the implications of risk and to maximize their own response to the changes in the work. The risk management mechanisms of the leader help the staff normalize risk and more easily engage it.

The leader creates a safe space for the professional to delineate the work, define it, undertake it, and evaluate it. In addition, the leader enables the professional to undertake the risk and effort necessary to advance successful work. This means essentially that the clinical leader must always be prepared to create the context, conditions, and organizational circumstances necessary to facilitate the ownership of the work and the delivery of the work at the point of service by those who own that work. In short, leaders can't ask others to behave and perform in a manner in which the leader him- or herself does not behave and perform.

All effective leaders are comfortable with ambiguity and can lead within the context of the potential. This potential occupies the space between what is and what will be. The capacity of the leader is to be able to observe, assess the environment, predict the trajectory, and identify the adaptive characteristics necessary to thrive in the context of what is coming next that both changes work and impacts performance (Porter-O'Grady & Malloch, 2010). This living in the potential is a critical skill set for contemporary leaders that requires the ability to incorporate this adaptive and predictive capacity into the role and expression of leadership. This capacity informs the creation of context and becomes the primary work of the contemporary leader.

Context frames action. As a leader more clearly articulates the appropriate contextual framework that responds to shifts in the environment and necessary changes in the organization, this leader creates positive conditions for staff investment and engagement. This capacity on the part of the leader prepares the groundwork for the action of the professional staff as they begin to move into new, enhanced, transformative experiences associated with the content and quality of their work and the impact of their work on those they serve. The dynamic changes, adjustments, shifts, and contemporary challenges to the current work of the professional staff should be anticipated by the predictive and adaptive capacity of the leader who uses that skill to discern the impact of the changing context on the character and content of professional work. From this role and the perspective that it brings, this leader is able to prepare the staff in a way that is congruent with the demand for change, the shifts in the environment, the requisite changes in the system that ultimately impact their own work, and calls them to deeper investment in those changes.

All of this requires a certain level of risk. Here, the clinical leader must demonstrate a personal willingness to incorporate and confront the vagaries of change and work transformation. In doing so, this leader models the behaviors that must ultimately be exemplified by the professional staff in their own practices. In the leader's effort to make it safe for staff to reach out and embrace risk, the leader makes risk confronting the normative and creates in the staff a level of trust that the vagaries and the noise embedded in undertaking risk will not result in punitive, negative, or constraining behaviors on the part of the organization (Malloch, 2010).

In dynamic organizations there is a deeper understanding that it is neither possible to eliminate risk nor is it appropriate to do so. However, because of the nature of health care and the fear of negative impact on patients, risk has been given a contextual framework that represents danger, fear, and limitations. Like all leadership capacities, risk is an essential constituent of human effort. While negative risk must be limited at all costs in terms of its impact on patients, the risks inherent in creating the conditions of safety, appropriateness, innovation, and creativity on behalf of patients in a way that advances their interest should not be limited or diminished (Hueth & Melkonyan, 2009). Indeed, in organizations if risk is eliminated, the life of the organization would end.

Risk is a sign of the continuous and dynamic reach of the human experience in new directions in new ways, often without a compass, exploring new territory in a way that advances that human experience and improves it in important ways. Risk cannot be eliminated, but it can be well managed (Figure 14-7).

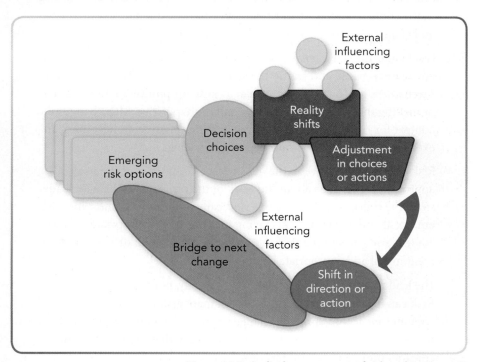

Figure 14-7 Cyclical engagement of risk and acting on it

The more effective a leader becomes in understanding and managing the nature and incidence of risk, the better able the professional staff in the organization is in predicting it, using its energy, and designing appropriate strategies and responses to adapting it and making the necessary changes it demands. The good clinical leader is able to dissipate the potential for risk, the degree of risk inherent in the change, and predict the appropriate level of response with a high degree of accuracy. By creating a safe space for staff to deal with risk, the leader actually helps the staff develop a positive affiliation with the elements and character of risk in a way that allows them to grapple with its implications, maximize the potential for meaningful change, and adapt their own practice responses to its demands in a creative and role-enhancing way. So, for the leader there are particular risk terms of engagement that are essential to guiding appropriate risk response and creating the conditions for managing it well:

- Effective risk relates directly to the practice work currently being undertaken, and it must have an influence either on positive work processes or clinical work outcomes in order to ensure that it is both legitimate and useful.

- All meaningful change encompasses some level of risk. This risk can often be found in the noise of the uncertainty embedded in change and in the confrontation of past rituals and routines, often upsetting them and challenging their validity and continuance.

- Risk and error can often feel synonymous. Mistaking risk for error can create uncertainty and fear in the staff. Positively calibrating error as a mechanism for learning rather than a cause for punitive action is a part of making the risk experience safer and more positive. This changes the context for risk and prevents the potential for error from becoming an excuse for failing to confront meaningful change.

- Risk calls leaders to live in the question and to push staff to raise appropriate questions about the work of the profession. The wise leader stops the trajectory of practice periodically in order to spend time with emergent and apparent risk, placing the risk in an appropriate change context and causing the staff to explore its potential in driving them to meaningful and appropriate changes.

- The leader works to manage risk appropriately, not to eliminate it. Risk can be anticipated and can be well managed. Risk is the essential content that accompanies all change processes. Risk brings attention to the notable variables in the change dynamic that require thought, consideration, and careful response.

- The leader demonstrates in her or his own relationship to risk its value, contribution, and impact on deliberation, action, and evaluation. The leader attempts to make risk a normative part of all intentional action and ensures that the team addresses the elements of risk as carefully as they address the components of the change process.

Accountability is always represented in the ownership of action, but not just any action. Action related to work reflects the professional's need to have a meaningful impact or make a difference on those the profession serves. Accountability always causes the professional to ask questions of meaning and of impact, causing the worker to think of personal action in light of its value and the effect it has on the service provided by the person and the profession. This real strong fit between action and value is the clearest and strongest indicator of the presence of accountability embedded in the role of the professional. The effective leader consistently addresses the issues of accountability and sets time aside with professional staff to help them reconnect with questions of meaning and value in their professional work. In this way, the leader keeps them focused on purpose and value as the driver of their work so they do not become captured by the functions and activities of work. Failure to take this focus and to be reminded of it periodically and regularly can often result in the loss of meaning reflected in the work of the professional. The vagaries and demands of day-to-day activity can often overwhelm issues of meaning and value and cause individuals to be subsumed by the activities of the work rather than the purpose and the impact of that work. It is the leader's obligation to prevent this potential for burning out. Burnout is often buried under the rituals and routines of daily activity and is evident in the failure to represent and access the meaning and value that drives the work and informs its content. The leader and the professional staff focusing on value is the one thing that can continuously distinguish the action and impact of accountability and its centrality in driving the effectiveness of the work and its impact on the health of the community.

CRITICAL THOUGHT

Ambiguity is the enemy of accountability. It is essential that performance expectations be clear and understandable at the outset or performance will always be negatively affected. Some basic elements for role clarity are as follows:

- Precise language that states role in terms that are clear
- Performance factors relate well to role tasks and functions
- Terms of reference are precise and expressed as single items
- Competence factors are clearly enumerated as role foundation
- Clearly state factors that will comprise evaluation of the role
- Tie together individual performance with team performance

Accountability and Performance

Although accountability is not complicated, it is demanding. It requires of the clinical leader a deep commitment to its expression and an understanding of its meaning for the individual professional and for the profession as a whole. Accountability reminds the leader of the central component of the differentiation of professional work from other kinds of work. The sum of accountability of the individual and team is about making a difference and producing meaningful outcomes (Figure 14-8). Accountability acts as the cornerstone of the profession's commitment to the persons and the communities they serve. It is the articulation between the social trust of the people for advancing health and the profession's responsibility to act as the agent of that trust. Therefore, the central characteristics of accountability that are nonnegotiable for the profession represent the following principles:

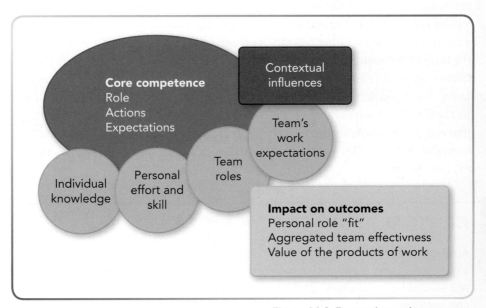

Figure 14-8 Factors impacting outcome

- Accountability generally reflects the individual professional commitment to performance and to action. It is this individual ownership of the profession's work that is necessary in order for action to be accountable.

- Personal accountability is the prerequisite to collective team effort and its ability to achieve and sustain desirable outcomes. Individual accountability and team action are one, and the effectiveness of the convergence of their effort is reflected against the level of sustainable health of those they serve.

- Accountability demands a dynamic convergence between ownership, action, impact, and outcome. The individual professional and the clinical team must link all of these in order to create sustainability in the service they collectively provide.

- Individual accountability cannot be sustained if the system structure does not allow it to be legitimately expressed by those who own it and the infrastructure fails to create the frame for enabling partnership, equity, ownership, and accountability.

- The clinical team has a right to expect that each professional member understands his or her unique contribution, performs that contribution to the fullest extent of his or her competence, and demonstrates that the collective skills of the team members link and integrate well to advance effective group processes and meaningful clinical impact.

Clinical excellence requires the engagement, accountability, and ownership of all stakeholders in the collective in a common effort that exemplifies the needs and demands of those they serve. Excellence cannot be obtained or sustained by the professions without a significant clarity of accountability and the contributions that clarity makes to the work of each discipline that makes up the collective work of the clinical team. Excellence is a demonstration of accountability in action. Excellence is impossible to sustain without a clarity of accountability and the delivery that represents full performance of that accountability. Therefore, it is the centerpiece of professional action and must be evidenced in the life and activity of every professional provider. Accountability is a demonstration that professionals have coalesced their efforts in the clinical team in a way that results in a positive impact on the health of those they serve.

CHAPTER TEST QUESTIONS

1. Accountability relates to designing good clinical processes that demonstrate individual competence and a deep understanding of the work. True or false?

2. Accountability means delegating responsibility to others who are competent to do the work and allowing them to do it well. True or false?

3. Nursing care is as old as human history, but the science-based professionalization of nursing has existed only for the past 100 years of nursing. True or false?

4. Professions are membership communities that establish standards of performance and membership requirements and provide a code of ethics. True or false?

5. One of the unique characteristics of a professional is the recognition of the intensity of the fit between the person as an individual and the person as a professional. True or false?

6. Leaders construct teams and allow them freedom, with a hands-off philosophy, while the team is working. True or false?

7. Individual ownership implies the commitment to engage with others in their learning and development and in mentoring and sharing in the learning process. True or false?

8. On-boarding interviews are not nearly as important as exit interviews because the staff and leadership get more accurate information regarding the work environment and how satisfied staff members are with their work experience. True or false?

9. Evidence-based leadership means demonstrating to the staff how well the leader knows the role and can work well in it. True or false?

10. Individual accountability cannot be sustained if the system structure allows it to be legitimately expressed only by those who own it. True or false?

WWW

For a full suite of assignments and additional learning activities, use the access code located in the front of your book to visit the exclusive website: http://go.jblearning.com/leadership. If you do not have an access code, you can obtain one at the site.

References

Bonvillain, N. (2007). *Women and men: Cultural constructs of gender*. Upper Saddle River, NJ: Pearson Prentice Hall.

Bowles, C., & Candela, L. (2005). First job experiences of recent RN graduates: Improving the work environment. *Journal of Nursing Administration, 35*(3), 130–137.

Buhler-Wilkerson, K. (2001). *No place like home: A history of nursing and home care in the United States*. Baltimore, MD: Johns Hopkins University Press.

Cope, Z. (1958). *Florence Nightingale and the doctors*. Philadelphia, PA: Lippincott.

Cowen, P. S., & Moorhead, S. (2011). *Current issues in nursing*. St. Louis, MO: Mosby Elsevier.

Dossey, B. M. (2005). *Florence Nightingale today: Healing, leadership, global action*. Silver Spring, MD: American Nurses Association.

Fitzpatrick, J. J., & Whall, A. L. (2005). *Conceptual models of nursing: Analysis and application*. Upper Saddle River, NJ: Pearson Prentice Hall.

Gebbie, K. M., Rosenstock, L., & Hernandez, L. M. (Eds.) (2003). *Who will keep the public healthy? Educating public health professionals for the 21st century*. Washington, DC: National Academy Press.

Goodnow, M. (1938). *Nursing history in brief*. Philadelphia, PA; London, England: Saunders.

Group, T., & Roberts, J. (2001). *Nursing, physician control, and the medical monopoly: Historical perspectives on gendered inequality in roles, rights, and range of practice*. Bloomington, IN: Indiana University Press.

Hein, E. C. (2001). *Nursing issues in the 21st century: Perspectives from the literature*. Philadelphia, PA: Lippincott.

Hueth, B., & Melkonyan, T. (2009). Standards and the regulation of environmental risk. *Journal of Regulatory Economics, 36*(3), 219.

Jameson, J. (2009). Nursing policy research: Turning evidence-based research and health policy. *Choice, 46*(10), 1973–1974.

Kleinpell, R. M. (2009). *Outcome assessment in advanced practice nursing*. New York, NY: Springer.

Lagemann, E. C., & Rockefeller Archive Center. (1983). *Nursing history: New perspectives, new possibilities*. New York, NY: Teachers College Press.

Malloch, K. (2010). Creating the organizational context for innovation. In T. Porter-O'Grady & K. Malloch (Eds.), *Innovation leadership: Creating the landscape of healthcare* (pp. 33–56). Sudbury, MA: Jones and Bartlett.

Malloch, K., & Porter-O'Grady, T. (2009a). *Introduction to evidence-based practice in nursing and healthcare.* Sudbury, MA: Jones and Bartlett.

Malloch, K., & Porter-O'Grady, T. (2009b). *The quantum leader: Applications for the new world of work.* Sudbury, MA: Jones and Bartlett.

McDonald, L. (2010). *Florence Nightingale at first hand.* Waterloo, Ontario: Wilfred Laurier University Press.

Moanojovich, M. (2005). Nurse-physician communication: An organizational accountability. *Journal of Nursing Scholarship, 23*(2), 72–78.

Oliver, R. W. (2004). *What is transparency?* New York, NY: McGraw-Hill.

Pollard, E. F. (1911). *Florence Nightingale, the wounded soldier's friend.* London, England: Partridge.

Porter-O'Grady, T. (2004). Accountability and action. *Health Progress, 85*(1), 44–48.

Porter-O'Grady, T., & Malloch, K. (Eds.). (2010). *Innovation leadership.* Sudbury, MA: Jones and Bartlett.

Stacey, M. (2009). *Teamwork and collaboration in early years settings.* Setauket, NY: Exeter.

Tilley, D. (2008). Competency in nursing: A concept analysis. *The Journal of Continuing Education in Nursing, 39*(2), 58–65.

Werhane, P. H. (2007). *Women in business: The changing face of leadership.* Westport, CT: Praeger.

Zedeck, S., & American Psychological Association. (2011). *APA handbook of industrial and organizational psychology.* Washington, DC: American Psychological Association.

Appendix A

Individual Role Accountability and Team Performance

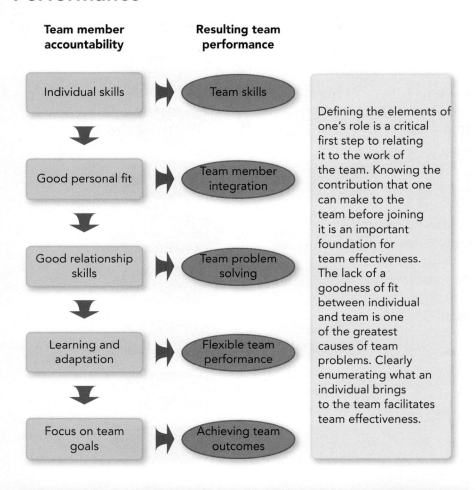

Team member accountability

Resulting team performance

Individual skills	Team skills
Good personal fit	Team member integration
Good relationship skills	Team problem solving
Learning and adaptation	Flexible team performance
Focus on team goals	Achieving team outcomes

Defining the elements of one's role is a critical first step to relating it to the work of the team. Knowing the contribution that one can make to the team before joining it is an important foundation for team effectiveness. The lack of a goodness of fit between individual and team is one of the greatest causes of team problems. Clearly enumerating what an individual brings to the team facilitates team effectiveness.

Appendix B

Fitting Individual and Team Goals Together

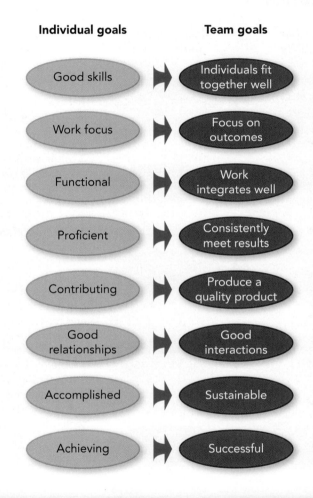

Appendix C

Creating the Culture of Accountability

Bring people on board with the clear understanding of their roles and contributions as members of the team.

Make sure everyone knows that participation is not optional and that every member of the work community must contribute.

Include participation and ownership behaviors in the performance assessment process; review at least quarterly.

Identify skill levels and developmental needs and make sure they are addressed as a part of the individual's growth plan.

Advise all members that accountability is about the achievement of outcomes, not just good work performance.

Identify and resolve interpersonal conflicts early; the later they are engaged the less likely they can be resolved satisfactorily.

Appendix D

Revisiting Invitation and Expectation

In a performance-driven organization, it should be clear to all participants that contribution, commitment, performance, and participation are expected. Team members should feel that they must be invited into ownership and participation in decisions and actions that represent the obligations of the team. Invitation indicates that accountability is optional. In effective team configurations, this is simply untrue. Membership implies ownership and accountability, and each team member must represent that in his or her role.

Invitation	Expectation
• External orientation	• Internal orientation
• Passive engagement	• Active engagement
• Other directed	• Self-directed
• Functionally driven	• Purpose driven
• Process oriented	• Outcome oriented
• Job mental model	• Role mental model
• Task fixed	• Relationship based
• Event based	• Journey based
• No ownership	• Full ownership
• Past active	• Proactive

Appendix E

Responsibility Versus Accountability

Responsibility (20th Century)	Accountability (21st Century)
Process	Product
Action	Result
Work	Outcome
Do	Accomplish
Task	Difference
Function	Fit
Job	Role
Incremental	Sustainable
Externally generated	Internally generated
Quality effort	Quality impact

The terms *accountability* and *responsibility* are frequently used interchangeably. However, these terms and the dynamics to which they relate mean entirely different things. Perhaps the most important distinction between responsibility and accountability relates to their orientation. Responsibility focuses on the work, the competence of the worker, the effectiveness of the processes, the quality of the effort, and the excellence of its application.

Accountability, on the other hand, focuses on the products of work rather than the processes of work. Accountability relates to issues regarding the impact of the work, the products or results of work, a difference the work makes, and whether the work mattered in relationship to performance and expectations. Quite simply, accountability focuses on issues of outcome and calls attention to the effects of the work rather than the processes related to the work itself. Today, questions of accountability have become increasingly important as the relationships among work effectiveness, outcome, and work process become important.

Appendix F

Accountability and Impact

Accountability always asks, what difference
does the work effort make?

Accountability focuses the effort of the worker on the
products of work rather than the processes of work.

In accountability, the discipline is focused on creating
a goodness of fit between work effort and results.

Accountability suggests that evaluation and comparison
occur between work and the products of work.

Accountability implies that quality improvement focuses
on work as a reflection of the value of its products/result.

Accountability seeks to identify what specific elements
of work make the key difference in its results.

Accountability requires an internal generation or motive
for excellence, not merely an external demand.

Appendix G

Role Clarity and Accountability Model

Individual performance skills and talents

Aggregated team-based talents, skills, and actions

Organizational need to fit work with product and to sustain

Central role obligations and definitions for the exercise of the role

Changes and Shifts in: society economics technology

Performance expectations and outcomes to which the effort of the role is directed

External influences that are constantly challenging the content of the role

Shifting demands that change the expectations and products of work

Appendix H

Accountability and Locus of Control

Accountability reflects the individual ownership of the decisions that attend to a particular role. A role holds decisional authority not so much because that authority is assigned to it but more because it is legitimate to the role because of the role's opportunity and obligation to directly affect outcome. The necessity to act in a certain way to effect a related, defined outcome is the authority basis for determining location and making decisions related to a particular work effort. A role is empowered to make specific decisions because of its direct relationship to the specific decisions and actions that result in the fulfillment of the purpose or products of the work. An accountability-driven organization has an infrastructure that supports and recognizes this approach to accountability and performance.

Accountable Decisions and Action

Role:
- Location
- Accountability
- Performance
- Competence

Accountable decisions flow from individual roles through the actions necessary to directly achieve outcomes and sustain an effective work–outcomes relationship.

Decisions:
Authority
Autonomy
Competence
Applicable

Actions:
Applied
Appropriate
Implemented
Good process

Outcomes:
Evaluated
Good fit
Effective
Sustainable

Accountability reflects the location of power in the hands of those who ultimately undertake the actions that produce results. Ownership of accountability is necessary to the achievement of sustainable outcomes. Without this dynamic interaction, all work is, at best, incremental and short term.

Appendix I

Ownership: The Center of Accountability

The central theme of accountability is the ownership of work. There is much controversy and disagreement about the locus of control for decisions and actions related to the work of organizations. In a private enterprise system, it is often assumed that the owner of the enterprise owns the means and processes associated with the organization.

In truth, however, this is an incomplete view of the work relationship. Although the organization owns the products of work and influences the processes of work, unless a real partnership exists between those who do the work and those who own the means and products of work, there is no sustainable, consistent, and accelerating outcome.

The challenge here is to incorporate the understanding that workers also have an ownership capacity. Because outcomes generate from the efforts of the worker as well as the resources of the owner, a fundamental partnership exists between them. When this partnership is well described and shared, the processes and products of work have the potential to be continually effective and sustainable.

The wise leader understands this fundamental relationship and does everything to clarify its elements and to better describe the contribution that both people and resources make to the achievement and sustainability of the organization. This leader continually balances the needs of workers and demands of the organization in a mosaic or dance of effort that ensures the energies of the worker (human capital) and the resources (financial capital) of the organization continue to contribute to success.

Balancing Ownership and Resources

Ownership of Work	Resources
Internally generated	Externally generated
Skill based	Adequate
Continual improvement	Relate to need
Conscious contribution	Cost–benefit value
Full engagement	Shared with workers
Good processes	Gain shared
Effect on outcomes	Return on investment

Note: So often workers feel or sense value if they accomplish a job or do good work. The problem is that simply accomplishing work or doing a job is not real value; making a difference with the work is a stronger indicator of real value.

Appendix J

Volume Versus Value

So many times the professional worker will indicate that the amount of work done should be evidence of the importance of work. Of course, nothing could be further from the truth. The amount of work one does has nothing to do with its meaning or value. Value is found in the effect of the work, or with its outcome. The inputs of work relate directly to the outcome and should advance or increase the value of the outcome at a faster rate than the cost associated with the input. There is no positive value if this exchange of the relationship between input and outcome is negative. Increasing one's work does not increase value. It just increases the effort. Value is better represented when there is an expenditure of just the right amount of effort to maximize the products or outcomes of the work and not an ounce more. In most effective workplaces, this relationship is important enough to be constantly defined and measured as a way of obtaining as much value as can be derived from the work effort.

Volume and Value Indicators

Volume of Work	Value of Work
Task focused	Results focused
Functional	Action based
Process oriented	Outcome oriented
Focus on the work	Effect of the work
Task completion	Achieving expectations
Many processes	Goodness of fit of effort
Worker centered	Making a difference
Immediate	Sustainable
Short term	Renewable

Appendix K

Some Risk-Dealing Rules of Engagement

Risk must relate directly to the work being undertaken and have an influence either on positive work processes or work outcomes in order to be legitimate and useful.

Risk usually accompanies all change and can be found in the noise or uncertainty of a change of past rituals and routines, upsetting them in ways that challenge their continuance.

Risk often first appears as error, creating uncertainty or fear. Error is simply a form of risk that needs to be placed in context rather than become an excuse for not confronting change.

Risk calls leaders and staff to question. It is wise to stop and spend time with the apparent risk, placing it in appropriate context and exploring what it is pointing out to all.

Leaders cannot eliminate risk. It can only be anticipated and managed. Risk accompanies all change processes and demands attention to the variables that affect the implementation of change.

The leader creates the attitude that determines how staff will respond to risk. The more normative the leader can make the presence and experience of risk, the better staff will deal with it.

WHAT COULD BE WORSE THAN BEING BLIND? THAT WOULD BE SEEING AND HAVING NO VISION. —HELEN KELLER

CHAPTER OBJECTIVES

Upon completion of this chapter, the reader will be able to do the following:

» Understand the requirements of linking and integrating leader learning in a way that can be effectively applied.

» Define the basic elements of leadership and translate them into situations and scenarios that require leadership application.

» Enumerate the components of a leadership challenge or problem and the steps and processes associated with its resolution.

» Outline the approaches to issue identification and selection of appropriate strategies to reflect on the issue and to construct mechanisms for its resolution.

» List at least five major components of each chapter leadership focus and the impact it has on the role of clinical leadership.

» State personal leadership growth and developmental needs that define the individual journey and trajectory of leadership and create a guide for personal leadership development.

Integrating Learning: Applying the Practices of Leadership

This chapter serves as a comprehensive summary of the work of this text and as a tool for synthesizing the foundational leadership concepts that will inform the reader's leadership practices. The ability to use tools to express leadership capacity and to apply principles is the best indicator of leadership success. Keep in mind that this work is directed to the emerging clinical leader who does not intend to become a manager but needs the insights and tools necessary to express real leadership in the clinical environment. Less than 1 percent of bachelor's of science degree in nursing graduates will become managers, but most will aspire to excellence in practice and clinical leadership. How well the clinical leader does is completely dependent on his or her ability to synthesize the capacities of leadership and apply them successfully to practice problems and human relationships that lie at the foundation of clinical practice. Be sure to review previous chapters for key concepts and behaviors that can and should be integrated into your discussions and creation of new and better solutions for health care.

In the Era of Health Transformation

Perhaps one of the most important roles of the leader is evidenced in the capacity to anticipate and predict future expectations and translate them for those he or she leads (Maxwell, 2010). Nothing is more important than helping the staff to anticipate change and to translate it into a language that colleagues can understand and, more importantly, actively engage in. These insights about the direction of the work journey are critical because they encompass people's hopes and the desire to improve or make things better, and they demonstrate a capacity to make a difference that will sustain over time.

At the same time, it is important for the leader to be able to exemplify for the staff the ability to own the changes that accurately lead to these opportunities in ways that will enhance both the work experience and the patient experience. Life is not static, and if it is not positively pressed forward, it inevitably falls backward, contracting opportunity and growth in ways that create the conditions and circumstances of decline and contraction.

The leader essentially provides a beacon on the pathway to the future that illuminates the path itself and enlightens fellow travelers to what they will find and what it will require of them to continue their own personal journey.

The Context of Healthcare Reform

There are a host of reasons that every nurse needs to be aware of the implications of the impact of healthcare reform. The demand for reform has been long in coming, even though the real noise and activities associated with actually implementing it have demonstrated the fear generated by implementing a change in the status quo (Phillips & Bazemore, 2010). The implications for practice are staggering and require the leader to be fully engaged in identifying and translating the particular changes embedded in the activities of reform to staff colleagues regardless of their practice arenas.

CRITICAL THOUGHT

The leader always stays in the question. The leader constantly recognizes that he or she does not own other people's problems, and the leader's role is to help them own their problems and develop the skills for resolving them.

The most significant reality shift for providers is the radical move from a volume service framework to a value-driven model of both delivering and paying for healthcare service. For years nurses have been objecting to the heavy dependence on the volume rubrics embedded in tasks, functions, procedures, and protocols without any real alignment of them to the values or outcomes to which they were intended or relate. In the emerging healthcare system, value drivers almost exclusively emerge as the sole frame of reference for health care. Unless the practice language changes to match the values perspective, our very practices become the impediment to moving and engaging the systems and structures that could compete with them and be tempted to create fixes or superficial remedies that are inherently inadequate and not currently open to improving our practice.

The full script for American health care is currently being completely recalibrated. It should be clear even to the most casual observer of the healthcare crisis that our traditional approach to service is nonsustainable; even if a new political administration didn't like the prevailing place for changing health care, he or she would have to begin at a zero point to transform a system that does not serve the country well. Eliminating the present does not return us to the past. Instead, it creates a new demand for making the system work effectively to fulfill the mandates to which it is directed.

REFLECTIVE QUESTION

Because work cannot provide meaning—instead, it demonstrates how meaning is present—how does the leader help others discern the meaning that drives their work so they do not lose touch with it?

A good leader recognizes the need for good policy and relevant direction (Hazy, Goldstein, & Lichtenstein, 2007). There must always be a good fit between the work of a system and its purpose. Indeed, when purpose is sacrificed on the altar of work, the work loses direction quickly and becomes devoid of meaning that should be guiding work. The leader will constantly be bombarded with people who are addicted to the energy of activity just for the sake of the activity and will be unable to alter their vision or change their practice. Ritual and routine inure people from both ownership and value, and they can be observed descending into the morass of functionalism of ritual and routines. Tasks and functions become their reason for being and subsume all their energy and creativity. We should not diminish the value of effort and work, but the leader does need to keep in mind that there are many who have entered into the ritual of work and have surrendered their attachment to good judgment, critical reflection, and a search for real value. The leaders must know these characteristics when he or she sees them and be prepared to identify and address them in ways that create sufficient change to make these sanctuaries of the historic places that are both untenable and unacceptable.

There are several drivers in healthcare reform that change the landscape of health care and require the leader to reconfigure both work and roles in the health system:

- Value drivers means that impact and outcome are more important to good and sustainable healthcare service than is good process and task. Process and task focus on the work; value focuses on outcome and impact. For the leader, much of theory in this script is helping colleagues deconstruct function and work as well as replace it with definers of what making a difference looks like and what it will take to get there.

- User-driven healthcare service means that the patient is the driver and that providers are respondents to that equation. This essentially means that providers have much to do to surrender ownership of health decisions to users and to help make them competent with the decisions they now own and that guide them in making effective healthcare choices.

- Digital technology is now the predominant means of communicating and interacting with patients. It is no longer optional for a provider to claim technological noncompetence in the course of her or his practice. It is simply impossible to practice and to prepare for the future of practice without sufficient technological competence to drive the digital clinical journey.

- In professional practice, collective wisdom is infinitely more valuable than unilateral action. If any practitioner sacrifices the products of collective wisdom on the altar of individuated practice, he or she is simply proclaiming to peers and patients that his or her personal judgment about standards of practice and the protocols that express them is more valid and appropriate that those established through the collective mind of the profession as a whole.

- Anything effective in healthcare reform will be constructed and will be the product of the work that addresses an inadequacy or limitation in practice. Practice relevance will be the reflection of the goodness of fit between what is considered normative behavior and that which lies at the periphery of human behavior, and indeed it may serve as a catalyst for changing the health priorities when a lack of goodness of fit becomes glaringly apparent.

Healthcare reform simply serves as the stimulus for rethinking and reconfiguring health care in a way that reflects real value for achieving objective measures of health and advancing the level of health of whole categories of health resource users (Berwick, Nolan, & Whittington, 2008).

CRITICAL THOUGHT

Value always has as one of its components the reduction of inputs driving the maximization of output.

The Management of Conflict

Principles of conflict management are essential to navigating the landscape of transformation and change, if only for confronting the divergent views and differences among stakeholders that have a genuine and positive commitment to advancing health care. These differences must be managed in a way that moves individuals and groups toward consensus and agreement that will inform and guide subsequent action. As indicated in this text, conflict is a normative dynamic and one that serves as a centerpiece in the leadership armamentarium. At every corner of the system and in almost every work process, the leader confronts differences that must be addressed and conflicting notions and processes that must be resolved. Applying the principles of good conflict management will be an essential skill set that will often be the difference between positive movement and stagnating immobility.

A few principles of sound conflict management to keep in mind are as follows:

- A good conflict process includes identifying conflict in its earliest stages. The sooner conflicts can be addressed, the easier they are to resolve. Conflicts ignored or left too long can become intransigent and waste untold resources in their negative effect and in the work to correct them.

- Conflict resolution is a dynamic process that has method and technique attached to it that must be addressed and utilized in a systematic and progressive manner. Through many years of application and research, the critical stages of conflict resolution and the activities associated with its success have been developed. Faithfulness to this process and consistency with its application bears positive results and helps the mediator ensure successful resolution.

- Human behavior can be widely variable and sometimes unpredictable, especially under duress or stress. The conflict leader must always be prepared for the potential of behavioral excess and emotional drama in the mediation of conflicts. Emotion is a legitimate component of real problems and when ignored can have a devastating effect on progress and resolution. The mediator must develop both comfort and skill with addressing emotional expression as a part of the resolution process so that the positive work of mediation can bear the fruit of resolution.

- Resolution means the achievement of a mutual solution that meets the needs of all the parties to a conflict. It is not accidental that the mediator role is often referred to as neutral. The mediator has no agenda other than meeting the participants' needs and discovering a mutually derived solution. As soon as the mediator has a position, he or she becomes a part of the conflict, so the effectiveness of the role dissipates and the conflict never really gets resolved.

- Conflict resolution and mediation are learned and developed skills that come with practice and application. A good mediator deals honestly with his or her own uncertainty and difficulty with conflict working to resolve whatever personal barriers might exist in effectively handling other people's conflicts. Good mentorship and practice improve the comfort and skills of the mediator in ways that ensure a meaningful and valuable experience for those experiencing conflict and who are working to resolve issues that keep them from mutually meeting their own needs and the needs of the patient.

A facility with conflict marks the strength and character of good leadership (Boulle, Colatrella, & Picchioni, 2008). In no other area of leadership are the skills of problem solving so critical. The vast majority of organizational problems are relational or interactional. A leader who is able to confidently confront these with a high level of skill is an asset to people and organizations beyond ordinary value. Furthermore, the effectiveness with managing conflict translates to so many other leadership skills that its utility is invaluable.

The Centrality of Accountability

Perhaps there is no greater challenge to professional performance and impact as that which relates to the personal expression of accountability. Accountability is the cornerstone of professional expression (Tilley, 2008). There are some scholars who believe that it is the cornerstone of professional practice and one cannot be a professional without it. While there is much conversation as to whether nurses actually behave as professionals, there is little doubt that accountability is the best indicator as to whether professional behaviors are at work in the clinical environment.

Accountability is not as amorphous and ambiguous a notion as many are led to believe. In fact, accountability is a very precise notion with particular characteristics that mark it as a unique expression of human action (Connors, Smith, & Hickman, 2004). Three essential characteristics enumerate the content of accountability and are essential to its definition. Accountability needs autonomy, authority, and competence in order for it to be properly expressed. Autonomy indicates the right to make decisions and take action. One cannot be accountable for that over which they have no right to decide and to act. Having a right is critical to accountability that no matter where a decision might be made, if accountability does not exist in that place, the right to decide and to act doesn't either, and any decisions and actions that occur there cannot be fully realized and the outcome cannot be sustainably achieved.

Authority as related to accountability addresses the assurance that the necessary power to decide and to act is located in the place where the right (autonomy) to decide and to act is located. Accountability has no value if it has no power. Not only does it need expressive power, but that power also must be expressed by those who have the right to decide. In short, power must be located in the same place as the right to exercise it. The further away a decision is made from the place it is exercised, the higher the cost, the greater the risk, and the lower the sustainability of the outcome related to it.

The third component of the definition of accountability is that which relates to the competence to decide and to act. While anyone can be given both the autonomy and the authority to act, there is no guarantee that they will do so competently. This notion of competent decision making and implementing is a critical component of successful decisions and actions. Having the capacity to make good decisions and to set the table where those decisions can be planned and acted upon is foundational to the action of accountability.

CRITICAL THOUGHT

There is no accountability if there is no autonomy to decide and to act, if there is no power to act, or if there is no competence to knowledgably exercise accountability.

Other elements of accountability that are essential to its exercise are as follows:

- Accountability cannot be delegated. It is internally generated and embedded in the professional role. While responsibility for tasks and functions can be delegated, the accountability for their fulfillment and the impact they create is held by the professional who is accountable for the results.

- Accountability is invested in individuals, not groups. It is a personal expression and attends to the action of the person, and it is in persons that accountability is expressed and in those same persons that its obligations are embedded.

- Accountability is about the products of work, not the processes of work. Accountability is demonstrated in what is achieved, not what is done. The action of work and how well it is accomplished is the demonstration of the fulfillment of responsibility. The impact of work and the difference it makes is the expression and evidence of accountability.

- Accountability implies change. The positive impact of accountability suggests that a positive and desirable change has resulted and the fulfillment of the goal to make change has been satisfied. There is no accountability if a change has not occurred because a positive change is the only demonstration of the action of accountability.

- There is no accountability without consequence. There are two consequences that imply the action of accountability: negative and positive. Accountable professionals are continuously asking the questions of accountability. What happens with the expression of accountability and what difference is made? What happens if the accountability is not achieved?

Accountability is the cornerstone of professional action. It is the essential core of the expression of the role of the professional and is demonstrated by its positive performance and the achievement of desired outcomes. Without accountability, there is no promise to perform on the part of the profession and no commitment to advance the trust and interests of those served upon which others can depend. It is essentially a part of the role of each professional and provides the best evidence of the value they have and the difference they make.

Structure, Organizations, and Professionals: Creating Context for Practice

Professional practice is as strongly supported by sound organizational structure as by standards of excellence. A poor organization and supporting infrastructure for practice can create a negative framework for the practitioner and ultimately negatively impact the kind and quality of care he or she provides.

Knowledge workers (professionals) need a very specific organizational context in order to facilitate good practice and positive outcomes (Porter-O'Grady, 2009). Organizational structure and professional practice models are underaddressed in the influence they have on creating a professional practice environment. The question as to whether nursing is a profession is best answered by those organizations that demonstrate their commitment to professional practice by providing a different way of doing business that best represents what both professional practice and professionals need.

Knowledge workers are intrinsically motivated. Their work is more than simply a job. Professional knowledge workers are generally licensed by the state and therefore are its agents in the performance of work that reflects a competency base and a particular kind of academic preparation. Society then entrusts these specially designated individuals with requisites for managing essential life processes in a way that acts in the best interests of society. Registered nurses are considered one of these groups.

 REFLECTIVE QUESTION

What is different about knowledge workers, from other employee work groups, that requires the relationship between them and the organization to be structured differently? How does shared governance create the structure for framing this relationship between professionals and the system?

Being a professional does not guarantee that individuals will behave that way. Without an expressed code of ethics and standards of membership and performance, there would be no indicators related to the unique trust society has for these individuals. These codes of conduct and performance standards outline the particular expectations to which the professional is held. Members of a profession express mutual accountability for their membership and demonstrate that in the performance of theory of the discipline.

But professionals also govern themselves differently from other work groups. Professionals have a level of self-direction and shared governance that gives them the obligation to manage the work of the profession and the relationship of professionals with each other and their interaction with those they serve (Styer, 2007). Because of the unique character of professional work and the charter the professionals hold with society, they generally create a structure that affirms their unique obligation and empowers them with exclusive control over the work, its quality, and the competence necessary to do it to the level of satisfaction the peers would define and require of their members.

It is this structure that creates the context for sustaining a high level of competent professional practice. The historical context for the work of nursing did not have this enabling structure, and the advancement of the professional and professional practice suffered as a result. Research over the past 2 decades has revealed that both a context and standards reflecting staff ownership of professional practice work in concert to create the conditions that both advance and sustain the work of the profession and produce the ground for performance excellence and high levels of provider and patient satisfaction.

There are some well-validated essentials that evidence a good fit between supporting infrastructure and the capacity for sustainable professional practice:

- Professionals organize around decisions, not positions. Hierarchy means little to professions, and a structure that enables and supports horizontal relationships and interactions is an essential foundation for establishing professional practice. Decisions should always be generated by those who own them. Decisions should be made by the right person, in the right place, at the right time, for the right purpose.

- Decisions are driven from the point of service, requiring that 90 percent of decisions are made at the heart of the organization where professional services are provided. This means that most content-based decisions are made by the practicing staff, and the design of the structure demonstrates the locus of control for content decisions that are in their hands.

- A grid of accountability demonstrates the locus of control for all decisions in the system and clearly identifies where decisions should be made and by whom. This clear enumeration of decisions in the structure clearly acknowledges the content of decisions and their legitimate owner and provides the structural frame to ensure those decisions are made where they belong and by those who are accountable for their exercise.

- Clarification and distinction of decisions that are *a priori* management driven and owned and those that are staff owned are important distinctions of accountability in professional organizations. The professions own exclusive accountability for decisions regarding practice, quality, and the competencies required to do the work of the profession. The management accountabilities relate to the management of the human, fiscal, material, support, and systems resources that provide the context for the work of the profession. Each cannot do the work of the other, but both work in concert to support the mission of the organization, exercise stewardship over its resources, and fulfill the requirement and expectations of the professional service and care provided. This mutuality is the bond between the profession and organization and is the strongest demonstration of their partnership in meeting the healthcare needs of their community.

CRITICAL THOUGHT

The central principle of shared decision making is ensuring that the right decision is being made by the right person, in the right place, at the right time, for the right purpose. Structuring for professionals is built around this centerpiece.

The integration of the social requirement to transform health care, resolve the conflicts that challenge that obligation in the day-to-day expenditure of the work of organization and professionals, express the accountability to make a difference in the health and lives of the community, and advance the work of the profession is critical to building the profession and making a sustainable difference. Together, these conditions and activities best demonstrate the potential and commitment of the professional nurse to ensuring the advancement of truly sustainable health (Institute of Medicine, 2010). The emerging leader must see these as foundations or cornerstones of the work of the leader and work to advance them as a part of personal clinical leadership capacity and demonstrate them within his or her own practice every day. Leadership is a dynamic and continuous work in progress and is a never-ending exemplar of the commitment to excellence and to making a difference in the world.

Resource Management in Health Care

CRITICAL THOUGHT

America has the best doctors, the best nurses, the best hospitals, the best medical technology, the best medical breakthrough medicines in the world. There is absolutely no reason we should not have in this country the best health care in the world. —Bill Frist

Without people, physical settings, equipment, supplies, computers, and financial resources, the healthcare system would nearly stand still. Ensuring that caregivers have the appropriate resources at the right time is complex and dynamic and requires proactive involvement from caregivers. Key issues specific to each of the categories of resources are highly interrelated within the system and are continually impacted by ethical challenges, professional role accountability, national and state legislation, and the evidence for increasing or decreasing resources. What is certain is that the allocation of resources is seldom a black-and-white decision; it is a decision of multiple considerations and exchanges of ideas to get to the best decision at a particular point in time.

Ethical Behaviors

The challenges of doing the right thing in health care cannot be underestimated. Multiple factors are continually interacting, changing, and impacting the processes of patient care. Perhaps the single most challenging issue is figuring out what the value of each participant in the discussion is and how those participants will impact the decision. While it is believed that the values of the patient drive the decisions, this is not always the case. Further exploration is necessary whenever there is doubt that the patient's wishes and values are not driving decisions. The importance of truth telling becomes paramount in getting to the best resolution of ethical dilemmas.

Also important are ethical issues specific to caregivers who are involved in errors. No longer is punishment following an error the expected action. Rather, the goal is to understand human fallibility and the influences of complex systems on practice breakdown. Remediation is always the goal when there is absence of intentional wrongdoing or a pattern of negligent behaviors.

CRITICAL THOUGHT

It is critical to synthesize all of the knowledge, skills, and abilities of nursing into an integrated whole that moves nurses from task completers to an overall demonstration of compassion and caring.

Thinking of nursing first as a job of caring and making a difference as well as the work of giving meds on time, checking an X-ray to see if the doctor needs to be called, or taking an admission at 2:00 a.m. with a smile on our faces reminds us of the synthesized whole of nursing work.

Moral courage is a critical professional competency that continually needs to be strengthened and role modeled. The inherent risks in speaking up, challenging unethical decisions, and standing one's ground are significant and require collaboration and support for moral courage to be a reality.

Staffing Effectiveness

Achieving staffing effectiveness 100 percent of the time is the desired goal for all caregivers. Understanding staffing effectiveness measures and outcomes provides clear and objective guidelines for caregivers and leaders as well as the incredible challenges in achieving goals 100 percent of the time. Numerous strategies are available to impact staffing processes at various levels and times in the process of staffing. Nurse–patient ratios, patient classification systems, legislative requirements, and different skill levels all enter into the equation for staffing effectiveness. Knowing that many professionals are attempting to reduce the staffing process to mathematical algorithms to simplify the process should be cause for serious concern. Mathematical forecasting provides but a portion of the picture of patient care needs and nurse qualifications; the art and humanity of juggling staffing assignments in real time based on events of the moment are still essential for staffing effectiveness and nurse satisfaction. Both the art and science of staffing and scheduling are essential.

SCENARIO

As changes emerge based on healthcare reform, one must wonder if things will be better or worse—will nursing be more humanitarian and respected as a profession or will it become depersonalized in our attempts to increase access to all citizens and decrease costs?

Discussion Question

In a small group, make two lists: one in which health care will become more depersonalized and another in which human suffering will be diminished. Include specific healthcare reform actions to support your two lists. Be sure to include the rationale for your categorization.

Change and Innovation

Nothing ever stays the same! Learning how to thrive in the presence of continual change requires both art and science in the healthcare environment. Nurses need to know personal attitudes, competencies, and values specific to change and innovation as a primary requisite for participating in change work. In spite of both obstacles and facilitators to change and innovation, there is no escaping the reality of change.

As individuals become comfortable with embracing change and innovation, it is equally important to recognize that not all change is urgent or value laden. Some good ideas just don't need to happen—unless there is evidence and rationale for the change.

Policy Making

Policies are made at the national, state, and local levels; each impacts the direct caregiver in different ways. Policies are also the backbone of private organizations and agencies. Knowing the source of policies that impact patient processes is an essential first step in understanding the goals of the policies, the appropriate avenue for feedback, and supporting metrics to determine the value and impact of the policy.

In addition to knowing the source, content, and consequences of healthcare policies, it is also important to recognize the role of the professional in providing feedback to policy makers when policies are no longer effective or achieve the desired goal. Too often, ineffective policies continue when there is sufficient evidence to terminate the policies. Speaking up and providing input is consistent with ethical and professional practices.

Delegation

No individual can do everything for everyone. Complex patient care requires multiple levels of caregivers at different times to provide the necessary services including surgical interventions, treatments, medications, therapy, nutrition, housekeeping, record management, and a host of other services. From the chief executive officer level to the patient, multiple caregivers interact with each other and oversee and direct different levels of caregivers. Nurses collaborate with medical providers, therapists, pharmacists, and nutritionists and oversee licensed practical nurses, nurse assistants, clerical staff, and often housekeepers. The importance of effective delegation cannot be overestimated. Effective delegation ideally distributes the workload equitably and effectively.

Career Management

A career in nursing provides an incredible opportunity to continually advance into numerous avenues and job roles. Proactively understanding and managing one's career requires not only a current license, but also continuing competence, participation in professional organizations, and mentoring nurse colleagues as they advance in their work. No individual should ever put his or her career on autopilot expecting that little will change over time and reentry into the workplace will not require updating and skill confirmation. The nursing career is both an incredible asset and an incredible obligation to the public.

 REFLECTIVE QUESTION

In the 1800s nurses like Florence Nightingale and Clara Barton believed nurses no longer wanted to accept things the way they were; instead they wanted to learn from past mistakes and improve the future of nursing.

Do you think this is the overall feeling of nurses today? Why or why not?

Concluding Thoughts

Learning and challenging our assumptions of the past is never-ending, sometimes overwhelming, but mostly energizing in that this work is a reflection of our vitality and abilities to create a better future and impact how the future evolves. The scenarios in the appendices of this chapter are intended to challenge your thinking, be outrageously creative, and push the walls of what we currently know and do in very special ways. The future relies on those nursing professionals continuing to learn creatively and take rational risks in pushing new ideas, projects, and initiatives forward quickly and effectively. Finally, the contemporary professional nurse is not afraid of failure—rather when an idea or project or initiative does not work as intended, the work of course correction has already begun! Best wishes on your journey. The healthcare world desperately needs your energy, wisdom, and passion for excellence in patient care.

CRITICAL THOUGHT

There is no medicine like hope, no incentive so great, and no tonic so powerful as expectation of something better tomorrow.
—Orison Swett Marden

> **www**
> For a full suite of assignments and additional learning activities, use the access code located in the front of your book to visit the exclusive website: http://go.jblearning.com/leadership. If you do not have an access code, you can obtain one at the site.

References

Berwick, D., Nolan, T., & Whittington, J. (2008). The triple aim: Care, health, and cost. *Health Affairs, 27*(3), 759–769.

Boulle, L., Colatrella, M. T., & Picchioni, A. P. (2008). *Mediation: Skills and techniques.* Newark, NJ: LexisNexis Matthew Bender.

Connors, R., Smith, T., & Hickman, C. (2004). *The Oz Principle: Getting results through individual and organizational accountability.* New York, NY: Portfolio Hardcover.

Hazy, J., Goldstein, J., & Lichtenstein, B. (2007). *Complex systems leadership theory: New perspectives from complexity science on social and organizational effectiveness.* New York, NY: Vintage Press.

Institute of Medicine. (2010). *The future of nursing.* Washington, DC: Author.

Maxwell, J. (2010). *The 21 irrefutable laws of leadership.* Nashville, TN: Thomas Nelson.

Phillips, R., & Bazemore, A. (2010). Primary care and why it matters for US health system reform. *Health Affairs, 29*(5), 806–810.

Porter-O'Grady, T. (2009). *Interdisciplinary shared governance: Integrating practice, transforming healthcare.* Sudbury, MA: Jones and Bartlett.

Styer, K. (2007). Development of a unit-based practice committee: A form of shared governance. *AORN Journal, 86*(1), 85.

Tilley, D. (2008). Competency in nursing: A concept analysis. *Journal of Continuing Education in Nursing, 39*(2), 58–65.

Appendix A

Exercise in Leadership: Advancing Evidence-Based Practice

SCENARIO

Michele is chair of the practice council. There has been much discussion on the unit about implementing evidence-based practices in all of the nursing practice protocols. However, the staff know little about the foundations and principles of evidence-based practices to understand the implications of changing practice patterns to reflect the related principles and applications into every nurse's role.

At the same time, Michele has been noticing a number of members of the practice council have expressed negative feelings about changing to incorporate evidence-grounded practices into their roles. In fact, one of them asked, "If what we are doing isn't broken, why fix it?" This person has managed to get a couple of the other members of the council to support her opposition. The nursing manager is insisting that the council seriously undertake this work because it is a "mandate" from the nurse executive and the unit manager's "reputation is on the line."

Michele has some concerns with the process of implementing changes as a response to a mandate from above. Their organization has been operating within a shared governance structure for some time. For Michele it appears that the move to evidence-based practice should be a staff initiative and come from the wider nursing division practice council rather than as a mandate from the nurse executive.

For Michele, evidence-based practice reflects a fundamental principle of accountability on the part of the staff. She feels that staff should want to validate their practice choices and application with data and demonstrate best practices in their clinical performance. She has noted that there have been some questions as to what the level of understanding and commitment is to personal accountability in all members of the staff. Michele knows that if evidence-based practice is to succeed it will need the support of leadership and staff throughout its implementation.

This scenario exemplifies a situation that will draw on the learning and skills enumerated in a number of related chapters in this text. Constructing a team of no more than five members (in each team), explore the issues presented in this scenario and use the principles and elements outlined in this text as your source for addressing Michele's leadership issues and resolving her questions and problems.

The following are some questions designed to focus your deliberations and problem solving:

1. What preparation does Michele need to do in relationship to her knowledge base about evidence-based practice before she brings the issue to the unit practice council? What information will she need to gather and provide for the council members before they meet?

2. How will Michele present the concept to the council, and what will she need to do to help them engage the concept and work to make it happen?

3. Michele has some conflict issues regarding evidence-based practice with council members. How will she address the conflict? What approaches will she need to use to help those who are opposed to the idea embrace and work with the council to make it happen?

4. Michele has some concerns with evidence-based practice being a response to a mandate. In keeping with the principles of shared governance, where does legitimate accountability lie for generating evidence-based practice? Where should the direction come for requiring its implementation, and what shared governance mechanisms should be used to drive it? What is the legitimate role of the manager in the requirement for and the process of implementing evidence-based practice on the unit?

5. Michele has expressed concerns with staff accountability. Because evidence-based practice depends strongly on staff personal accountability for successful implementation, what will Michele need to do to generate interest and accountability in the staff for practicing in a way that demonstrates evidentiary foundations for practice? How will she know when accountability is present?

6. Do a mind map or visual graphic presentation of the problems and issues Michele must address and how she should deal with them as she leads implementation of evidence-based practice on the unit. Share your indicators of success for each element of the process that will demonstrate that you are making successful progress in making it work on the unit.

Appendix B

Exercise in Leadership: Increasing Capacity

SCENARIO

John is an experienced critical care nurse in a 12-bed unit. The facility is new and equipped with the latest technology. In general, the unit is well respected and attracts highly committed, professional nurses. Teamwork is above average, and nurse–physician relationships are quite good.

The strategic planning analysts for the organization have determined that the census for the critical care unit will triple in the next 12 months based on the anticipated increase in patients requiring care as a result of health-care reform. There is neither time nor resources available to build more patient rooms.

The organization has determined to double nurse–patient assignments (from two patients per registered nurse to four patients per registered nurse), decrease the length of stay by 50 percent, and maintain quality outcomes at the 90th percentile. Currently, the outcomes are at the 95th percentile.

As a respected and competent clinical leader, John is asked to lead a team of clinical caregivers to create a new delivery model that meets the identified needs for the future. John is also encouraged to include any other stakeholders, including patients, to be on his team.

The key concepts to be considered are change, innovation, staffing effectiveness, policy, ethical issues, delegation, healthcare reform, and professional practice. The plan is to include the following 12 items for presentation to leadership of the organization and interested community members:

1. John's assessment of his competence with change and innovation

2. An assessment of other team members' competence with change and innovation

3. Identification of the who, what, when, and where of the change process

4. A list of supporters and nonsupporters of the change and the reasons for their positions

5. Ethical issues that could arise and how they will be managed

6. Changes in the staffing plan for days and nights

7. Nonregistered nurse staffing additions and rationale for increase

8. A list of rational risks that will be taken

9. Plans to address potential policy violations

10. A list of evaluation criteria and metrics to monitor the change

11. Completion of a performance demonstration document by each member of the team identifying his or her contribution to the project and supporting patient care in the new model

12. A timeline for implementation and evaluation

Appendix C

Exercise in Leadership: Clinical Technology Management

 ### SCENARIO

The use of clinical monitoring, documentation, and communication devices is at an all-time high in the oncology unit. Nurses have individual communication devices, portable tablets for documentation, badge locators for movements, and internal phones for special team assignments. Patients are linked to smart pumps, smart beds, cardiac monitoring, forehead stress monitors, and the communication system to call for assistance, order meals, and access television and movies.

Recently feedback from patients has indicated a decrease in satisfaction and specific comments that more attention is being paid to electronic monitoring than to the patient. Given that the Hospital Consumer Assessment of Healthcare Provider Systems (HCAHPS) scores specific to patient satisfaction are now linked to reimbursement, there is an expectation that the issues will be addressed.

A request has been put forth for direct caregivers to volunteer to form a team, select a facilitator, and develop a strategy to effectively address this complex issue. The expectation is that the wisdom of an effective solution will come from experienced caregivers who are knowledgeable about the effective working of the systems and oncology care excellence. Participation on shared leadership committees is a preferred prerequisite.

The key concepts to be considered are technology management, change and innovation, ethical issues, healthcare policy, resource management, professional nursing practice role clarification, and the infrastructure for practice.

The team is asked to identify the following:

1. Change and innovation competence of each team member
2. The primary issues causing the dissatisfaction
3. Key stakeholders required to address the issues
4. Ethical issues specific to care of the oncology patient, reimbursement, and technology use

5. Issues related to professional nursing practice, use of technology, and compliance with regulatory mandates

6. Team dynamics including conflict, agreements, and challenges in addressing the issues

7. A plan to address the issues

8. A communication plan to inform key stakeholders of any changes

9. A list of evaluation criteria and timeline for evaluation

10. A timeline for implementation

Glossary

Accountability—A demonstration that professionals have coalesced their efforts in the clinical team in a way that results in a positive impact on the health of those they serve. An obligation to account for or explain the events.

Accountability Care Organization—Networks of providers that are rewarded financially if they can slow the growth in their patients' healthcare spending while maintaining or improving the quality of the care they deliver. The Accountable Care Model emphasizes population care, value-driven outcomes, emphasis on the point of service at which patient care occurs, protocols for effective hand-offs, and inclusion of the family.

Analysis—Breaking down the components of a problem or issue into parts or elements.

Assignment—The distribution of work that each staff member is to accomplish in a given time period. Assignment occurs when the authority to do a task already exists.

Attitude—The manner, disposition, or inclination as to how one approaches and reacts to situations.

Authority—The legal source of power; the right to act or command the actions of others and to have them followed.

Balance sheet—A financial statement that includes assets, liabilities, and equity. It is a snapshot of the organization's financial position at a specific point in time.

Bargaining—The phase of negotiation that emphasizes the give and take related to the variety of positions at the table. Bargaining is the work of exchange. There are a number of different bargaining approaches.

Betrayal—A person's words or actions that indicate he or she lacks good intentions toward another; the breaking or violation of a presumptive contract, trust, or confidence that produces moral and psychological conflict within a relationship among individuals, between organizations, or between individuals and organizations.

Bottom line—What an individual most needs or wants from the negotiation process.

Cash flow operating activities—A financial report that shows the cash inflow and outflow activities or financial stability of the organization.

Chunking—Instead of summarily reaching a point of broad generalized agreement, the final agreement may actually be the aggregation of smaller agreements that, when looked at comprehensively, satisfy the needs of the participants.

Classification—The ordering of entities into groups or classes on the basis of their similarity, minimizing within-group variance and maximizing between-group variance.

Coach—One who assists others to develop viable solutions, prioritize them, and then act on them.

Code of ethics—Guiding principles that enumerate the expectations of members of the profession and the personal and performance standards that represent what is best in the work of the profession.

Complex adaptive system—A densely linked, intersecting, and interacting connection of agents, each making their own contribution and acting both independently in making that contribution and interdependently in linking that contribution to the independent but related contributions of other agents.

Conflict—A metaphor for difference. It is more normal than it is exceptional.

Core schedule—An aggregated average number and skill mix required for patient care, which includes caregivers, shift length, and calendar days.

Critical thinking—Active, purposeful, organized thinking that takes into consideration focus, language, frame of reference, attitudes, assumptions, evidence, reasoning, conclusions, implications, and context when deciding what to believe or do.

Dashboard—A combination of graphics and numbers to quickly display important data elements.

Decision making—A complex cognitive process that involves choosing a particular course of action from among alternatives. Decision making is an essential component of the problem-solving process.

Deep dive—A tool to advance change and innovation in which a particular area is selected for observation in multiple ways. Workflows, photos, interviews, and observations are gathered by a team to analyze current processes and brainstorm new ways of doing the current work processes.

Delegate—The individual staff person receiving the delegated task.

Delegation—The transferring to a competent individual of the authority to perform a selected nursing task in a selected situation.

Delegator—The individual making the delegation.

Developmental stretch assignments—Assignments to improve employee satisfaction and engagement through autonomy and leadership practices.

Directed creativity—A tool to advance change and innovation in which a situation is proposed to encourage and advance new ideas.

DRG—Diagnosis-related group. A system used to help clinicians and hospitals monitor quality of care and utilization of services. It has been used by Medicare to pay hospitals.

Emergent—Conditions that are driven by new sociopolitical realities, economic changes, technological advances, evidence of best practices, and a host of related shifts that demonstrate that holding onto current practices is an impediment to better engaging work processes in the best interests of those they serve.

Employee recognition—Acknowledgment of outstanding behaviors, communication, accountability, valuing diversity, delivering excellence, and teamwork.

Employee rounding—Regular rounding in work areas to identify employees' most critical needs, safety issues, and clinical concerns.

Equality—A measure of condition.

Equity—A measure of value.

Evidence-based practice—Practice based on facts and truth. The integration of the best research evidence with clinical expertise and clinical values.

Evidentiary dynamics—Nursing practices based on research that is conducted so that evidence may be presented.

Federal Register—The official daily publication for rules, proposed rules, and notices of the federal government and an unbiased source of information.

Fidelity—Duty to keep one's promise; the quality of being faithful.

Healthcare economics—A branch of economics focused on efficiency, effectiveness, and behavior in the production and consumption of healthcare goods and services.

Income statement—A financial statement that includes information about revenue sources and expenses at a specific point in time.

Individual accountability—Knowing the requirements and behaviors of effective delegation.

Leader—A person who coordinates, integrates, facilitates, and provides a context for the performance of the people in the organization.

Manager—An organizational position and function. Managers have subordinates and a vertical relationship to those they manage.

Mediator—A person who manages the conflict resolution process.

Mentor—A wise and trusted advisor who guides others on a particular journey. A mentor provides support, challenge, and vision.

Mentoring—The process of a more accomplished person assisting others to develop expertise and learn new skills based on the mentor's personal, untapped wisdom, reinforcing their self-confidence, supporting real-life situations, and sharing personal experiences when appropriate.

Mind mapping—A tool to advance change and innovation in which software is used for collecting, organizing, and synthesizing large amounts of data in layers with complex relationships.

Negotiation—An attempt to identify, enumerate, and undertake a process that clearly establishes needs and wants and where all parties work to reconcile their interests in a way that results in mutual advantage or value.

Onboarding—The early processes of socializing nurses into the workplace to achieve optimal employee engagement.

Organizational accountability—Providing sufficient resources, staffing, appropriate staff mix; implementing policies and role descriptions; providing opportunity for continuing staff development; and creating an environment conducive to teamwork, collaboration, and client-centered care.

Patient acuity—The level of need or dependency of an individual patient.

Patient care delivery model—A method or system of organizing and delivering nursing care, including the manner in which nursing care is organized in order to deliver the care necessary to meet the needs of the patients. The delivery system encompasses work delegation, resource utilization, communication methodologies, clinical decision-making processes, and management structure.

Patient classification system—A tool to improve the clarity and objective identification of patient care needs. The goal of the system is to provide the most valid and reliable information specific to work that needs to be done for patients.

PICO approach—A methodology used to form a clinical question, in which P is patient or problem; I is intervention; C is comparison intervention; and O is outcomes.

Profession—An expression of a role and its relationship to the world, representing a social contract and reflecting high expectations for its exercise from those who will depend on it.

Professional boundary—The limits of the professional relationship that allow for a safe therapeutic connection between the healthcare provider and the client. These include, at a minimum, time, location of patient care money, exchange, favors or gifts, self-disclosure, and physical contact.

Research—The systematic examination of an idea using rigorous principles of experimentation and measurement.

Research utilization—The use of knowledge that is typically based on a single study.

Responsibility—Reliability, dependability, and obligation to accomplish work.

Right choices—Those choices that conform to ethical norms or principles, and others can know whether or not one has made a right choice.

Scheduling—The long-range plan that combines your organization's goals, legislation, regulation, and accreditation requirements and planned patient demand.

Setting the table—Knowing how all the decisions need to be served, what talent or expertise needs to be gathered, the size of the team in relationship to the issues it will be addressing, and what particular gifts and skills will be present to the team as they deliberate the questions before them.

Shared governance—A structural format for nursing to implement a more horizontal locus of control and practice power enablers that are essential to professional self-governance. This framework provides support of the professions, their interaction, and their collective obligation to advance the interest of health care.

Social networking—Specific social activities to support team building, seasonal challenges, and common needs.

Staffing—The real-time adjustment of the schedule based on census, acuity, and the mix of available resources.

Statement of purpose—A statement that serves as an anchor for the work of a team and indicates the direction for team activities.

Supervision—The provision of guidance or direction, evaluation, and follow-up by the delegator for accomplishment of a task delegated to another; to watch over a particular activity or task being carried out by other people and ensure that it is carried out correctly.

Synthesis—The act of combining and integrating numerous complex elements or components of the system in order to view it as an integrated whole.

Terms of engagement—General rules of relationship and interaction that the team adheres to as a way of maintaining a positive communication and interaction environment within the context of the team as it completes its work.

Trust—One individual's willingness to be vulnerable to another based on the belief that the other is competent, open, concerned, and reliable, thus rendering risk taking more rational and realistic.

Utilitarianism—The principle of utility or the greatest happiness principle; actions are chosen that will produce the greatest amount of happiness for the greatest number of people.

Veracity—Truth telling, or the duty to tell the truth.

Workforce management—A comprehensive system that includes patient classification, scheduling, staffing, and budgeting systems.

Index

Page numbers followed by *f* or *t* indicate figures or tables, respectively.